Phantom Illness

Phantom Illness

....

SHATTERING
THE
MYTH
OF
HYPOCHONDRIA

....

Carla Cantor
with Brian Fallon, M.D.

HOUGHTON MIFFLIN COMPANY

BOSTON • NEW YORK

1996

For information about permission to reproduce selections
from this book, write to Permissions, Houghton Mifflin Company,
215 Park Avenue South, New York, New York 10003.

For information about this and other Houghton Mifflin trade
and reference books and multimedia products, visit The Bookstore
at Houghton Mifflin on the World Wide Web at
http://www.hmco.com/trade/.

Library of Congress Cataloging-in-Publication Data
Cantor, Carla.
Phantom illness : shattering the myth of hypochondria / Carla
Cantor, with Brian Fallon.
p. cm.
Includes bibliographical references and index.
ISBN 0-395-68988-0
1. Hypochondria. I. Fallon, Brian, M.D. II. Title
RC552.H8C36 1996 95-26084
616.85'25 — dc20 CIP

Printed in the United States of America

Book design by Robert Overholtzer

QUM 10 9 8 7 6 5 4 3 2 1

The Illness Attitude Scale on pp. 295–297 is provided
by the courtesy of the University of New Mexico,
and the University of New Mexico reserves all rights.

TO DAVID

for the love and loyalty
that sustains me,
in sickness and in health

CONTENTS

	FOREWORD	ix
	Prologue	1
1.	A Much Maligned Malady	14
2.	The Many Faces of Somatization	35
3.	Digging Beneath Symptoms	60
4.	Are Hypochondriacs Born or Made? The Nature-Nurture Debate	86
5.	Healthism: A Symptom of Our Time	111
6.	It's Never All in Your Head	131
7.	The Susceptibility Factor	156
8.	Family Ties — in Sickness and in Health	185
9.	Between Doctor and Patient	223
10.	The Steps to Successful Treatment	255
	Epilogue	285
	APPENDIX: A SELF-DIAGNOSTIC TEST FOR HYPOCHONDRIA	293
	NOTES	299
	ACKNOWLEDGMENTS	327
	INDEX	331

FOREWORD

Doctors typically treat hypochondriacs with disrespect. Derogatively referred to as "crocks," hypochondriacs are thought to be self-centered complainers who believe they are ill when they are not and who reject all help that doctors try to provide. Doctors find it frustrating to provide the repeated reassurance these patients crave, and many do not consider them to be truly troubled or medically ill.

In fact, hypochondriacs are severely troubled. Plagued by uncertainty and dread, the hypervigilant mind of the hypochondriac cannot rest. Minor symptoms become signals of deadly diseases. Unable to free themselves from escalating fear, hypochondriacs seek reassurance from family members or doctors. But the cycle never ends. The reassurance is never enough, and many of these patients endlessly pursue a diagnosis for their unexplained symptoms. Others live lives of quiet terror, no longer checking with doctors because they know physicians regard them with disdain or because avoiding doctors prevents the identification and confirmation of their feared disease.

New medical perspectives on hypochondria now suggest that hypochondriacs may in fact be physically ill. However, the illness is a result not of the disease they fear but of a neurochemical imbalance in the brain. Their inability to let go of the fear of disease may be mediated by this imbalance, which itself may be the result of multiple factors, such as severe stressors, genetic inheritance, and/or gradual environmental conditioning. This new medical perspective has important treatment implications and provides new hope for the patient with illness fears.

I became interested in hypochondria as a result of my encounter with Mr. A during my residency training in psychiatry at Columbia University. Mr. A was then a fifty-two-year-old stockbroker who suffered from a persistent pain in his head, which he feared was evidence of a brain tumor. He had consulted ten different medical specialists and had four brain scans in the preceding year. Despite the fact that all physical exams and all tests were normal, he was not reassured. How did he know that the doctors had done *all* of the necessary tests? How could he be certain that he had adequately explained the symptoms to them? Was it possible that these doctors weren't telling him the truth? He was almost certain he was dying of a serious illness.

Hypochondria invaded his home and work life as well. This patient's profound self-absorption caused his wife and children to leave him. At work, whenever there was a lull in the trading, his dread of illness returned. He became distracted, and fellow stockbrokers started to notice that his job performance was slipping. His job was in jeopardy.

During our first meeting, Mr. A demanded to know my credentials and then proceeded to tell me that I would never be able to help him. He asked, "How could you help me? I have a physical problem—I know I do. . . . The pain is there every day. I feel I have a serious medical illness, but the doctors won't tell me what it is. You are a psychiatrist. I don't want to *talk* about my problems. I don't care how well trained you are, you can't help me. I have a physical problem, *not* a mental one! The only reason I'm here is because Dr. Fink demanded that I see a psychiatrist—so I'm here for this one session and that's it."

This man's rage and distrust made me wonder if I would be able to help him. Although he expressed contempt for psychiatrists and distrust of doctors, the fact remained that he had come for help. What could I do?

I listened. The hypochondria had started ten years earlier, but he had been a worrier even before that. His childhood had been dominated by a mother who was filled with anxious worry about the health of her children. He had been in psychotherapy for eight years and taken numerous medications to treat anxiety and depression, all to no avail. He loved his family, but in the last three years his fear of a brain tumor had literally driven them away. He had lost most of his friends as well. Over the last year, the pain in his head had become more and more intense.

In order to learn more about the treatment of hypochondria, I looked in textbooks of psychiatry. The textbooks were unanimous in their pessimism. Unless the person had a concurrent major depression, there was very little one could do for the patient other than give support. This man did not have a major depression. He did not have panic disorder. He did not have obsessive-compulsive disorder. In other words, he did not have any of the major anxiety or depressive disorders that respond readily to medication or psychotherapeutic treatments. This man suffered from hypochondria. According to the textbooks, his prognosis was terrible.

Around this time, a revolution was occurring in psychiatry. A disorder previously thought to be one of the rarest of mental problems was discovered to be one of the most common, occurring in one out of every fifty Americans. This disorder — obsessive-compulsive disorder, or OCD — is characterized by obsessional thoughts and/or compulsive, ritualistic behaviors. Typical manifestations of OCD include intrusive thoughts that one has caused harm to others, fear of contamination by germs, horrifying violent images, and compulsive hand-washing, counting, or checking. Because people who suffer from this problem are often aware of the irrational nature of their fears, they may hide their behaviors and not reveal their horrific thoughts.

Whereas before the mid-1980s the treatment of obsessive-compulsive disorder was clouded in pessimism (as was true for hypochondria), clarity emerged after that time as specific and effective treatment strategies were identified. In particular, the discovery that medications affecting the serotonin neurotransmitters of the brain are very helpful in the treatment of OCD brought hope to a previously despairing, hidden mass of the population. Television news programs about such medications as clomipramine (Anafranil), fluoxetine (Prozac), fluvoxamine (Luvox), and sertraline (Zoloft) encouraged sufferers to come out of the closet and into psychiatrists' offices. As a result, knowledge about the biology and treatment of OCD has exploded in the last ten years.

What exactly have we learned about this disorder, and why is it relevant to hypochondria? Patients with OCD often suffer from the expectation of harm and the tyranny of doubt. They fear that any action might result in harm to themselves or others. In addition, they are often uncertain whether they have done enough to prevent harm — whether they have checked the gas stove sufficiently or washed their hands thoroughly enough. Like patients with OCD, people with hypochondria suffer from the expectation of harm and the tyranny of doubt. Benign bodily sensations become signs of severe harm; disease has infiltrated their body. To ward off the harm, they must then check. They check medical textbooks, magazine articles, AIDS hotlines. They check with family members and doctors about their symptoms. After checking, they may feel temporarily reassured — for hours or days — but then a new sensation once again causes the seed of uncertainty to germinate. How can I be sure the doctor did all the proper tests? How do I know that the doctor understood what I was describing? Racked by fear, hypochondriacs spend their waking hours consumed by obsessions about illness.

How does this relate to Mr. A? The phenomenological similarities between hypochondria and obsessive-compulsive disorder led me to wonder whether the new treatments for OCD might also help to reduce Mr. A's hypochondria. I had only a glimmer of hope for Mr. A. He had failed to respond to all prior treatments. In addition, I saw this man's hostility and distrust as a sign of a character problem, a personality flaw, that was not likely to change with medication. So, with guarded expectations, this man was given the serotonin reuptake inhibitor named flu-oxetine to take on a daily basis at the high doses necessary to treat OCD. Within six weeks, his life was changed. Although still aware of occasional bodily sensations, he was now able to let go of the irrational fear that momentarily became attached to the sensation. He experienced a liberation from the dread that had occupied so much of his life. In his words, "I wish I had had this medicine twenty years ago." Just as remarkable as the re-duction in his hypochondriacal concerns was the improvement in his overall personality. No longer hostile and demeaning, he readily expressed gratitude to me for his new state of health. This improvement was sustained over time.

Impressed by this man's remarkable recovery after years of misery, I decided to test this treatment strategy with other hypo-chondriacal patients. The results were promising. Many patients experienced dramatic improvement, and the success of my stud-ies of Heightened Illness Concern conducted at the New York State Psychiatric Institute started to become known outside the vicinity of Columbia University. As a result, Carla Cantor, the author of this book, and I met.

Carla's riveting personal story, her careful research into the history of hypochondria, and her thoughtful interviews with pa-tients and national experts make this book unique. I am pleased to have been asked to review the book for medical accuracy and to help shape its content. People who suffer from hypochondria, their family members, and health care providers will find much of interest in the pages that follow.

What will motivate a hypochondriac to read this book? Hope and courage: hope that he or she will be able to conquer this problem; courage to seek a new path to liberation from the stranglehold of illness obsessions. Many people with hypochon-dria have contributed their stories to this book. I hope that these eloquent stories and the promise provided by contemporary psychiatric approaches will persuade the reader that freedom from illness fears is possible.

BRIAN A. FALLON, M.D.

Phantom Illness

Prologue

It is easy to see how the condition is part of the psyche's apparatus of defense: unwilling to accept its own gathering deterioration, the mind announces to its indwelling consciousness that it is the body with its perhaps correctable defects — not the precious and irreplaceable mind — that is going haywire.

— William Styron on hypochondria, *Darkness Visible*

ONE WARM JUNE EVENING I found myself imprisoned, a patient on a psychiatric ward of a hospital a few miles from my New Jersey home. It was not at all what I had intended. I had come to the emergency room earlier that day in desperation: I *had* to talk to someone about the undiagnosed pain in my wrist, my thinning hair, and the unrelenting fear that I was morbidly ill. Physical symptoms had plagued me for nearly a year, the problems starting a few months after the birth of my son, Michael, in April 1990.

That spring had begun so beautifully; my husband and I were thrilled when our second child turned out to be a boy, a complement for his three-year-old sister, Danielle. One of each, we thought, the ideal family. But while I was nursing Michael, I developed an excruciating pain whenever I moved my left wrist. My internist said it might be carpal tunnel syndrome brought on by hormonal changes. He suggested that I stop nursing and give the wrist a rest. I consulted an orthopedist, who advised me to try a splint. When that didn't work, another specialist injected my wrist with cortisone. Nothing alleviated the pain, which had spread to my shoulder, and confusing the situation, tests that initially showed a borderline case of carpal tunnel syndrome— a benign though painful ailment—were now negative.

I felt betrayed by the medical profession. The doctors couldn't figure out what was wrong with me, nor did they seem to care. So I began to search for my own diagnosis, requesting sophisticated tests to rule out obscure disorders I had read about, like thoracic outlet syndrome and de Quervain's disease, tenosynovitis. All that showed up was a mild inflammation of the left wrist on a bone scan, a sensitive, expensive procedure used to screen for arthritis and cancer. The physicians didn't seem to find the laboratory results at all disturbing. Just a stiff wrist! One doctor prescribed physical therapy, which only made the pain worse.

Without any suggestion from a doctor, I settled on a diagnosis of lupus, a frightening, disabling autoimmune disease with an array of horrifying symptoms—arthritis, hair loss, skin rashes, mouth sores—and nearly as deadly as cancer. It was a disease with which I had some familiarity. Ten years earlier, after a traumatic breakup with a man I'd been living with, I had fallen sick with something doctors couldn't explain. As they prodded and prescribed, I pored over medical texts in the library—where I discovered this hideous, heartwrenching illness.

Each day during the winter of 1983 I'd catalog my lupus-like symptoms—joint aches, rashes, itching attacks, black and blue marks, exhaustion. I'd bring the list to doctors, begging them to confirm my diagnosis. I shook up one rheumatologist enough that he admitted me to a hospital for a five-day physical workup. It turned out to be just the right prescription. Tests, treatments, attention from visitors, time off from my demanding job as a newspaper reporter, a rest for mind and body. My discharge diagnosis: psychophysiological reaction/muscular-skeletal system.

Finally, I allowed the doctors to convince me that whatever was going on in my body was not symptomatic of a deadly disease, but the psychological dimension of the diagnosis had little impact. By the time I left the hospital, I was ready to put lupus and everything it signified behind me. Without realizing it, I'd spent months grieving for the loss of my relationship. I had recovered my sense of self and could function again. Although, on my doctor's advice, I consulted a psychiatrist—I had seen a social worker for a number of years but was not in therapy at the time—I resisted insight and went on my way, chalking up the experience to a "weird episode." I returned to my job, offering a vague explanation of my illness to colleagues, and began a new relationship.

Now, a decade later, lupus was back and *this* time it seemed my fears were justified. I was unable to bend my wrist without pain; my hair, which had turned brittle, was falling out; and I had sun allergies—on several occasions I had developed a rash in tropical sunlight—all markers for the disease. Tests were negative, but no matter how many doctors tried to reassure me that I didn't have lupus, I wasn't convinced. *I* knew about the bizarre and fluctuating symptoms that make lupus so tough to diagnose and that no test was entirely accurate in ruling it out. No one could offer a 100 percent guarantee that the disease wasn't in the early stages of the illness—and nothing less would do. Perhaps, I thought irrationally, the earlier episode had been its initial onset.

As months went by I became increasingly distracted and depressed as my husband grew resentful and impatient. My work as a freelance writer suffered and, worst of all, my children weren't getting the love and attention they deserved. Yet despite my conviction, no doctor would pronounce the diagnosis I dreaded but in some perverse way wanted. One young rheumatologist, in retrospect among the wisest doctors I consulted, hinted that this obsession with my wrist and well-being might be related to the birth of my son, a latent postpartum depression of sorts. He suggested psychological help, which I resisted.

My trip to the hospital was a last desperate plea for help. I was on the verge of a breakdown, though it wasn't clear to me why. Was it because of my intolerable symptoms? That doctors couldn't find what was wrong? Or was I possibly going crazy because I *was* crazy? . . . something I briefly and reluctantly considered. I picked a sweltering Friday afternoon when I had just completed a writing assignment and expected my in-laws from out of town for a visit. I knew that they would be supportive of my family and help my husband with our children should I be gone for some time. At the hospital I waited hours in the emergency room to see the physician on call, who after examining me sent in a third-year medical resident in psychiatry. This brash young doctor listened to my woes of the past year: the pain, the tests, the physicians, my exhaustive search for an answer. After a few questions, he looked at me squarely and said, "I believe you are suffering from clinical depression. I want to admit you to the psychiatric ward."

After the initial shock of hearing his words, I felt relief. My shoulders relaxed and my stomach stopped churning as I sat calmly at the edge of the examining table, waiting for a nurse to take me to my room. A pleasant male orderly asked if I was hungry and brought me a cup of tea and a sandwich, the first food I had eaten all day. Finally, my illness would be diagnosed! Doctors would examine my inflamed wrist, psychiatrists would listen to me talk about the psychic pain of the past year, and they would all figure out whether I was really sick or just plain crazy. Being in a hospital also seemed like a reasonable excuse for leaving behind the responsibilities and stresses that go with being a freelance writer and mother of two young children.

But when the nurse arrived with a wheelchair — hospital policy — things got a little strange. Riding up in the elevator with her, I hung my head to avoid eye contact. *What if I didn't have a disease? Maybe I really was a fraud!* Then I was wheeled down a dingy hall into a sterile, forbidding-looking place: the psychiatric ward. I sucked in all that was disagreeable at once: the drugged-out patients sprawled on vinyl couches, watching a communal television set mounted on the ceiling, the group and occupational therapy schedules posted on the wall, the No Visitors sign. This, I knew, was no Club Med.

"Let me see your bag, miss," said a stern-looking woman with a sergeant's voice. I watched in horror as she rifled through my pocketbook and pulled out a pair of eyebrow tweezers. "I need those!" I cried, an edge of hysteria in my voice. (Now they'll really think I'm nuts, I thought.) She replied, "You'll get these back, miss. Hospital policy. The patients can't keep any sharp objects."

"I want to go home," I said, feeling panicky. Any moment my husband, David, would arrive with my clothes. I asked the woman at the desk if I could leave with him. She furrowed her brow and dialed the telephone. Phone calls went back and forth and then came the bad news: I couldn't be released until the director of the program evaluated me in the morning. I was under their control and had no one to blame but myself.

It was after 10:00 P.M. when David arrived on the ward with a bag. I ran toward the doorway, a guard at my side. Patients were not allowed visitors, except for one hour during the day. As the guard collected my belongings, I blew a kiss to my baffled husband through the glass door. "I'll be home in the morning," I mouthed.

Such was my night on a psychiatric ward, my one and only, I pray. I spent it in a cold, bare room on an uncomfortable bed, talking to my roommate, a twenty-three-year-old woman who had been diagnosed with schizophrenia. This time she was in for six weeks. All I could think was how lucky I was and that I couldn't wait to see my children. Suddenly, my undiagnosed illness didn't seem so terrible. I could live with it. In fact, maybe, just maybe, I thought, there really wasn't much wrong with me after all.

Early the next morning I departed. I told the director it had all been a terrible mistake. What could he say? My husband came to get me and I walked back into my life with the joy and relief of waking from a nightmare. My kind, accepting in-laws asked no questions, and the children were overjoyed to have Mommy home.

It was time to take stock of my life. Perhaps the best thing to do was to leave the pain alone. Accept the symptoms, ignore them. After the hospital fiasco, I was able to do that for a while and there was a slight reprieve, but unwelcome and frightening thoughts intruded and the wrist was still stiff. I made the occasional visit to a doctor, getting a blood test for reassurance that never lasted long. Then one summer day I spotted a *New York Times* article headlined, "Patients Refusing to Be Well, A Disease of Many Symptoms." The subject was hypochondria, a preoccupation with the fear of having or getting a serious disease. I had never before read anything about the topic. The article talked about people who suffer from symptoms for which no cause can be found or whose complaints are inappropriate in relation to their symptoms. In the past such patients had been dismissed by doctors and left to shuttle from medical laboratories to specialists to emergency rooms. But an effort was under way in the medical community to identify these patients, whose problems ranged from cancer phobias to chronic pain, to help them find relief. Physicians were even giving them a less pejorative name—somatizers ("soma" from the Greek word for body), a term psychiatrists use to describe people who unconsciously convert emotions into bodily ills.

Suddenly something clicked for me. The myriad tests, the files of medical bills, the dozens of maladies for which doctors could never find a cause. There *was* something wrong with me, but not a deadly disease, which, in my more rational moments, I believe I had always known. And if studies were correct, the problem affected millions of others—I had read that at least 25 percent, if not 75 percent, of all patients who visit doctors' offices report symptoms that appear to have no medical basis. One in ten continue to be frightened of disease in the face of reassuring information. That meant I had nothing to be ashamed of. It meant I could get well.

Nervously, I picked up the telephone and dialed the number

of Dr. Arthur Barsky, then a psychiatrist at the Massachusetts General Hospital, whom the article mentioned as one of a handful of experts on hypochondria in the country. He returned my call right away. I told him I had just read the *Times* article about somatizers and stammered, "I think I might be one of them. Is there anyone in New York who works with such patients?"

Dr. Barsky suggested that I contact Brian Fallon, a psychiatrist at Columbia Presbyterian Medical Center in New York, who was evaluating the effect of Prozac, touted as the new wonder drug in the treatment of depression, on hypochondria. I spoke with Dr. Fallon about his research. He explained that his approach represented new thinking among psychiatrists, that hypochondria, which had long confounded physicians because of its recalcitrance to treatment, was in many cases linked to obsessive-compulsive disorders or depression with obsessional aspects and, indeed, might be caused by a biochemical imbalance within the brain. In his experiments, he sought to inhibit nerve impulses with fluoxetine, the generic name for Prozac, which has been successful in treating obsessions and compulsions to lessen the hypochondria. Dr. Fallon's work, in its early stages, appeared to hold promise. He suggested that I make an appointment to see if I was a candidate for the study, which was being funded by the National Institute of Mental Health.

At our meeting that fall, I spent an hour telling Dr. Fallon about my inflamed wrist, the hair loss, the photosensitivity, and the now wavering conviction that all these symptoms were signs of early lupus. He administered a psychological questionnaire to evaluate my problem and asked me to participate in the Prozac experiments. I never did take part in them. My husband and my parents, whom I had told of my troubles, were supportive and encouraged me to begin treatment with Prozac, but not as a participant in a double-blind study, in which I might be administered only placebos. So I established a relationship with another psychiatrist and began a trial of Prozac, my initial course on the drug lasting five months, less than the usual duration. Within weeks I felt better. The obsessive thoughts lifted; the pain and stiffness receded; the lost hair began growing back. After a year of misery I was happy and productive again.

I telephoned Dr. Fallon, who was delighted to hear of my progress and curious about my treatment. I couldn't explain why things were going so well. Had Prozac been a catalyst for change? Was it the working out of issues with my new therapist? Or had my growing recognition that for years I had been expressing emotions through physical symptoms finally reached a new stage? A former therapist had tried to convince me that my maladies and fears were symptomatic of other problems, but it hadn't sunk in. Or perhaps I wasn't ready to face my problems until now, even to consider that my intrusive thoughts could be related to deeper psychological troubles or biochemical imbalances.

Not long after my response to Prozac, I approached Dr. Fallon with the idea for this book. I had begun reading more about hypochondria, a subject well documented in academic and medical literature but rarely discussed in popular culture. It is an affliction millions suffer in silence and shame. I wanted to reach out to others who struggle with this mysterious ailment and share my experience and knowledge with them. I believed a book that could sensitively address a subject that is rarely discussed openly was needed. In living rooms, at parties, we talk candidly and with concern about topics like incest, bulimia, and rape. Why is hypochondria something we turn away from? Though our society is tolerant of the ill, hypochondriacs are sneered at, joked about, and ignored.

Hypochondria may not be as serious a condition as illnesses like schizophrenia or manic depression, but to be so terrified of disease or to feel symptoms so acutely that you get little pleasure from life can be just as disabling. Hypochondriasis, the medical term for the problem, officially recognized as a mental disorder by the American Psychiatric Association in 1980, is defined as "a preoccupation with the fear of having, or the belief that one has, a serious disease, based on the person's interpretation of physical signs and sensations." It isn't classified as a psychiatric illness unless unwarranted conviction about disease persists for six or more months despite medical reassurance.

The truth is that most who suffer from hypochondria do not need an "official" diagnosis to know that they have a problem. Like people with obsessive-compulsive disorder, who think the same senseless thoughts over and over, hypochondriacs tend to be painfully aware of the irrational nature of their fears. They are besieged by irrational beliefs pertaining to their bodies and ill health but feel powerless to dismiss them. Though preoccupations may range from mild to disabling, be episodic or unremitting, the fears are rarely delusional in intensity. And in the unusual case when health obsessions reach psychotic proportions, as I believe my lupus phobia came close to doing, the psychosis tends to be limited to this single aspect of experience.

A forty-five-year-old executive who struggles with paralyzing fears of cancer described hypochondria's vicious cycle. "When I get crazy over a symptom, I feel ashamed of my behavior and what it's doing to my wife and kids. My self-esteem spirals downward and the symptoms get worse. I try to stop. I carry on this elaborate debate in my head. C'mon Pete. You've had these fears dozens of times. They never amount to beans. But this little voice keeps reminding me of terrible things, for instance, my thirty-year-old cousin's dying of leukemia, the fact that one in three adults get cancer. It's easy for people to say don't think about it. But no matter how remote the chance that my headache is a brain tumor, the thoughts won't leave my mind."

As difficult a problem as it is at times, most sufferers from hypochondria, a perfectionist bunch, don't "crack up," have nervous breakdowns, or end up in mental hospitals. They function, even achieving great things, but often at a cost of happiness and intimacy with the people they most care about.

During the decade between the two lupus scares, I lived a highstrung but productive life: I attended graduate school, held jobs, was married, had children. But my existence was peppered with episodes of illness. When the going got tough, I'd get sick. Or just the opposite: when things seemed to be going well, I'd come down with a symptom, or at least what I interpreted as one. It might be stomach pain, dizziness, black and blue marks, swollen glands, an achy heel, anything. Whatever the symptom, I always interpreted it as a precursor of some crippling illness: leukemia, Lou Gehrig's disease, scleroderma. I knew just enough about most diseases to cause trouble. Eventually I'd get past each episode, but it always took time—the cure a mysterious concoction of enough negative tests, a lessening of symptoms, some positive change in my life. And when the event was over, the realization that I was healthy and wasn't going to die, at least not immediately, was like a high, a reprieve, a new lease on life. That is, until the next time. The two hospital stays—interestingly, one for the physical workup, the other a mental one—were like bookends; they represented the two times in my life when symptoms, regardless of whether they were labeled organic or psychiatric, did not abate, when the way I usually coped with life just didn't work.

Like some of the other sufferers I interviewed for this book, I was in talk therapy throughout most of these hypochondriacal years with a Freudian-oriented analyst. We did some terrific work together, but not during my "episodes." A symptom would pop up and I'd start running frantically to doctors and checking *The Merck Manual.* Others I interviewed recounted similar difficulties. As one woman complained, "I'd be telling the analyst about my breast lump and he'd want to know what I dreamt last night." That was how it was for me, too. To my therapist my symptoms were an intrusion, a resistance to treatment, an obstacle to insight.

Yes, Prozac has helped me quiet my intrusive thoughts, so much so that when I first began taking the drug I felt more like myself and freer than I had in years. It was as if all the wisdom accumulated in all that time in talk therapy suddenly came alive. The drug let loose the best in me, or perhaps the best me, the one without the internal battlefield. It restored my capacity for pleasure. I had symptoms, but they no longer terrified me. So natural did this new emotional balance seem, the side effects of Prozac so minimal, that I thought I was making it happen. Twice I went off the drug to try to do just that and was disappointed. Both times the preoccupations came back. Not always as fears about illness, but the same catastrophic thinking would manifest itself in other ways: in obsessions about my work, my ability to be a good mother, my relationships with my husband, my friends. Working with my psychiatrist, I came to realize that my style is an obsessional one. I worry, I fixate, and unwelcome negative thoughts intrude into many areas of my life. Hypochondria just tends to focus the worries in a particular direction.

With Prozac's help, I've learned to control my anxiety and phobic tendencies and keep hypochondria at bay. I've been back on the drug for nearly two years, and although it helps greatly in managing everyday life, I know that it's not a panacea. Many people, including myself, are leery about medication, especially of a relatively new drug whose clinical trials evaluating the effects of long-term use are still in the early stages.

Others resist medication because they find something dehumanizing, almost robotlike, about every day swallowing a pill that alters their way of feeling. Hypochondriacs, especially, hate being out of control and tend to fear chemical dependence. Many illness phobics I spoke with seem to possess a stubborn insistence on wanting to do it on their own, to nip the behavior without medicinal help. One promising alternative to medication is behavior therapy, a technique by which patients confront illness fears and learn to replace obsessive, maladaptive thought patterns with healthier ones.

For hypochondria, however, there is no simple regimen or pill that cures. In my personal odyssey, what has probably helped as much as anything is the realization that I'm not the only one fighting this battle. The knowledge that one is not alone—which dawned for me in reading the *New York Times* article—can be the first step toward self-acceptance and recovery. But because hypochondria is such a hidden and misunderstood problem, it can be hard to find support. Few resources exist whereby sufferers can trade information, share feelings and experiences, offer suggestions; in short, share the journey. Nationwide, there are more than seven hundred support groups, from gatherings of wounded daughters of remote fathers to victims of lightning, but not one for hypochondria. People I interviewed have told me what a relief and comfort it is to talk to someone who has been there and understands. It is wonderful for those who have long felt humiliated and isolated to see that hypochondriacs are not selfish, whiny complainers incapable of love but, on the contrary, are talented, able, and sensitive people whose bodily preoccupations and fears sometimes get the best of them.

When I first told friends and acquaintances that I was writing a book about hypochondria, a few eyes rolled; more than one person said with a laugh, "Don't get sick over it!" Yet, while a subject of ridicule, hypochondria also holds great fascination. Many I spoke with mentioned a friend or relative who they believed suffers from the problem. After hearing my story, a good friend, whose complaints I've always suspected might be hypochondriacal, confided in me that for years she has suffered from vague symptoms. At times she was convinced that they represented the onset of multiple sclerosis; several times a year she checks in with her doctors, complaining of tingling, numbness, and achiness in her joints. Each time she undergoes a battery of tests and nothing shows up. "While it's happening it's all so real," she told me. "I have these awful pains — once I could barely walk. But eventually, after enough doctors say there's nothing wrong, they go away. Only later do I look back — when I'm totally pain free — and wonder, Could that have been stress pushing its way into my body?"

Is my friend a hypochondriac? And if she is, does she deserve compassion or scorn?

This book is for all who, like my friend, are in pain. Not the pain of bodily illness, but the pain of bodily imprisonment, in which happiness, well-being, and, yes, health are threatened by destructive thoughts the mind can't control. I hope this work helps to bring hypochondria to public attention and gives courage to those who project emotions onto their bodies, or live with the morbid fear of disease, to look beyond symptoms and, if necessary, seek treatment. I hope it also helps the friends and families of hypochondriacs, who often lose patience, to become more understanding and supportive of their loved ones. Each day more is being learned about the dynamics of hypochondria, offering those afflicted better treatment and relief. Last, I hope the book helps physicians who, dedicated to healing the sick, find themselves angry and frustrated with "patients who refuse to be well."

Confronting hypochondria may mean uncovering unpleasant truths about yourself. It may mean giving up a way of life, an elaborate set of defenses, a method of coping. But living with the terror of catastrophic illness or unbearable physical pain is no way to exist. It is a formidable barrier to happiness and fulfillment, which may indeed destroy the chances for both. Digging beneath symptoms and learning new ways of managing stress and emotions require time, determination, and above all, courage. But as someone who wasted precious time being terrified of death and disease, obsessed with every ache and pain, I truly believe that once you make the choice to be well, both in body and spirit, you'll cherish your health. You'll *never* want to take flight into sickness again.

CHAPTER ONE

A Much Maligned Malady

> I have always felt the obscurity in the question of hypochon-
> dria to be a disgraceful gap in our work.
> — Sigmund Freud, in a letter to Sandor Ferenczi

YOU HEAR THAT A COLLEGE friend has died of lymphoma
and for days, even weeks, you worry. In the wee hours of the
morning you wake up in a sweat. You reach for your neck. Are
those swollen glands I feel? As you toss and turn, dark ruminations play over and over in your head. Why have I been so tired
lately? . . . I really should get a checkup. Then the thoughts
become more frightening: What if I really get sick? How will
my family manage without me? Never before have you been
so aware of your mortality. Never before has death seemed
so close.

Psychiatrists call this transitory hypochondria, the bodily preoccupations and health fears with which just about every adult,
and a smaller number of children and teenagers, has had a brush.
Though the reaction occurs most frequently in patients recovering
from acute illnesses, it can be triggered by almost anything—
the death of a friend, media hype over a new ailment, even a cancer brochure. Nearly three quarters of first-year medical students
experience heightened health anxiety while learning about dread
diseases. The response isn't necessarily unhealthy and doesn't

mean one is destined for a life of worrying about illness. It may simply be a reaction to stress, a method of incorporating new information. As with the fear of flying, which even seasoned travelers develop after reading about a particularly horrific airline crash, most people get over this mild and temporary form of hypochondria quickly.

But for millions of otherwise normal, often highly functioning men and women, intense preoccupation with illness is a fact of life, a central feature of their identities. Many people experience baffling, terrifying physical symptoms that doctors are unable to diagnose. Or their complaints are given conflicting diagnoses, none of them satisfactory. They run from physician to physician in search of a cure, or even, a name for what ails them. Or afraid of what doctors might find, they avoid them altogether. Their friends and family members are soon turned off by their endless recitations of aches and pains. The word *hypochondriac* is spoken, often in a whisper.

To be thought of as a hypochondriac is a crushing experience. At best, the hypochondriac is a figure of fun, like fussy Felix Unger in *The Odd Couple* with his irritating, chronic complaints; or neurotic, self-absorbed Woody Allen; or George of *Seinfeld* fame, who tackles illness phobia with self-deprecating humor. At worst, a hypochondria sufferer carries a terrible stigma: someone who feigns medical problems for attention, a crank, faker, or fraud whose problems are "all in his head."

The caricature of the whining, self-involved complainer who frets endlessly about imagined ailments is the longtime staple of the humor industry. Meet Fred, a prototypical hypochondriac and the subject of much hilarity in a satirical *New York* magazine essay, "Listening to Advil." (The title plays off Peter Kramer's 1993 best-seller, *Listening to Prozac*.) The author, David Blum, seems to take much glee in describing the foibles of Fred, his patient, like the time the silly man convinced himself that he'd contracted smallpox on the subway. For this disease, Blum writes, "he wanted me to fly him to a medical conference in Wales, where he could participate in some longitudinal studies, and maybe become the subject of a touching Oscar-nominated short film." When during a session Fred demands reassurance that the throbbing sensation at the front of his head isn't a brain tumor, Blum comfortingly assures him that among brain tumor patients, "one was likely to observe other signals besides low-grade head pain—such as, for example, death." Blum eventually cures Fred's hypochondria by giving him Advil.

To those who have never experienced it or been through the problem with a loved one, hypochondria—which involves unremitting fears about disease and preoccupation with bodily symptoms despite medical reassurance—may seem comical, the very definition of nonsickness. But, in fact, the malady is responsible for much human misery and billions of dollars in unnecessary medical tests and procedures. Though people make fun of hypochondria, the problem can be debilitating, and in the extreme, a serious psychiatric illness that disrupts every facet of life. Mental health experts employ the diagnosis, and the medical term "hypochondriasis," but cautiously; they reserve it for a category of people who suffer not merely unexplained physical ailments but an almost phobic concern about their health.

Some interesting facts about hypochondria:
- It is experienced by men and women equally.
- It most commonly surfaces in one's twenties or thirties.
- Six to 10 percent of those who visit physicians' offices have some degree of the problem. (These figures reflect research conducted within medical populations and do not include the many sufferers who avoid doctors or turn to alternative therapies.)

Hypochondriacs tend to fall into two groups: those who have a medical illness but are plagued by constant worry about it even if their condition is stabilized, and those who perceive themselves ill despite diagnostic tests and examinations to the contrary.

Yet despite hypochondria's prevalence in our culture, few

hypochondriacal patients ever receive a true diagnosis—or assistance. General practitioners, who resist the term because of its negative connotations, have almost completely overlooked it—the standard two thousand–page medical text still devotes less than a page to the subject—leaving befuddled, frightened patients to make their way through the medical maze. And though psychiatrists have long been intrigued by the phenomenon, hypochondriacs have generally shunned them, preferring to seek help from internists, cardiologists, and neurologists, doctors who have no time, inclination, or expertise to deal with them.

Some of the reluctance of physicians to become involved is understandable. For one, hypochondria is a tough call to make. Ruling out an organic cause for physical complaints can be risky, and doctors have good reasons not to go out on a limb—not the least of which is fear of malpractice suits. Hypochondria is also a touchy subject and hardly the diagnosis most patients want to hear. People who feel sick do not really want psychological answers, and in many cases hypochondria may serve as a cover for, or be symptomatic of, other emotional troubles.

In times of a medical crisis it can be difficult to be a hypochondriac's friend, lover, or doctor. Nothing reassures hypochondriacs; they become so involved with the symptoms that they seem to think of no one else. Yet contrary to popular myth, they do not derive perverse pleasure from their illnesses. They suffer miserably and, in many cases, go to great lengths to conceal their anguish. That makes the stigma of hypochondria doubly cruel, because people often turn unconsciously to sickness not just to avoid confronting their own emotional problems but to "protect" their loved ones. They choose to express suffering and conflict by producing symptoms of illness rather than through nastier forms of acting out, such as hitting their children or abusing alcohol and drugs.

But the climate for hypochondriacs may at last be warming as the malady begins to emerge from a long period of disregard and neglect. Promising new treatments and a renewed interest in the mind-body phenomenon, combined with recognition that the dismissive attitude is translating into dollars and cents, are causing the medical community to take the problem more seriously. During the past two decades, a small but growing group of psychiatrists and general practitioners has been attempting to unravel the mysteries of hypochondria, identify hypochondriacal patients, and get to the underlying causes of their pain. "Hypochondria carries with it an implication of exaggeration, as if the problems were within a person's control. That somehow they aren't real," says psychiatrist Arthur Barsky, a leading expert in the field. But hypochondriacs are not malingering or pretending to be sick. Their pain and anguish, he says, is "as genuine as it is intense."

Ten years ago, Dr. Barsky, a Harvard professor who directs psychosomatic research at Brigham and Women's Hospital in Boston, took a break from academia to write *Worried Sick*, a book about America's preoccupation with health. His goal was to educate physicians and the public about hypochondria and get out the word that hypochondriacs really suffer. But the stigma has been difficult to erase. After the book was published in 1988, Barsky found that its message often elicited a reaction opposite to the one he'd aimed for. "I'd go on television talk shows and the response I'd often get was: 'How can you waste your time with these people when there are real tragedies out there—people suffering from cancer and AIDS?' "

A HISTORICAL PERSPECTIVE

Hypochondria is not one of medicine's success stories. Over nearly two millennia, the nature and cause of this elusive disorder has remained a matter of confusion and controversy. From Hippocrates through Freud until today, attitudes and interpretations have shifted, and the malady has gone in and out of fashion, along with medical theories and sentiments of the day.

One British researcher surveying the medical literature collected eighteen different usages of the term. In the words of Donald R. Lipsitt, chairman of the Department of Psychiatry at Mount Auburn Hospital in Cambridge, Massachusetts, "Perhaps no other word in medical and lay language is more confounded or abused."

Just how hypochondria acquired its pejorative label isn't entirely clear. Its history is a long and tangled one—the modern characterization of hypochondria as an emotional illness involving morbid preoccupation didn't crystallize until the early nineteenth century—and the term has traveled far from its original meaning. The concept, as old as medicine itself, dates back to ancient Greece. During the fourth century B.C., Hippocrates, who came to personify the ideal of the Western physician, used the term "hypochondrium," a transliteration of the Greek words *hypo* (under) and *chondros* (cartilage of the ribs), as an anatomical concept. In the earliest medical literature, hypochondria was linked to digestive disorders affecting the soft organs under the ribs, particularly the liver, gallbladder, and spleen.

The key to understanding hypochondria's metamorphosis from a part of the body to a phantom of the mind is to understand the history of medicine itself. It is important to realize that the notion of hypochondria was born of a different philosophy and time, in an era in which, unlike the present, physiology and psychology were virtually inseparable. What happened in the body also happened in the mind, the events united, indivisible, and mutually influential. So close was the interaction of psychic and physical states in the classical view that the notion of an "all in the head" or psychosomatic malady would have been absurd.

The speculation among modern psychiatric researchers that hypochondria is not an imaginary ailment but a complex condition that bridges both body and soul has its seeds in ancient medicine. Greek physicians believed that good health was an expression of a harmonious balance among internal and external forces and that, by some mechanism, psyche and soma communicated with each other in sympathetic discourse. Disease reflected a disharmony of these elements. As early as the second century A.D., the physician Galen, the Roman Hippocrates, described a condition, *Morbus hypochondriacus,* which had both physical and psychic manifestations—bodily pain, digestive troubles, sleeplessness, irritability, malaise—symptoms we now recognize as anxiety and depression.

The classical view of health and disease prevailed until the seventeenth century, when it was refined in the doctrine of "humors." This prescientific theory held that the body was composed of fluids, or humors, which shaped both physical constitution and disposition. Specific diseases, many of which we call psychiatric, were associated with imbalances in body chemistry caused by "humoral" abnormalities, a concept not so different from today's biochemical theories of neurotransmitters. Depression or melancholy, for instance—hypochondria later became synonymous with morbid depression—was caused by too much black bile, mania by an excess of yellow bile.

The objective was to deplete the offending humor that was acting on the brain, and physicians favored such therapies as bloodletting, purging, and potions designed to make patients sweat, salivate, and evacuate their bowels. Such remedies, however, were probably of less curative value than the humane treatment patients received. In the Hippocratic tradition, Renaissance physicians were both healers and moral guides, offering sympathetic hand-holding along with their prescriptive advice.

During the seventeenth century in England, hypochondria, or "hyp," as it was called, became a popular complaint. The Elizabethans linked hypochondriacal troubles with melancholy, a sentimental, self-pitying, mildly discomforting affectation that had swept in from northern Italy, and both men and women were soon addicted to what in England was relabeled the English malady; in France it was called *la maladie du français.* A trip to the spa for "vapours," "perturbations of animal spirits," and illnesses of "the spleen," all synonyms for hyp, became a chic therapeutic activity, and hypochondria a symbol of civilization. For in spite of hypochondria's vague character—the Renaissance scholar Robert Burton described its symptoms as so "ambiguous" even the "most exquisite physicians cannot determine of the part affected"—a diagnosis of "hysteric and hypochondriac affections" was something not only patients, but also physicians took very seriously, no doubt fueling its popularity.

The Elizabethan attitude toward melancholy and hypochondria was one of resigned acceptance: they were wretched conditions, but not at all shameful. Some modern scholars have linked the vogue of intellectual melancholy to the temper of the age. The late English Renaissance was a period marked by conflicts in religion and politics and tumultuous social change, and melancholy seemed to offer an avenue of escape from a confusing, disheartening world. By the mid–eighteenth century, the melancholic temperament had become a signature not just of the intellectual elite but of the middle classes. The physician George Cheyne, author of *The English Malady*, claimed in 1733 that one third of his countrymen suffered from nervous afflictions, primarily hypochondria and hysteria.

Whatever the reason for the popularity of these ailments, the English, fond of recording their distress, left a legacy of suffering and diseases in literary form. Burton's classic composition *The Anatomy of Melancholy*, published in 1621, may be among the best known confessional journals. The encyclopedic work has been called by the eminent physician Sir William Osler "the greatest medical treatise written by a layman," and it often reads like an early textbook on psychiatry. Much of the text is an attempt to clarify the melancholy's various guises. Burton describes a category of hypochondriacal melancholy, called windy or flatulent because of humoral vapors believed to be gaseous and hot. Its symptoms include "sharp belchings, fulsome crudities, heat in the bowel, wind and rumblings in the guts . . . sudden tremblings . . . suffocation, and short breath."

Though Burton viewed hypochondria primarily as a constitutional disorder, he believed it could be triggered by such emotions as fear, grief, and "some sudden commotion or perturbation of the mind . . . in such bodies especially are as ill disposed." Clearly, Burton recognized the mind as a key player in health and disease. His metaphor of the human body as clock — "If one wheel be amiss, all the rest are disordered, the whole fabric suffers" — harks back to the tenets of Greek medicine. But the idea that emotions and thoughts have a powerful influence on health, as opposed to the narrow biological interpretation of disease as a faulty functioning of some organ, is also quite modern, anticipating the mind-body approach to medicine that has become so popular.

Another well-known hypochondriac lived in the next century. James Boswell, the great Scottish biographer, watched public hangings to divert himself from an obsessive fear of venereal disease. He chronicled his lifelong struggles with hyp in seventy essays called "The Hypochondriack," which were published anonymously in the *London Magazine* between 1777 and 1783 and later collected in a book.

Boswell's more celebrated subject, Samuel Johnson — essayist, poet, and lexicographer — was tormented by ill health and paralyzing self-preoccupation. His physical disabilities seem to have been nervous in origin. He had a variety of twitches, moved awkwardly, and in later years his limbs shook frequently. Boswell felt that many of Johnson's eccentricities were "of a convulsive kind," and there is some speculation that he may have suffered from a type of obsessive-compulsive disorder. (The latest thinking about OCD is that in some forms it may overlap with hypochondria. Psychiatrists often have a difficult time telling the two apart when the behavior involves thoughts of illness and contamination, repeated requests for reassurance, or a compulsive checking of the body for signs of disease.)

Other notable creative people who have waged battle with hypochondria include the French novelist Marcel Proust, the

Russian author Leo Tolstoy, the American poet Sara Teasdale, England's poet laureate Alfred, Lord Tennyson, and the naturalist Charles Darwin. Darwin, whose controversial theories of evolution put him at odds with the church, suffered from intestinal troubles, headaches, and fatigue. Some biographers believe that he unconsciously used his ill health to avoid public speaking and that his ailments were rooted in the guilt he felt about toppling religious canons. Tennyson, in contrast to Darwin, suffered less from symptoms than from illness fears, particularly of going blind, though he lived into his eighties with tolerable eyesight.

Closer to our own time, E. B. White, author of *Charlotte's Web* and *Stuart Little*, struggled terribly with health anxiety—and Alzheimer's disease—as he grew older. "He was always in the grip of some ailment, missing out on some important event—Christmas, his granddaughter's wedding—because of his health; and his self-absorption could be depressing," writes Linda H. Davis in an essay published in *The New Yorker*. "Now and then, he would spend a night at the Blue Hill Inn— if he was feeling lonely.... If he felt especially ill, he would check himself into the Blue Hill Hospital for a day or two—a unique arrangement."

But hypochondria is far from an affliction of just the brilliant or famous. Most of the people who struggle with illness terror, or are possessed by symptoms no doctor can explain, are ordinary folk—secretaries, laborers and businessmen, journalists, lawyers, and physicians, men and women, old and young. In the course of research for this book, I've commiserated with a professor haunted by fears of death from a sudden heart attack, who takes his blood pressure behind locked doors and hides his medical bills from his wife. I've shared the anguish of a young Lebanese woman, a recent immigrant and mother of four, who can't get through a weekend without a panicky trip to an emergency room. I've sat over coffee with a graduate student plagued by fears of cancer who avoids physicians practicing traditional

Western medicine, but is fanatic about his regimen of vitamins, acupuncture, and homeopathic remedies.

Hypochondria Falls Out of Fashion

Somehow, within a period of less than two hundred years, hypochondria stopped being a point of cultural pride. After engaging scholars and physicians for centuries, the disorder was largely dismissed and ignored in our time, lost in a no-man's-land between the disciplines of medicine and psychology. How did hypochondriacal complaints, which once affected perhaps one third of England's population and continue in the modern era, fall into disregard and neglect? How did this malady move from its status of cultural acceptance to one of stigma?

Susan Baur, a historian and psychologist, explores these questions in *Hypochondria: Woeful Imaginings*. Her explanations for hypochondria's mysterious unpopularity lie largely with the arrival of Freudian psychoanalysis and the idea that the vague, confusing symptoms of hypochondria and hysteria arose not in the body but in the mind.

The departure from humoral theory and the dichotomizing of disease into physical and mental, a notion introduced into Western thought by the French philosopher René Descartes some five hundred years ago and popularized by the psychoanalytic movement at the turn of this century, dealt hypochondria a crippling blow. Cartesian dualism fostered the myth of the body as a machine governed by physical laws, tilting the focus of medicine away from more naturalistic explanations of healing to physiology. Human anatomy was mapped, circulation of blood described, and diseases classified, while the more obscure behavioral and environmental aspects of health faded into the background.

Then along came Freud with his idea that unconscious conflicts could be expressed as physical symptoms. Psychoanalytic theory, while resurrecting the importance of the mind, dealt hypochondria its second blow: the notion that the mind could be a major culprit in some diseases but play no role in others. This opened a whole new world of illnesses—those which could be all in the head—and paved the way for the division of medicine into two camps: the mind and the body specialists.

Freud, a neurologist by training, based his new practice of psychoanalysis on studies of hysterical women. Hysteria as a woman's illness was not a new concept; it had been around since the time of Galen, and the word derives from the Greek term "hyster," which means "womb." Until the eighteenth century, when it became known as a neurological disorder, the condition was widely believed to be associated with problems of the uterus, in contrast to hypochondria, in which the offending organ was thought to be the spleen. Over time hysteria came to be regarded as the female counterpart of hypochondria.

By the mid-nineteenth century, hysteria had become pandemic. Women were showing up at doctors' offices exhibiting a kaleidoscope of bizarre symptoms: fits, tremors, tics, fainting spells, convulsions, and paralysis, among the most usual. Rarely did medical therapies work; as soon as one symptom cleared, another popped up. Frustrated and threatened by refractory symptoms, physicians could offer patients little more than rest cures, although some doctors resorted to savage surgeries, such as oophorectomy (removal of the ovaries) and cauterization of the clitoris.

Physicians began to loathe hysterics, viewing them as vain, whining, and histrionic, far from the Victorian ideal, and regularly suspected them of faking their illnesses. As David Morris writes in *The Culture of Pain*: "Any woman whose symptoms did not respond to conventional treatment—especially if her doctor judged her too emotional, too theatrical, too self-centered, too moody or oversexed—might soon be classified and implicitly condemned as hysterical. Hysteria provided a convenient diagnostic box for imprisoning women whom male doctors were unable to cure."

Then in 1895, Sigmund Freud and Josef Breuer published *Studies in Hysteria*, presenting the case of Anna O., the first hysteric in psychoanalytic literature. Freud had solved the mystery of the disorder, interpreting hysterical symptoms not as signs of disease, but as symbolic expressions of hidden sexual fantasies and repressed childhood trauma. So the word went out: hysteria had been officially declared a neurosis, a mental disease. No longer were its symptoms legitimate in the eyes of medicine, so women stopped having them. Fits and paralysis, which had spread epidemically since the Middle Ages, came to an end. By 1930, the medical diagnosis of hysteria had virtually disappeared.

But what about hypochondria? Freud, in devoting his prodigious skills almost exclusively to intrapsychic conflict, did much to add to the confusion and neglect of the disorder that would follow. Unlike the metaphoric, almost poetic character of hysteria — a woman suddenly goes blind struggling to repress memories of sexual molestation by an uncle — which Freud viewed as a pure example of mental illness, or psychoneurosis, hypochondria was labeled an actual neurosis, that is, a neurosis with a physical basis. Freud theorized that in hypochondria an increased blood supply from pent-up libido produced changes in the internal organs, a hypothesis of which he himself was never entirely convinced.

The theories of Freud and his followers left hypochondria in therapeutic oblivion, rejected by the psychoanalysts for being too much of the body and disdained by the medical establishment as being too much of the mind. As Susan Baur aptly puts it: "Toward the end of the nineteenth century hypochondria turned a corner, historically speaking, and nearly dropped out of sight."

It is ironic that Freud, whose discoveries opened the inner world of the patient, would instill in hypochondriacs a horror of self-knowledge and insight. But once psychoanalysis came into play, patients would shed the symptoms the new mental health practitioners called psychosomatic in hope of finding new ones that physicians would label genuinely organic. The Canadian historian Edward Shorter, author of *From Paralysis to Fatigue: A History of Psychosomatic Illness in the Modern Era*, writes: "Consultation with a psychiatrist . . . now became tantamount to 'seeing a shrink,' lying on a couch attended to by *New Yorker*–style cartoons of little men with pointy beards and thick accents, and learning 'it was all in one's head.' "

What the psychoanalytic movement essentially did was erect an unbridgeable divide between the brain and the mind, pinching all other budding forms of psychotherapy and isolating psychiatry from the mainstream of medicine. Shorter believes that hypochondria's ultimate assignment to psychiatry represented "a fateful chapter, from the patient's viewpoint, in the history of psychosomatic illness." It did not dissolve the peculiar mix of emotional and physical problems that society once readily accepted as "hypochondriac and hysteric," but instead transformed them. Many believe that these problems have made their way into more socially acceptable illnesses, what Shorter calls "fashionable" diseases, which are comprised almost entirely of symptoms still puzzling to medical science: among them, fibromyalgia (pains all over), chronic fatigue syndrome, temporomandibular joint syndrome, total food allergy, and a heightened cultural sensitivity to chronic pain — a controversial notion with which many sufferers of these ailments would undoubtedly take issue.

Freud may have done little to further the cause of hypochondriacs, but that doesn't mean his theories aren't valuable or important. The relevance of his work to our time lies largely in his insights into the darker aspects of sexuality and trauma and appreciation for the healing power of the therapeutic relationship. In *The Illness Narratives*, Arthur Kleinman, a Harvard psychiatrist and anthropologist, suggests that Freud's model of inner turmoil expressed as a physical event — for example, the case of a patient who is literally unable to walk because he can't resist his father's dominance—has proved useful to a limited degree. (Here, in what is called a classical conversion, the physical symptom is a symbolic expression of an unconscious conflict.) But for the most part, the narrow psychoanalytic approach to the interpretation of illness meanings, Kleinman says, has become "an extremely difficult path to follow, a torturous lane, which, for all its fascination and promise, leads to a dead end of speculation and an absence of research."

Still, he credits Freud for an important contribution to medicine, which was to "authorize the interpretation of the biography of the patient and the interpersonal context of disorder as appropriate components of the practitioner's craft." Unfortunately, Freudian doctrine placed mind-body problems in the domain of psychiatry, leaving physiology to biological science, which led to dead ends on both levels. As Kleinman points out, "A single-minded quest for psychoanalytic reality can dehumanize the patient every bit as much as the numbing reductionism of an obsessively biomedical investigation." For Kleinman and many practitioners it is time to bring the best of both approaches together. And for an understanding of hypochondria, which stands at the crossroads of physical and mental illness, this is essential.

BACK INTO VOGUE

Today, as medicine struggles to develop a unified theory of how organic and psychic processes coexist, the study of hypochondria is being resurrected; and this most ancient, intriguing disorder is once again captivating the minds of physicians and the lay public. Renewed interest began during the 1970s with the revolution in biopsychiatry, in which psychiatric researchers began to recognize the enormous power a new generation of drugs could wield on brain chemistry and over mental illness. Not only could these substances help to alleviate general mood disorders, like anxiety and depression, they also appeared useful in treating a host of other psychiatric conditions — eating disorders, panic attacks, obsessive-compulsive behavior, and phobias, to name but a few.

The first of this new class of drugs was discovered in the 1950s by Swiss scientists looking for a cure for the common cold. The drug, imipramine, did nothing for the sniffles, but it remarkably boosted the supply of neurotransmitters, the signaling molecules that shuttle information between nerve cells in the brain. Once science had pointed the way to a neurological basis for mood disorders, research in the neurosciences exploded, culminating in the 1970s discovery of selective serotonin reuptake blockers (SSRIs). Prozac was the first of this new generation of "wonder drugs" (followed by Zoloft, Paxil, and Luvox), which could selectively target the neurotransmitter serotonin, a powerful brain chemical that regulates a slew of bodily functions and emotions, including anger, depression, and impulsivity.

Until the arrival of the SSRIs, hypochondria was considered refractory to therapeutic treatment. The legacy of Freud, that hypochondria was basically unanalyzable, remained, and without a neurotic conflict to uncover, hypochondria wasn't thought to respond to talking cures. (Even today's *Merck Manual*, the physicians' official compendium of illnesses, speaks of a poor prognosis: "Only a very small proportion of patients — perhaps 5% — recover permanently.") Behavior therapy, which teaches patients new ways of responding to unsettling stimuli, was beginning to be touted in the 1970s as an effective treatment for patients with obsessions and compulsions like hand-washing and "checking" rituals, but therapists hadn't yet thought of applying it to hypochondria.

Now there was hope of a cure. If obsessive-compulsive disorder was indeed caused by a biological glitch in the brain, perhaps hypochondria was, too. With interest in the disorder rekindled, psychiatrists became eager to investigate new treatments. But there was a problem: they didn't know many hypochondriacs. These types of patients, who weren't under psychiatric care, were shuttling from doctor to doctor, lost in the confusing maze of general health care. So, backed by university and later federal grants, a core group of psychiatrists interested in treating hypochondria as well as applying psychiatry to problems in physical medicine set out to find the "worried well" and determine just how many were seeking medical treatment.

What they discovered was truly astounding: patients with symptoms for which there was no apparent cause—and a subgroup who suffered from illness fears that didn't respond to medical reassurance—made up the bulk of the patient population! This didn't come as a surprise to Nicholas Cummings, a psychologist hired in the 1950s to develop a mental health program for the Kaiser-Permanente Health Plan in California, the first managed health care network, which is still among the country's largest. Examining patient records, Cummings discovered that 60 percent of visits to physicians were by people with no discernible illness. Their chart code, NDA, no discernible abnormality, actually meant hypochondriac.

Cummings says, "These were the patients doctors made fun of," the GOMERs (Get Out of My Emergency Room), Crocks, Thick Charts, and Turkeys. At first Cummings, a former president of the American Psychological Association who now heads the Institute for Behavioral Health, thought there was something about the health maintenance organization (HMO) approach that encouraged this type of patient to enroll. (Unlike the fee-for-service system, HMOs tend to cover medical care regardless of whether a "physical" diagnosis is recorded.) Then, in 1976, representatives of the American Medical Association testified before a U.S. Senate health committee that "in the United States on any given day, 60 to 70 percent of the patients who are waiting to see the physician either have no physical disease but are somatizing stress, or stress is impeding the treatment and healing of a physical condition."

Epidemiological research would confirm these early findings.

Over the years, various studies have shown that between 25 and 75 percent of those who visit doctors are suffering primarily from psychological and social problems, not medical illnesses. The majority of these patients are troubled by at least one symptom with no obvious organic cause; one in ten patients has no signs of any physical disease whatsoever but doesn't respond to medical reassurance.

Indeed, the symptoms people most frequently complain to doctors about—back pain, chest pain, headache, fatigue, constipation—rarely have a clear-cut organic basis. Of one thousand patients seeking help from internists at a San Antonio medical center, the most common complaint, chest pain, signified a medical problem in just 11 percent of the cases. Fatigue, the next most frequent, had a medical cause in only 13 percent of the cases, and dizziness in 18 percent. A study of 685 patients at two Montreal clinics found that 180 patients, or 26 percent, had symptoms doctors couldn't explain—nearly a third of this group suffered from anxiety or depressive disorders and a quarter displayed hypochondriacal behavior, that is, they had no signs of a serious medical illness to justify their extreme worry.

To the health care industry the most significant findings have not been the percentage of people who seem to define emotional problems as medical, but their expenditures. Studies have shown that those who somatize distress consult physicians four times as often and have medical bills ten to fourteen times higher than the national average. A conservative estimate of the burden to the health care system—through extensive and repeated workups, needless operations, doctor-shopping and overmedication—is about $20 billion a year.

As early as the 1970s, psychiatric researchers realized that they needed a broad conceptual framework to account for the vast array of people who complained of physical symptoms but had no biological markers to explain them, one that wouldn't discredit the patients. The concept had to encompass a wide spectrum, from the patient whose back "goes out" under certain types of stress to patients with complicated histories of multiple ailments to others terrified of a specific disease. They chose to call the phenomenon somatization, which refers to the notion that mental anguish not consciously acknowledged can be expressed as a physical complaint. Coined by the Viennese analyst Wilhelm Stekel, who used the term as early as 1924 to connote "a bodily disorder that arises as an expression of deep-seated neurosis," it was still virtually unknown to the public, so the feeling was that it would be free of pejorative connotations. However, finding a name for the problem wasn't enough; the researchers knew that proper treatment of these patients depended on slotting them correctly, and the psychiatric profession went to work formally categorizing their behaviors. The result was the creation in 1980 of a new classification of mental illness, the somatoform disorders.

Textbook Cases

Psychiatrists today classify hypochondria as one of a type of behaviors collectively known as the somatoform disorders. What
these conditions have in common is that sufferers feel physical
symptoms for which they seek medical attention in the absence of
a detected organic disease or which are out of proportion to a
given ailment.

Depending on symptoms and behavior, "somatizers" fall into
one of several categories:

Somatization disorder: "My body is falling apart." This is a serious, debilitating malady in which the patient is focused on multiple physical complaints and on an often chaotic attempt to find a
cure for them. The trouble usually begins before age thirty, persists
for several years, and includes a history of lifetime symptoms—
nausea, bloating, pain in the head and abdomen, sexual indifference, and pseudoneurologic symptoms are among the most
common. A milder ailment, with fewer symptoms and of shorter
duration, is termed either "adjustment disorder with physical
complaints," or if it persists for as many as six months, "undiffer-
entiated somatoform disorder."

Hypochondriasis: "I have a brain tumor." People with hypochondriasis are less focused on their symptoms than on what they
believe the symptoms signify; no amount of medical reassurance is
capable of permanently removing their nagging fears that a serious or perhaps fatal disease is present or lurking. Whereas people
with somatization disorder just have the symptoms, the hypochondriac says, "I know something is seriously wrong with my
bladder" or "I've got colon cancer."

Body Dysmorphic Disorder: "My face looks weird." Normal-
looking people are preoccupied with an imagined ugliness or a
physical deformity. Men may become obsessed with the size of
their penis, women with their breasts. Noses, lips, and wrinkles are
other target areas. Sufferers frequently consult plastic surgeons
and submit to multiple surgical procedures.

Conversion disorder: "I can't walk." Here the relationship between a trauma and the related physical disability is sometimes
transparent; a person unable to have a child develops symptoms

of pregnancy, called pseudocyesis, or a soldier who cannot bring himself to kill may find his hand paralyzed.

Pain disorder: "Nothing helps." A preoccupation with pain in one or more parts of the body that is thought to have been induced or exacerbated by psychological factors. It's diagnosed after examinations either fail to uncover a biological explanation or the complaint is grossly in excess of the physical findings.

CHAPTER TWO

The Many Faces of Somatization

> To some, ill health is
> a way to be important,
> others are stoics,
> a few fanatics,
> who won't feel happy until
> they are cut open.
> —W. H. Auden, "The Art of Healing"
> In Memoriam, David Protetch, M.D.

THE NAME SOMATOFORM DISORDERS is really just a new designation for old clinical problems. Though the classifications may have seemed like a radical idea when first proposed, all modern psychiatry did was take the old constructs of hypochondria and hysteria and divide them into seven discrete categories: hypochondriasis, body dysmorphic disorder, somatization disorder, pain disorder, conversion disorder, and two others that more or less serve as catch basins for less severe symptoms or those which don't fit into any group. All these disorders share some common features: symptoms suggestive of a physical illness but without a diagnosable medical disease, or other psychiatric condition, to fully account for them; there is evidence, or at least a strong presumption, that the symptoms are linked to psychic or emotional distress.

When psychiatric researchers set out to distinguish among the various kinds of somatizers, they had no idea how many different candidates there might be, or how long the process would take. They faced both theoretical and logistical hurdles. Research was scattered all over the place: Washington University's School of Medicine in St. Louis was the hotbed for the study of Briquet's syndrome, the earlier term for somatization disorder, while psychiatrists in Australia and Great Britain were investigating the morbid fear of disease. There was the additional barrier of ferreting out sufferers, the majority of whom frequented general medical settings, thus representing a subset of their own: patients who sought traditional care.

As it was, medical patients alone made for an unwieldy group. There were hypochondriacs who were truly sick but excessively worried and those who were well but afraid. There were individuals who were preoccupied with physical appearance; who focused on headaches or bowels; who were embarrassed by their preoccupations; and those who relished discussing them. Some were aware of deeper problems, but most were oblivious of anything else being wrong. Then there were patients with true organic disease. Did a medical condition rule out the possibility of hypochondria? As Ian Pilowsky, the Australian psychiatrist credited with devising one of the first questionnaires to detect hypochondriacal beliefs, remarked, "There is obviously no reason why a patient with advanced carcinoma should not show abnormal illness behaviour."

Though the somatoform disorders made their clinical debut in 1980, in the third edition of the *Diagnostic and Statistical Manual of Mental Disorders* (DSM), the American Psychiatric Association's compendium of mental illness, the uncertainties about their usefulness and validity are far from resolved. Partly because the categories are so new and medicine so far from unraveling the mind-body puzzle, they tend to be subject to professional controversy.

In one camp are the "splitters," who endorse the somatoform classifications. They argue that because the vast majority of mental disorders cannot be detected by laboratory tests, grouping patterns of behavior that predispose people to psychiatric distress is the most promising method psychiatry has to predict the course, severity, response to treatment, and outcome of an illness.

The "lumpers," on the other hand, criticize the classifications as overlapping, arbitrary, and needlessly stringent, preferring the umbrella type concept of somatization, the broad notion that emotions can masquerade as bodily complaints. For example, if someone has a hypochondriacal belief that lasts for five months, his problem would fall under the category of somatoform disorder not otherwise specialized; add another month to the suffering and he'd be classified a hypochondriac. Moreover, the lumpers argue, somatic symptoms are so common and widespread that it is nearly impossible to separate psychiatric illness from, say, a temporary retreat from conflict or stress. They contend that somatoform disorders should be looked at not on their own, but as secondary symptoms of other psychiatric illnesses, like anxiety and depression. Some fear that psychiatry, in its zealousness to classify, is making the same mistake many claim biomedicine has made, forgetting to make people well.

This tension has made for some heated arguments. One debate involved the definition of somatization disorder itself. For diagnosis, the 1987 version of DSM required a patient to have a history of thirteen unexplained medical complaints from a list of thirty-five over the major part of adult life. As a result of a lobby by a group of psychiatrists to lower the symptom threshold, researchers in charge of creating DSM-IV conducted analyses of data from a large number of patients with somatization disorder to determine which symptoms were reported most frequently and whether a shorter list would be sufficient to diagnose patients. The search led to the conclusion that a diagnosis based on eight criteria was sensitive and specific enough to correctly identify patients.

One controversy that has not been resolved involves hypochondria: whether the presence of physical signs or sensations is a necessary yardstick of the disorder or whether hypochondria can be diagnosed on the basis of phobia alone. For example, would a person with fear of AIDS, but lacking physical symptoms, be considered a hypochondriac? According to DSM-IV, such an individual could not be labeled hypochondriacal, a perspective with which not all psychiatrists agree.

Yet despite such disagreements, many believe the creation of the somatoform disorders represents an important step toward addressing the needs of patients and bringing a new perspective to primary care. Perhaps more valuable for overall description than specific diagnosis, the classifications give researchers a vision of a population that is vital to future investigation and provide clinicians with a common language for communicating about problems for which they have professional responsibility.

The *Diagnostic and Statistical Manual* is not a catechism, and few practitioners adhere to its guidelines strictly. Diagnostic boundaries tend to become blurred in the everyday practice of medicine. Because most people don't come in the distinctive flavors of DSM, a doctor doesn't say to his patients, "Gee, you don't fit under a label. I can't help you." As the editors of DSM point out, the manual "doesn't classify people; it classifies the disorders that people have."

Nor are these classifications written in stone. DSM is very much a work in progress intended to keep pace with developments in psychiatry and medicine, a barometer of social change as well as a diagnostic tool. The manual lends clarity and order not only by defining psychiatric illnesses, but helping clinicians distinguish them from other mental and physical conditions. Since its first edition was published in 1952, psychiatry's official reference book has been overhauled three times, although critics accuse its developers of promoting "syndromitis," inventing quasi-medical categories to suit almost any deviation from the norm. Diseases listed in the most recent revision, DSM-IV, published in 1994, have grown to more than 300 from an original 106.

From the perspective of hypochondriacs, one of the most important achievements of the new classifications is that they separate somatoform ailments, which by definition *never involve conscious intent*, from factitious disorders, in which there is a deliberate fabrication of illness, two quite different phenomena that have tended to be confused in public and medical consciousness. Factitious disorders come in two types: malingerers who feign illness to achieve some end, for example, to avoid work, win a lawsuit, or obtain drugs, and Münchausen's patients, who falsify symptoms or laboratory results for a less tangible goal. In Münchausen's syndrome, playing sick seems to be an end in itself.

The irony is that physicians in residency training spend more time relating the bizarre tales of "professional" and "surgery addicted" patients, as Münchausen's sufferers are referred to, than learning how to care for the hypochondriacs or other somatizers, patients with whom they will undoubtedly have more contact and whose prognosis is infinitely more hopeful. Münchausen's syndrome is certainly tragic, especially the subset of sufferers who make their children sick—a related disturbance called Münchausen's by proxy. Of course, people who inject themselves with pus or feces or contaminate children's urine samples lend themselves to juicier, more sensationalistic news stories than garden variety somatic sufferers. Perhaps these all-too-common fears and symptoms hit too close to home.

THE PATIENTS SPEAK

More revealing than the listings of manual writers are the stories of real people, many of whose voices I heard in the course of my research. The material is organized so that the first three people you meet struggle with hypochondria as psychiatrists define the malady today. Their symptoms vary and each grapples with the problem uniquely, but they share a common enemy: a morbid fear of disease that greatly interferes with happiness.

The remaining cases represent variations on the somatizing theme. These four short clinical vignettes, based on the stories of real people, depict body dysmorphic disorder, somatization disorder, pain disorder, and conversion disorder.

HYPOCHONDRIA

For all the puzzlement surrounding this condition, its DSM definition is fairly unmysterious and straightforward: "a preoccupation with fears of having, or the idea that one has, a serious disease based on misinterpretation of one or more bodily signs or symptoms." For a person to be considered a hypochondriac today, her unwarranted fear or belief of illness must persist for at least six months despite the failure of repeated examinations and diagnostic tests to uncover a medical condition that can fully account for the concerns or symptoms, although a coexisting medical condition may be present.

During the 1960s, the psychiatrist Ian Pilowsky, noting the myriad ways in which morbid thoughts and body sensations could intermingle, identified three dimensions of hypochondriacal behavior, which are still generally accepted. They are bodily preoccupation, disease phobia, and disease conviction in spite of medical reassurance. As the cases that follow suggest, for most individuals these dimensions tend to overlap. But they can exist on their own or any one of them may predominate.

Bodily Preoccupation

ABIR: FROM BEIRUT TO BROOKLYN

"Ears clogged, loss of appetite, fatigue, chills up and down spine, muscle aches, twitches, pins and needles on forehead, dizziness, fluttering of eyelids, forgetting all the time, itchiness, rashes, vaginal inflammation, no enjoyment of sex."

This laundry list of complaints appears to reflect the concerns of an eighty-year-old, but Abir, a tall, attractive Lebanese woman, was only thirty-two. She had responded to an advertisement seeking participants for Dr. Fallon's Heightened Illness Concern study and enrolled at once. Abir had come to the clinic, fittingly called Freedom from Fear, because she was desperate; she felt sick and afraid all the time, sure something awful was going to happen. "I can feel it in my body. It's just not right," she explained during a therapy session. "Maybe I'm going to have a stroke. I feel numbness always on my left side. Like pins and needles, a heaviness. It's crazy the way it comes and goes."

She and her husband, Ali, had four children, twin ten-year-old girls and two younger boys. The couple worked for the same car service in Manhattan, trading shifts so one of them could be at home with the kids. Most of the time she was too busy to think, but come the weekend she'd start feeling terrible — dizzy, nauseated, certain she was on the verge of a stroke. Her husband had to take her to an emergency room several times; sometimes she'd go by herself. "Each time they'd do tests. My blood pressure is good, they'd say. My blood is okay. I have mildly elevated cholesterol, but that's all." One day a doctor told her this was anxiety and advised her to get psychiatric help. "Why not, I thought. If this is my problem, I'll do it. I went to the psychiatric clinic the doctor recommended, and they asked me there if I thought about killing myself. When I told my husband, he was angry because he didn't think the place was for me. He said, 'It's for people who are sick on alcohol and drugs. You just make a big deal of things.' That's what he says is my problem. I exaggerate. 'You're not going to die,' he says. 'You're strong.' "

Growing up in Beirut, Abir remembers being nervous and high strung. Her fears, however, were based on something quite real. It was a civil war, and Lebanon was under siege. No one ever knew when a bomb would fall. At least once a month, her parents, six sisters, and two brothers would leave their three-room apartment and run from an explosion to a nearby sewer or an underground shelter a mile away. But Abir always felt different from the rest of her family. None of them liked the war, but they accepted it as the way life was. "If I heard the slightest noise, I'd be the first one out the door. 'Hurry up,' I'd say. 'We're going to die.' They'd laugh at me—a lot of times it was a false alarm."

She met her husband, Ali, as a teenager, and when Beirut was invaded by the Israeli army in 1982, she fled with him to Syria, hiding out in the mountains, sleeping in the woods, and eating bread and water supplied by the Lebanese militia. "You could hear the sound of warplanes and missiles in the valley," she recalls. She worried about the family she left behind, later learning that her fifty-year-old mother had died trying to escape and a sister had been shot and paralyzed in one leg. She never had the chance to say good-bye. Abir and Ali fared better. They befriended a soldier who smuggled them into Syria, then moved to Jordan so that Ali could serve in the army. Abir gave birth to the twins there. As a mother, she felt purposeful, even healthy. The family was happy in Jordan, but after five years, the economy went sour. It was time to go.

Not speaking a word of English, Abir arrived at Kennedy Airport in 1989 with her daughters and a six-month-old baby in tow. She had $200 in her pocket and the address of a mosque in Brooklyn. The Arab community befriended her, and when Ali arrived a few months later, friends helped him find a job as a security guard. Abir enrolled in a community school to learn English and taught herself to read; after a year of typing and filing for an Arab businessman, she decided she wanted more. Her interest in medicine led her to a nurse's aide course, but as soon as she enrolled she knew the decision was wrong. She began looking up diseases in the dictionaries and encyclopedias. "I'd read them and have chills all over. I felt the symptoms applied to me." During her hospital training period, she'd see the sick patients in the wards and they terrified her. She didn't want to be home alone. "I kept asking my husband, 'What's this bump? What's this rash?' Then the symptoms got worse. I was sick all the time. I'd lose my temper with the kids. I'd cry and I didn't know why."

For a year she fought off fears that she might be HIV positive and became convinced that her son had contracted the virus three years earlier from a baby-sitter she thought might have had it. "Every time I turned on the television, AIDS was there, like it was out to get me." She gave up the nursing course, thinking it would solve the problem, but her trips to the hospital increased. "I'd be in my apartment and would get so anxious and upset I'd just have to go. I'd pay only thirteen dollars at this one clinic, but still my husband got mad. Not only about the money, but because I wasn't taking care of things at home."

Dr. Fallon's study, Abir says, saved her life. She began a trial of what she thought was Prozac—it turned out that she was given the placebo—and spent about six months in therapy. "For the first time in years, I felt relaxed. I'd sit and talk with Dr. Fallon and he'd try to help me with my problems. I thought the medication was the reason I was doing better. I was able to stay in my apartment without feeling I had to run to the emergency room. The anxiety was better, the symptoms too, and I didn't have so many fights with my husband."

Life is still hard, money is tight, and driving wealthy people around New York can make her testy. But Abir is happier than she has been. "In the Arab community, no one likes to talk about mental illness. If you have a problem, you solve it. The people at Freedom from Fear understand that you can't always do it yourself. They made me realize I'm not crazy. And even if I am sometimes, there's a place I can go."

Disease Conviction

JULIE: "I'M NOT MY MOTHER!"

Julie, a fifty-year-old writer, tells people that a spell was cast over her as a child. "My mother was an artist, bright and witty. When I was seven, she got sick with something mysterious. She had pains in her legs and terrible fatigue. At thirty-six, she took to her bed in our small Boston apartment and conveyed her fears to me, her only child: 'All the women in our family die young'—Julie's grandmother had died of a heart attack at forty-three—'and it's going to happen to me,' she said. And because she was Mommy, I believed her."

For two years her mother's illness became the focus of Julie's life. Her father withdrew, going out for drinks after work and leaving Julie alone with her mother most nights. "Dad didn't want to hear about her ailments. His attitude was 'I'll pay the doctor bills. Tell me when you're cured.' " After school each day, Julie wrote in her diary. Page after page said essentially the same thing: Mommy had a bad day. Mommy had a good day. Mommy's worse.

Her mother died early on a Sunday morning. Her father ran into Julie's room, yelling, "Go get help. Mommy's not breathing." Julie ran to get a neighbor, but it was too late. Detectives came to the house. They took pictures. Julie remembers their confiscating a jar of photography developing fluid. Later police told the family she had inhaled a chemical that had killed her. And that was that. "Dad didn't have the passion to find out much more. It was never termed a suicide and we never talked about it. Our story was that Mommy got sick and died and we don't know why."

Julie grew up, fell in love, and married at twenty-two; she gave birth to three children. "I was really into babies—natural childbirth, breast-feeding, carrying them in Snugglies, the whole bit." Her first child was a boy, and after the second, a girl, was born, she remembers breathing a sigh of relief: "Now I'm definitely not my mother." But at thirty-five, pregnant with her last child, she developed a fear of dying in childbirth. The morbid thoughts disappeared after she came through the birth with flying colors, but looking back, she realized that it was around that time she began to obsess about her health. A doctor friend later told her he was concerned about the way she focused on disease and needed constant reassurance.

During that period Julie decided to satisfy some questions about her mother's death. For $40 she obtained a copy of the autopsy report and learned that the pathologist had found a small quantity of chlorinated hydrocarbon in her mother's brain and stomach. "Somehow, as I stared at those words, I felt I knew my mother," she says. "I understood how it was possible to be so afraid of death that you could take your own life, and it terrified me."

After that "all hell broke loose." In her early forties, Julie began to have terrible chest pains and difficulty breathing. She became convinced that "bad genes" would cause her to die of a heart attack, just as her grandmother had. Clutching her mother's autopsy report, she went to see a cardiologist. "He gave me some tests, then opened a drawer and said, 'Take your pick, Halcyon or Xanax. You'll feel better. There's nothing wrong with your heart that I can find.'" Eventually she found her way to a cardiologist who practiced homeopathic medicine. The doctor was gentle. He diagnosed a slight arrhythmia, but said it was nothing to worry about. He explained the mind-body connection, how alarming thoughts can set off panic, which can lead to changes in breathing and cause physiologic changes in the body. "We talked about diet, exercise, and relaxation techniques. He told me in a sensitive way that I wasn't sick. I wasn't dying. It was something I needed to hear."

Julie turned to Eastern medicine. She began taking courses at the Himalayan Institute, learning about biofeedback, yoga, and vegetarian cooking. As her kids got older, she had more time to pursue outside interests; she enrolled in psychology and computer courses, joined a writers group, and began to freelance. Then out of the blue came another episode. Swollen glands, debilitating fatigue, pelvic pain. She noticed a bizarre smell under her left armpit that wouldn't go away no matter how clean she was. It had all started again, the downward spiral of pain and fear. Julie vowed not to let it affect her family — "I didn't want to cut myself off as my mother had done" — but she became depressed and couldn't help herself. She locked herself in her room, let things go in the house, and started making the doctor

rounds. A blood test showed a slight abnormality, and she became convinced that she had rheumatoid arthritis or lupus. Two
rheumatologists assured her she didn't, that it was only an in-
significant immune deficiency. "My husband, a tough-it-out
person who has never been sick in bed as long as I've known
him, would blow up at me. We have only catastrophic insurance
and the bills were killing us. He'd be hurtful, then remorseful."

Once when Julie was at her computer, she logged on to an on-
line discussion about fibromyalgia, also called fibrositis. It's a
diagnosis many patients, 90 percent of them women, have received, a rheumatic syndrome characterized by muscular-skeletal
aching and stiffness as well as "trigger points" — spots on the
body tender to touch. Whether fibromyalgia is a "real" disease
is controversial, as one of the hallmarks of the syndrome is normal lab tests. Julie researched everything there was to know
about fibromyalgia and took the literature to her internist.
There were support groups for the problem, she told him, with
people described as feeling like "being run over by a truck." She
asked her doctor if she could have the syndrome, and he said it
was possible. Finding the diagnosis seemed to snap Julie out of
her troubles. Since the best treatment for fibromyalgia is healthy
living, it was time to get back to emotional stability. Vitamins,
herbs, regular exercise, yoga. She also began reading about menopause and it dawned on her that its approach could be contributing to her physical symptoms and mood swings. Whether
it was hormones or fibromyalgia didn't matter; the flare-ups,
she knew, were exacerbated by stress. "I used to think the symptoms came out of nowhere, but I now see a pattern. The tension comes first, then I feel sick, then I start obsessing about
a particular illness. Now I try to stop the cycle at the tension stage. I make a huge effort to think pleasurable thoughts.
I go to bed early, meditate, get a grip on myself, do construc-
tive work."

One positive change in Julie's life has been establishing a relationship with an internist she trusts. "He's not an alarmist," she
says. "I can talk to him about my fears and my constant need

for reassurance and he understands." She doesn't run to doctors because she's already had so much radiation from testing. Another motivation to work on having a more positive view of health is the impact her problems have had on her middle daughter, who has "too many" physical ailments. "She's hypersensitive, sensitive to changes in her body, sensitive to light. 'What's this, Mom?' she asks. 'Don't worry,' I tell her. I think about my dear mother, the grandmother my daughter never knew, and I'm determined. It's up to me to break the chain."

Disease Phobia

PETER: MARKED FOR DEATH

Successful and bright, a partner in an advertising firm and the father of three, Peter is painfully aware of his hypochondria. So why can't he beat it?

Peter's first memory of being overly concerned about disease was at about the age of thirteen, when his best friend developed lymphoma. It happened suddenly. There were blood transfusions, then he was gone. As a teenager, Peter, now in his mid-forties, recalls the horror of finding bruises on his legs and rushing to see his internist father, who would see patients six days a week and even on Sunday nights. "Dad was a very professional, cold, and formal man. His patients had a lot of confidence in him. Basically, his life was all work. For him, children were to be seen and not heard."

Of course, it now makes sense to Peter that producing symptoms might have been a way of relating to Dad and being nurtured by him. His father was the primary physician for Peter and two sisters, so if Peter felt tingles in his arms and legs, he'd make an appointment at his father's office, talk to him about multiple sclerosis, and be comforted. Thinking he was thirsty too often, he'd ask Dad to test him for diabetes. When his father died—at eighty of a noncancerous intestinal blockage—Peter got a look at his own records. There were notations like "Peter needs reassurance"; "Peter is unsure of his physical state."

Peter was not surprised. When he was first married, his wife teased him that he had a brain tumor every six months. "At least twice a year some frightening symptom would pop up and I'd see my Dad for reassurance. I'm sure she thought it was a joke at the beginning." But to his wife, Susan, the health preoccupations were less and less funny, and as time passed, they became much more serious. Before his marriage, he could hide them, even from himself, but within a family he could not. "The feeling I got from my wife was the same one I'd gotten from my parents: I am a pessimist. My fears are ridiculous and I should just stop." The trouble was, he couldn't stop no matter how he tried.

Things got particularly bad after a beloved younger cousin became ill with leukemia. He was with her during the whole process, donating blood, watching her platelet counts go up and down. "It was a terrible thing to see, the debilitation and wasting away," Peter recalls. She died at thirty-two, and from then on the thoughts of cancer became relentless. Death didn't frighten him, it was dying miserably. He wasn't afraid of a heart attack. "You have it, and with luck you're gone." Most terrifying was having "the knowledge that you are incurably sick and that each day could be your last."

Peter's fantasies usually involve cancer, but not of one type. There's leukemia, colon cancer, pancreatic cancer, brain tumors, melanoma. Ironically, it was a phobia about skin cancer, the least deadly form of cancer, that got Peter into psychotherapy. Nine years ago, when he was in the doctor's office for a routine stress test, a physician looked at his arm and said, "You've got a little skin cancer there." It was Friday, the day most hypochondriacs know not to get a biopsy, and he remembers the interminable wait until Tuesday for lab results. Even though most skin cancers are curable, he was sure he had the most deadly kind. "I practically wrote my will that weekend," he says. When the test came back benign, he made the doctor recheck it. Over the next week, he saw other spots and wanted them checked out. He had four biopsies altogether. He promised himself that if they came out okay, he'd get help.

Shortly after that, he began therapy. "My wife told me how frustrated she was: she didn't know how to handle me anymore, and the hypochondria was destroying our family." He called mental health associations seeking someone who specialized in hypochondria but reached a dead end. He decided to see a social worker, and for three years talked a lot about symptoms and his childhood. He achieved some insight. "My father was distant, my mom an alcoholic. Both were unavailable, so I never felt I was okay. I always had to be checked out and have somebody say, 'You're all right. You're going to live.' There was also an aspect of masochism and punishment, though for what I'm not sure. Being a hypochondriac is like being an alcoholic. You're running away from terrible feelings. You can't stop yourself. You hate yourself in the morning. Getting reassurance is kind of like getting a high, one that never lasts. Each time I have a biopsy or a test and it's negative, I dodge the bullet, but sooner or later that bullet is going to hit me."

Self-knowledge helped, but it didn't stop the obsessions, and after a few years of getting nowhere with the problem, the social worker advised him to take a more dramatic approach and to see a psychiatrist. Peter spent two years under the care of a Freudian analyst whose cold, clinical approach he despised. "I had the feeling he was very judgmental. He intimidated me. I finally couldn't take it anymore and left in the middle of a session." As he walked out the door, the therapist said, "Go ahead. That's what you've always done, avoided things." "I'm certain," says Peter, "that my negative reaction had something to do with my father, but I felt I needed someone who was kinder."

Next someone recommended he try behavior therapy and for a while it was a nice change of pace. The psychologist he saw was funny and interactive. "His approach was basically you have to be able to say fuck it. Don't spend time thinking about dying. Get on with your life. He wouldn't let me go to doctors.

He'd ask me, 'If it isn't death you're so afraid of, only suffering, why not take a pill and commit suicide?' Sure, it made rational sense, but it didn't fit emotionally. I knew I'd never have the courage."

Peter swears he gave the method a chance. He tried role-playing, creating scenarios in which he'd be diagnosed with cancer and pretend to go through the emotions. The psychologist asked him to read books on cancer and visit a hospital cancer ward. But Peter wasn't buying this desensitization technique, which of course he'd read all about. "I had enough of cancer in my everyday life. I didn't want to focus on it more. I couldn't stand the thought of these books. Plus, I saw through the approach. It seemed phony." So he dropped behavior therapy and got worse. He saw his internist, who prescribed Prozac, 40 milligrams a day.

Prozac didn't work either. "The only change was that I developed headaches, which I thought were a brain tumor," Peter says. His wife, however, saw improvement. "He still had the episodes, but they were less frequent and he got over them more quickly. He was also warmer to me and the kids, less preoccupied." Peter pooh-poohed Susan's talk of progress. Susan says that from the minute he started the drug, he was looking for an excuse to get off it. "He didn't give Prozac a chance, just as he never gave reassurance a chance," she says. Peter then stumbled on a *New York Times* article citing a Canadian study that found that antidepressants hastened the growth of malignancies in mice and pigs. And that was it. If Prozac had caused blindness or the loss of the use of an arm, that would have been okay. But it caused the very thing he'd been trying desperately to avoid.

Yes, Peter has heard it all. You can't live worrying about sickness. You're wasting your life. You're already dead. You've been dying for thirty-five years. "They're right. But it doesn't make it any easier. There's something so stubborn about the world view I cling to. Now that I'm getting older, the reality of death and cancer seem all the more likely and less and less irrational." He wonders if hypochondria isn't a protective device from the truth of life, that we all have to die. "If I'm not happy," he says, "then it won't be so bad when it's over."

What gets him so angry are those who say, "You don't have to be this way. You can control yourself. You're hurting other people." "Hardly anyone understands hypochondria. Unless you have it yourself, it's looked upon as a character flaw. If a reason for hypochondria is self-punishment, it doesn't help to make you feel you are injuring others. Hypochondria is not something you can admit to anyone. It's so embarrassing. No one at work knows. I rarely take sick days. I never talk about my ailments or fears at the office."

A year ago Peter tried to start a self-help group for hypochondriacs, but it didn't go anywhere. "I advertised, but the people didn't come forward. My feeling is that if I could get a group going, something like this would help me. It would be nice to see how other people function with it. To talk about the various approaches. What do you do when this happens? This has helped a lot of alcoholics get over their problem. It also might help our relatives understand. People with hypochondria feel less worthy, that they are doing something terribly wrong. Like alcoholics, they have a lot of guilt. I've heard people who have been through AA say that without one another they'd be dead."

BODY DYSMORPHIC DISORDER

Also called dysmorphophobia, this disorder has been described as the "beauty hypochondria." Sufferers do not fear disease or believe they have one but are convinced that a part of their body is deformed or ugly. The condition is associated with mirror checking or avoidance, time-consuming grooming activities, and requests for reassurance. These people do not look like the elephant man: the so-called defect, which typically involves a "large" nose, "thinning" hair, or minimal acne, is generally not noticeable to others. Most sufferers of BDD are aware of and embarrassed by their fixations and may keep them secret, even from family members and friends.

Although the precise gender ratio is unknown, men and women appear equally likely to suffer from BDD. The classification has been used only since 1987, when the disorder was accorded a separate diagnostic status.

Megan's Nose: Imagined Ugliness

Since fourth grade, Megan, twenty-eight, has been obsessed with the size of her nose. It began with a classmate's taunt of "Pinocchio," and after that she'd constantly examine her profile and, in public, self-consciously cover her nose with her hand. "I had this strange sensation that my nose was tingling, growing a little every day."

Megan was so unhappy that when she turned seventeen her parents encouraged her to get a nose job. Despite surgery, she still hated her looks and acquired other bodily obsessions — for one, about losing her hair. In college, new ruminations appeared. She worried that all the reading she was doing would cause her to go blind. She couldn't enjoy herself at concerts, afraid the loud music was damaging her eardrums. She knew the thoughts were senseless, but they wouldn't go away. To hide her fears, she adopted a "manicky, up personality." But the charade took all her energy. She saw herself as repugnant and felt tortured by her continuing thoughts. She began to drink to cope with the anxiety. Eventually, she dropped out of school and moved back with her parents. Megan sought help from a psychiatrist, who diagnosed her with BDD. "As soon as I heard that my problem had a name, I felt a huge weight had been lifted off my shoulders."

Under her psychiatrist's care, she has tried many medications. On most, she has been able to cut her "episodes" from a dozen to about six a week. The drugs help for a while, then seem to lose their punch. "I think I'm a very tough case," Megan says. "I've resigned myself to the fact that I was born with this strange bodily focus. I look at my family—there's alcoholism on both sides—but I really can't blame anyone. I have a married brother who's a doctor, and as far as I can tell, he's totally normal."

SOMATIZATION DISORDER

Sufferers have been sickly most of their lives, beginning usually in their teens and early twenties, with recurrent and vague multiple medical complaints. For diagnosis, patients must at some point have had four unexplained pain symptoms, for example, headaches, joint pain; two gastrointestinal symptoms apart from pain, for example, nausea, bloating; one sexual symptom, for example, sexual indifference, erectile dysfunction; and one pseudoneurological symptom, for example, impaired coordination, paralysis. Women's complaints are frequently related to the menstrual cycle.

Somatization disorder is relatively rare, affecting between 0.2 to 2 percent of the population, and mental health professionals have begun to screen for an abridged version of the problem, which they dub somatization syndrome. During the mid-1980s, epidemiologists set out to document the true dimensions of somatization in this country by literally knocking on doors and questioning people about their long-standing unexplained physical complaints. The investigation, part of a giant effort sponsored by the National Institute of Mental Health to examine the magnitude of mental disorders, interviewed a sample of nearly twenty thousand Americans not only in medical settings but in private homes, hospitals, and prisons. Across the nation researchers sought individuals with a history of four to six recurrent, unexplained medical problems. (The ailments had to be severe enough to interfere with life or work, cause sufferers to seek medical attention, or to take medication more than once.)

The symptomatic picture of somatization syndrome was found in 12 percent of the sample.

Edward: One Hundred Doctors

As an infant, Edward had scarlet fever and a mild form of epilepsy, from which he recovered. By school age, he was complaining of stomachaches and joint pain and often missed school. There were many doctors but no dire diagnoses: Edward was healthy, but many commented, a somewhat lonely and serious little boy.

Through high school and college Edward capitalized on those traits, achieving high grades and going into the insurance business. At forty-five, he is plagued by mysterious symptoms — heart palpitations, dizziness, indigestion, pain in his shoulders, back, and neck, and fatigue — and lives with his parents. His physical disabilities have made it impossible for Edward to hold on to a job, and his engagement was broken off. He remains on disability and spends much of his time in and out of hospitals undergoing various tests and procedures.

Edward has all the typical "suspect" diagnoses: temporomandibular joint syndrome (jaw pain known as TMJ), fibromyalgia, tinnitus (ringing in the ears), and chronic fatigue. "I'm very astute when it comes to what I have," he remarks. He claims to have been to nearly one hundred physicians and adds, "I know more about medicine than they do."

PAIN DISORDER

The symptoms, which may be present in one or more parts of the body, must persist in the absence of physical findings to account for their intensity. In most cases, pain is either incompatible with lab findings or can't be adequately accounted for by organic pathology. Patients may visit physicians frequently to obtain relief, use analgesics excessively, request surgery, and assume the role of invalid. In many cases, the problem develops after an accident or physical trauma, but psychological factors are judged to play an overriding role in the onset, severity, exacerbation, and maintenance of the pain.

Interestingly, chronic pain specialists don't exactly embrace the concept of somatoform pain. Though the idea supports the legitimacy of the pain their patients feel, the somatizing diagnosis still carries the stigma of a mental disorder. "That's something the chronic pain movement has been trying to get away from," says Robert Dworkin, a psychologist with the Pain Treatment Center at Columbia Presbyterian Medical Center. Even in pain cases that appear primarily psychogenic in nature, Dr. Dworkin prefers to make two separate diagnoses, one describing the pain and the other addressing a psychological state such as depression. In chronic pain cases, he says, it's nearly impossible to differentiate between cause and effect. "It's the chicken-and-the-egg dilemma—Did depression and anxiety cause the pain, or is the person depressed and anxious because he's in pain?" To a certain degree, this chicken–egg problem is specific to all the somatoform diagnoses, including hypochondria.

Daniel: Rebuilding Life after a Fall

Daniel, a high-flying thirty-year-old Wall Street banker, had a beautiful girlfriend and lived in a spacious loft in Soho. One night he returned to his apartment, stepped into the elevator, and fell down the sixteen-foot shaft. He was lucky to survive, having fractured the lumbar portion of his back and ravaged his ankle so badly that doctors had to install a metal plate.

His surgeon believed that the injuries would heal with time, but three years later Daniel was still racked by severe back pain. He gained seventy-five pounds, became addicted to narcotics, slept poorly, and was quite depressed. "I ended up being a person who avoided contact, didn't answer the phone, let the answering machine pick up."

That's when he decided to sign up for an inpatient pain program offered at a New York hospital. "I'm not a pain wimp," Daniel says. "But after the accident, I viewed the pain like I did everything else in my life: If I applied myself I could beat it and win." Pain, however, wasn't an easy foe. Daniel had to face the chance that unpredictable back pain had become a part of him, something that might never go away. That's where the psychological component came in. "I couldn't forgive myself for not beating the pain," Daniel says. "I felt so sorry for myself that I couldn't separate which part of the misery was physical and which was mental. All I knew was that I didn't recognize the bellyaching, self-centered wretch I had become."

During the three-week treatment program, Daniel learned breathing and relaxation exercises, biofeedback, techniques of sitting and standing—healthier methods for managing pain. Psychotherapy, which he credits with helping him reclaim his days, was also important. Daniel's role model for pain had been his father, a man who had come home from World War II on a stretcher with shrapnel in his body. To this day, he never talks about the experience. For Daniel, that approach doesn't work. "My view of the world had been black or white, sick or well. It's now a few good days, then the inevitable bad one or two."

In fact, since the accident Daniel has become an entirely new person. Perhaps a little more vulnerable and dependent on others, but, he's beginning to think, a nicer one.

CONVERSION DISORDER

This condition, originally called hysterical neurosis, has historical interest because it was the founding problem for psychoanalysis. Freud based his new theories on his experience with hysterical symptoms, which he described as the somatically expressed compromise between forbidden impulses and the defenses against them.

In conversion disorder, individuals suffer some form of impairment. They may have difficulty seeing, hearing, walking, or moving a limb; the loss of function suggests a physical disorder but is an expression of psychological conflict. In some cases the symptoms may offer a solution to a problem or keep an internal wish or need, like dependency, from becoming conscious. The handicap often has symbolic value—a concert pianist, afraid to perform, develops paralysis of her hand; a spouse, full of rage at her husband, loses her ability to talk.

Conversion symptoms, which are two to ten times more common in women than men, most likely involve a single symptom related to extreme psychological and social stress and do not necessarily cause permanent damage. When overcome, they may sometimes serve as a catalyst for monumental change.

Mary: A Nun's Story

When Mary, a mother superior of a group of nuns, was thirty-six she inexplicably became blind in one eye.

On graduating from high school, Mary decided to enter a convent and by the age of twenty-one had taken her vows of poverty, chastity, and obedience. This came as a shock to her family who, although they were practicing Catholics, had been far from religious. "I had a great need to help people and do something spiritual and good," Mary recalls. "But I think that if there had been such a thing as the Peace Corps back then, I would have been a volunteer."

For the first decade she enjoyed the sense of community and the studious aspect of convent life. She earned a bachelor's degree and a master's in education and was appointed principal of a parochial high school where she taught literature. But as time went on she became disenchanted with the church, which she felt was "out of touch with real people." She found herself counseling pregnant high school girls against abortion, when she thought abortion seemed to be the most reasonable alternative. Though she tried to work within the system, she was seen as too way-out, too liberal. "The church required blind obedience and no disagreement."

Mary began feeling nervous and anxious. She was rarely sick, but one day developed soreness in the back of her eye. Every time she moved it, she'd feel pins and needles. She splashed cold water on her face and took aspirin, but the pain wouldn't go away. By the fourth day she couldn't see out of one eye. A neurologist said it was optic neuritis, a diagnosis for nerve inflammation of unknown origin. She was hospitalized and given cortisone, but her sight didn't improve. "Whatever it is that's bothering you, you've got to get a handle on it," the doctor told her.

Mary took a leave of absence and spent the good part of a year at a less stressful convent in the countryside. She began meeting regularly with a psychologist. They talked about her strange life of silent prayers in the morning, teaching all day, disillusionment, and conflict. "I discovered I was a perfectionist, overworking to avoid my growing doubts," Mary says. Her eyesight gradually came back, and shortly after that she left the church. "I had to make a clean break."

At the age of thirty-seven, she arrived in New York City with $300 and landed a college teaching job, working her way up to assistant dean. In 1971 she met a successful New York investor on an airplane, and they were married a year later, when she was forty-three and eight years out of the convent. She now has three stepchildren and a grandchild she adores.

Does it sound too rosy? Perhaps. But more impressive than the job or happy marriage is that, unlike many, Mary could rise above a bad situation and become the mistress of her destiny. "During that period in my life I was undergoing deep psychological trauma. I was so unhappy, and I literally didn't want to see," she says. "I believed then, as I do today, that the body was telling me something, and I had to listen to it."

These may be extreme examples of the mind–body connection, but with a bit of reflection all of us should be able to recognize some low-level somatizing in our own lives. You may know it by the name of sympathy pains, when we respond physically to a friend's misfortune or develop symptoms resembling those of a disease we've seen reported on television. Or think of occasions when you repress anger, sadness, or other emotions, and the very act takes a physical toll.

Each of us experiences and communicates discomfort both verbally and physically, and most of the time there is no need to tease the equation apart. Difficulties arise only when we lose our balance, when the discourse between mind, body, and the complicated lives we all lead gets out of sync. That's when mental anguish not consciously acknowledged can become a problem. But if you're lucky, distress will descend upon you in a neat somatoform label that someone, perhaps you yourself, will recognize, and that simple act of awareness will set you back on course.

....

CHAPTER THREE

Digging Beneath Symptoms

The sorrow that has no vent in tears makes other
organs weep.

> —attributed to Henry Maudsley, renowned
> nineteenth-century English anatomist

EVERYONE, IT SEEMS, has had the experience. You have a
fight with your spouse and end up with a pounding headache. A
make-or-break project is due and your muscles are tense. Somatic symptoms are the natural order of things, a part of being
human. They help us identify emotions that give meaning to our
lives. We may feel giddy with excitement. We become choked
up and know the depth of our sorrow. We blush and realize that
we're embarrassed. Symptoms, the language the body speaks,
can be a source of valuable information, providing one makes
the proper connections. For some a headache may be a signal to
slow down. Faced with a big decision, we're often guided by our
gut instincts.

When asked by researchers to keep a diary of their discom-
forts, average basically healthy adults record physical symptoms, such as fatigue, backache, cramps, coughing, headaches,
palpitations, on one out of every four days. Most of these symptoms are trivial, not worrisome or bothersome, unless we pay
too much attention to them. As Lewis Thomas wrote in *The*

Lives of a Cell, "The great secret . . . is that most things get better by themselves. Most things, in fact, are better by morning." The reason people feel on top of the world some days and laid low on others has less to do with the onset of a serious illness than other factors, for instance, whether they've had enough sleep, whether they're doing productive work, how well they're relating to others. And most people know this: the bulk of the population doesn't consult doctors about somatic symptoms or, for that matter, even minor illnesses.

Nevertheless, a percentage of the population seeks a great deal of medical attention—researchers call these people high utilizers—and the leading reason is not serious illness, but symptoms: back pain, fatigue, dizziness, and headaches unexplained by science. "A large portion of patients who visit physicians' offices are suffering from psychosocial stress, not medical problems," says Charles V. Ford, a psychiatrist at the University of Alabama School of Medicine. But they feel more comfortable talking about physical distress. "And the ticket of admission to a doctor's office is a physical symptom, not a depressive work situation or a bad marriage."

The fact that emotions can be expressed as physical symptoms is neither harmful nor problematic in itself. Somatization becomes a problem, however, when people consistently misinterpret and magnify normal expressions of psychic discomfort. Somatizers take what's troubling them emotionally and put it into the purely physical realm. They say "I'm sick, my stomach hurts," and act out their problem in the body, channeling it into physical pain. Hypochondriacal somatizers go a step further, infusing their symptoms with additional meaning. "They have the firm belief they are sick, so they reinterpret vague sensations like cold hands or a twitching eyelid as proof," Dr. Arthur J. Barsky says.

WHO FEELS SICK AND
WHO FEELS HEALTHY?

No two people respond to bodily sensations in the same way. Individuals with similar physical conditions react quite differently to their situations: some feel healthy and make the most of their capabilities and opportunities while others give in to their illness completely. Consider, for example, two men of roughly the same age who consult an orthopedist for back pain. Both have nearly identical X rays and are given the same explanation for their discomfort: a herniated disc, a common diagnosis in many over twenty, and, according to John E. Sarno, a professor of clinical rehabilitation at New York University School of Medicine, "no more pathological than graying hair or wrinkling skin." Yet while one man manages his problem by exercising regularly and taking Advil whenever he feels an ache or twinge, the other is incapacitated by back and leg pain. He gives up most physical activity and worries constantly about his condition.

A study conducted at the University of Virginia Medical School highlights the notion that how one feels has much to do with who one is. Of 208 patients in a Virginia medical practice surveyed about health attitudes, 62 rated themselves as sick, diseased, or unhealthy. By comparison, physicians examining the patients found only 23 to be in poor health; the other 39 appeared no sicker than the 146 patients who said they felt fine. Nevertheless, those who believed they were ill had more health worries, higher levels of depression, anxiety, and acute pain, more office visits and telephone calls, and higher medical bills than patients who perceived themselves as well.

During the throes of my own lupus fears, I came across a book that brought home to me the crucial role beliefs and attitudes play in creating the sickness experience. Suzy Szasz, a reference librarian in her early forties, diagnosed with lupus at age thirteen, wrote *Living With It: Why You Don't Have to Be Healthy to Be Happy* to encourage others with serious illnesses to live "competently, contentedly, and with as much self-determination as possible." I read of her remarkable battle against high fevers, incapacitating joint pain, hideous rashes, with a mixture of horror and awe. All that medication, surgery, and energy just to keep her body from attacking its own healthy tissue!

It didn't seem fair. But at the time I remember thinking, she's happier than I am. Though Szasz never denies the severe impact a life-threatening disease has had on her, she resists being defined by her illness. Szasz doesn't see herself as a victim. "Unlike the hypochondriac who wants to be accepted as a patient, I have always wanted to be accepted as a nonpatient," she writes. "For me, having a chronic illness for most of my life made shouldering such responsibility, perhaps paradoxically, easier. I could use my illness and the necessity to take care of it as a guidepost for taking care of my life as a whole."

THE SICK ROLE AND ILLNESS BEHAVIOR

The "sick role" as conceptualized by Talcott Parsons, a leading medical sociologist of the 1950s, provides a framework for looking at how illness can affect social and psychological functioning. Sickness is a departure from everyday life: to be sick is to be different, but in a role that is sanctioned by society. In our culture, being sick carries with it certain privileges: release from social responsibilities as well as support, reassurance, and care. Many writers have noted that there is something paradoxically exhilarating, even spiritually healing, about the illness experience.

The late critic Anatole Broyard characterized critical illness as "a great permission, an authorization or absolving." Among his many eloquent meditations on life and mortality in *Intoxicated by My Illness*, written during his battle with prostate cancer, from which he died in 1989, Broyard describes the intoxication he felt after learning of his diagnosis: "It's all right for a threatened man to be romantic, even crazy . . . All your life you think you have to hold back your craziness, but when you're sick you can let it out in all its garish colors."

Virginia Woolf, in her essay "On Being Ill," speaks of the sense of freedom illness confers. "There is, let us confess it (and illness is the great confessional), a childish outspokenness in illness; things are said, trusts blurted out, which the cautious respectability of health conceals . . . With responsibility shelved and reason in the abeyance — for who is going to exact criticism from an invalid or sound sense from the bedridden? — other tastes assert themselves; sudden, fitful, intense."

In *Illness as Metaphor*, Susan Sontag discusses the Romantic cult of disease as it related to tuberculosis in the first half of the last century. Sontag's theory is that the Romantic poets and philosophers invented invalidism as a pretext for leisure, enabling them to dismiss bourgeois obligations and live only for one's art. "It was a way of retiring from the world without having to take responsibility for the decision — the story of the Magic Mountain," Sontag writes. (In Thomas Mann's novel, the hero is diagnosed with tuberculosis and exiled to an exclusive sanatorium in the Swiss Alps, where he remains for seven years and is spiritually transformed.)

One of the major conscious or unconscious motivations of the people who somatize is to take on the sick role. The benefits — escapism, nurturance, dependency — can be so appealing that it isn't easy to give them up. (Psychological illness is still not considered a legitimate sick role. Just look at most health insurance policies!) For some, holding on to or exaggerating physical symptoms, even consciously or unconsciously fabricating them, may provide a better solution to life's problems than a return to health. But according to Parsons's social theory, society grants a legitimate claim to the sick role on two conditions: that the person strive to get well, and that he or she cooperate with healers in the recovery process, which Parsons called a common task. The expectation of relatives, friends, and physician is that the patient wants to recuperate and become more independent as recovery progresses, but with hypochondria and other somatic disorders, that's not what occurs.

Another medical sociologist, David Mechanic, introduced the term "illness behavior" to refer to the ways in which symptoms are perceived, evaluated, and acted, or not acted, upon by different types of people. It has become medically and psychologically correct these days to talk of the subjective "experience of illness," as opposed to the objective measure of disease. Illness is what happens to people, while disease happens to organs. Or as Larry Dossey, author of *Meaning and Medicine*, says, it is "disease plus meaning." Arthur Kleinman, in *The Illness Narratives*, describes illness as "the lived experience of monitoring bodily processes such as respiratory wheezes, abdominal cramps, stuffed sinuses, or painful joints." The term refers to how a sick person and the members of his family or wider social network perceive, live with, and respond to diagnosis, symptoms, and disability.

The dynamics of illness involves the appraisal of symptoms — as expectable, frightening, or requiring treatment — and our behavior and judgment about how best to cope with distress. Do we stay home from school or work? Change our diet or pattern of exercise? Seek medical attention? Our choices depend on a number of influences like personality, beliefs, culture, previous exposure to sickness, and upbringing; in short, what makes us tick. For example, a parent's response to a child's Monday morning stomachaches can shape illness behavior in adulthood. Perhaps you remember being sick, staying home from school, and having your mother all to yourself. She brought chicken soup and buttered toast to your bedside and read you stories. Your pattern of responding to illness might be different from that of someone who was raised in a household where sickness was minimized, to be suffered stoically and in silence.

A third, more controversial sociological concept is "abnormal illness behavior," a term coined by psychiatrist Ian Pilowsky. Whereas illness behavior is a neutral idea, abnormal illness behavior conveys a sense of acting inappropriately. Some clinicians believe that labeling patients' conduct abnormal can be misleading. It shifts the burden of responsibility onto the patient, while medical fashion, a troubled doctor-patient relationship, or even someone's level of insurance coverage may contribute markedly to behavior. Nevertheless, it can be a useful term when one talks about somatization. Abnormal illness behavior can range from the extreme of Münchausen's syndrome, in which a person derives emotional satisfaction from purposely feigning drastic disease, to the other extreme, in which a person unconsciously denies the signs and symptoms of disease, an illness behavior that can be self-destructive and possibly life-threatening.

CROSSING THE LINE: IS IT ABNORMAL ILLNESS BEHAVIOR?

The question of whether one is somatizing is not easily answered. There is no litmus test to tell you whether your perceptions about health, illness, and your body are appropriate. Somatizing is a matter of degree and comes in many flavors. It can be mild, transient, extremely distressing, or incapacitating. It can disrupt interpersonal relationships or be the glue that holds them together. What turns normal concern about health into a problem is preoccupation or worry so intense that it gets in the way of everyday happiness. When you find yourself dissatisfied with medical explanations, switch physicians frequently, and voraciously read medical literature that terrifies you, when you feel sick all the time and can't enjoy life, when you start missing out on important occasions, it's essential to figure out what's going on. At this point you have to ask yourself some questions: Do I really have a physical condition the doctors are missing? Could there be an underlying emotional problem? Am

I acting out illness behavior learned in childhood? Do I have a stake in being sick?

YOUR DOCTOR COULD BE WRONG

Misdiagnosis occurs. We hear about it on television and read about it in newspapers and magazines. I know, I collect the cases: one, Angela Farnum, thirty-eight, whose physician dismissed the uncomfortable twinges in her breast as fibrocystic disease, a benign condition. Later, when Farnum requested a mammogram, the doctor said there was no basis for the test and chastised her for her "hypochondria." Five years after her initial symptoms, she had an MRI (magnetic resonance imaging). The result: a virulent carcinoma had metastasized throughout her system. Then there's the Rhode Island laboratory investigated for misreading nearly two dozen Pap-smear slides. One woman, a teacher who suffered years of abdominal pain, died of cervical cancer after receiving four negative Pap-smear results from the lab in eight years. *The New York Times* reported that the woman had been told she was free of cancer as recently as three weeks before her malignant tumor was found.

Mistakes can and do happen; that possibility lies at the heart of hypochondria. The hypochondriac's fear is based on this persistent doubt; he can't convince himself, or be convinced, that a serious disease is not present. That uncertainty creates the continuing pas de deux between the hypochondriacal patient and the practitioner who, as medical detective, is trained to act as if she can never be entirely sure there is no hidden biological cause for the patient's symptoms. Also hanging over doctors is the scepter of a malpractice suit, which can strike if a patient gets sicker.

If you believe you are sick and the medical profession has let you down, there are avenues to pursue. Linda Hanner, a journalist who had a six-year bout with undiagnosed Lyme disease, wrote *When You're Sick and Don't Know Why: Coping with*

Your Undiagnosed Illness to help people manage the emotions of not knowing what ails them and to help them live with uncertainty. One physician told Hanner early in her illness that she had "too many symptoms" for a real disease and needed a psychiatrist. Some patients, dissatisfied with explanations, treat themselves to Cadillac workups at high-reputation, high-power medical institutions like the Mayo Clinic. Others have found relief in alternative medicine, which seems to know more than conventional medicine about the healing effect of paying attention. But if neither conventional nor alternative medical workups have provided the answers and you're still unhappily symptomatic, you may want to entertain the possibility that your symptoms have a more psychological root, or in the new lexicon, that the origins of your problem may be biopsychosocial.

MIND OVER MATTER: COULD SYMPTOMS BE PSYCHOLOGICAL?

Most who suffer inexplicable medical problems, I imagine, won't jump at this explanation and say, "Of course, that's the answer! I'm depressed, I'm anxious. Why didn't I think of that before?" More likely, this supposition will evoke a skeptical reaction. I remember during my lupus episodes, especially the second one, how vehemently I resisted any insinuation that my problems could be mental. I particularly resented the implication from my husband, who never called me a hypochondriac—at least not to my face—but whose lack of worry over my physical concerns made his thoughts transparent. Because I had spent a good part of the previous ten years in psychotherapy, I found it impossible to consider that the wellspring of my pain might be rooted in the mind. *I'd* worked that stuff out.

The hurt was too physically real. In fact, examinations had shown that I had lost some degree of flexibility in my wrist, and there was that slight abnormality on a bone scan, neither of which the doctors made much of. To this day I remain convinced that there was something genuinely wrong with me, perhaps precipitated by hormonal changes after childbirth or working on my word processor. But I now see that it was not the pain but my extreme reaction to not getting a physical diagnosis—and my fixation on lupus—that qualified as a psychological disturbance. And I tell you: I am *so* glad that my problem turned out to be primarily an emotional, not a medical disease—certainly not lupus.

The stigma associated with psychiatric problems continues to be enormous despite recent surveys which claim that as many as one of every two adults has had a brush with mental illness at some point in life. Being able to admit that something feels wrong about the way you are handling life is courageous, not a sign of personal failure. And considering a somatizing diagnosis doesn't mean that the sensations you are feeling aren't real. Emotional and physical troubles are often impossible to separate. Look at the classic symptoms of depression, which often underlies somatization: right up there with blue mood, hopelessness, guilt, and suicidal feelings come headache, back pain, constipation, sleep disturbances, loss of appetite. The constellation of symptoms depends on who's getting depressed.

WHERE DOES ONE BEGIN?

Digging beneath symptoms is tough work. Medical tests aren't accurate. Doctors aren't infallible. What might be considered somatization today could be diagnosable disease tomorrow. Lyme disease was an ailment, which, until technology came up with tests that could detect its presence, many sufferers were told it was all in their heads. Recognizing somatoform disorders is all the more complicated because the somatization process occurs in a wide spectrum of mental and physical illnesses and doesn't require the total absence of organic disease. Sickness and psychological distress often go hand in hand. Physical disorders can be aggravated by stress and emotional turmoil, just as disabling physical conditions can be ameliorated by a positive outlook. We've all known people with life-threatening illnesses who live happier, more fulfilling lives than some hypochondriacs.

The process of transforming mental anguish into physical complaints is a common, if not the most common, way for emotional disturbances to make themselves known. According to Charles Ford, a leading expert on the somatic illnesses, the presence of any somatoform symptom doubles the likelihood of an underlying depressive or anxiety disorder; somatic symptoms are linked to increased dysfunction—marital discord, lost workdays, and substance abuse. "Regardless of whether a patient is experiencing an actual disease, when it comes to unexplained or inappropriate symptoms, a warning bell should go off," Dr. Ford says. "Practitioners should be stopped dead in their tracks and consider the role of these symptoms in the context of the patient's life."

DOES ANYONE SUFFER FROM "PURE" HYPOCHONDRIA?

One of the most consistent findings about hypochondria is that although it can occur by itself, more often than not it accompanies a host of other psychological conditions. Various studies show, for example, that 25 to 60 percent of patients diagnosed with depression suffer from intermittent or chronic hypochondriacal fears. Conversely, research conducted at McGill University found nearly 30 percent of medical patients with entrenched hypochondria to be in the throes of a major depressive or anxiety disorder. Only 9 percent of nonhypochondriacal medical patients experienced such problems.

One way clinicians approach the problem of comorbidity, the psychiatric lingo for overlapping disturbances, is to distinguish between primary and secondary hypochondria. Some psychiatrists label hypochondria primary when bodily preoccupation and fear of disease dominate the clinical picture. Others identify patients as having a "pure" form of hypochondria only when no other psychiatric diagnosis can be made, which, in patients suffering from hypochondria, tends to be somewhat uncommon. In a study of forty-two hypochondriacal patients, Dr. Arthur Barsky found only 21 percent who did *not* have a concurrent psychiatric condition, the overlap particularly striking with depression and anxiety disorders such as phobias and generalized anxiety.

In investigations of the cause of nagging symptoms and health concerns, prevalence alone makes these psychiatric disorders a good place to begin. According to the National Institute of Mental Health, the following can be anticipated during the course of any given year.

Depressive disorders will affect as many as 11 million Americans. Nine million people—one man in ten and one woman in five—will experience major depression and 2.2 million manic depression (bipolar disorder). The rate is even higher if you include the 9.9 million who suffer from a low-grade, chronic form of depression known as dysthymia.

Panic disorder, an unanticipated surge of agonizing symptoms—heart palpitations, drenching sweat, dizziness, fear of impending doom—will affect 2 to 3 million people. One in ten Americans report having experienced a panic attack during the past year; a little less than 2 percent have symptoms severe enough to qualify for a panic disorder diagnosis.

Obsessive-compulsive disorder. Nearly 4 million Americans—one in forty people—will suffer from this debilitating anxiety disorder, which is characterized by senseless thoughts and rituals.

ARE YOU DEPRESSED?

You don't have to feel sad or blue to be depressed. Depression can be masked or hidden in many behaviors, for example, drug and alcohol abuse, overeating, compulsive shopping, and promiscuity. It can also be camouflaged in hypochondriacal complaints and symptoms. The biological markers for depression can run the gamut from insomnia and weight change to memory loss and sexual dysfunction. Fatigue, pain, weakness, appetite loss, headaches, dizziness, constipation, and stomachaches are also common. A study of people seeking help from internists found complaints of weakness eight times more common and constipation three to four times more frequent in those with undiagnosed depression.

Nearly 50 percent of patients with unexplained symptoms seen in primary care are depressed, and somatized depression, the clinical name for masked depression, goes unrecognized or misdiagnosed half the time. For some, to be depressed is to lose face. Such people may be perfectionists, highly critical of themselves and others, and intolerant of personal failure. They may feel that they don't deserve to be sad or needy. "Alexithymia," a Greek term meaning "no words of emotion," is another cause of somatized depression. People with alexithymic personalities find it difficult to sense, identify, and express emotions. The body becomes a substitute for what they cannot say.

Research has shown that the physical sensations of depression may have a biological base in the disruption of the metabolism of amines, a class of brain chemicals. When neural cells don't make the proper amount of this chemical messenger, a chronic mood disorder may result. In depression, sleep cycles change, libido plummets, appetite diminishes; daily bodily rhythms become upset. In addition, depressed people frequently have a higher than normal level of cortisol, a hormone associated with stress, though researchers remain uncertain whether these physiological changes are the result or the cause of depression.

Despite our growing knowledge about its chemistry, the clinical picture of depression hasn't changed much historically. As far back as the seventeenth century, when depression was known as melancholia, physicians and writers have made a connection between dark moods and bodily ills. A Viennese psychiatrist, in an 1860 textbook, ranked hypochondria among "the conditions of psychic depression"; the difference between hypochondria and melancholia, he said, was merely that while the hypochondriac was busily seeking out medical consultations, the melancholic was planning his suicide.

Novelist William Styron, in his affecting memoir, *Darkness Visible*, describes the pervasive hypochondria that afflicted him months before he knew he was suffering from depression. Styron had been a heavy drinker most of his adult life when, in 1985, when he was sixty, alcohol began to have a troubling physical effect. Small mouthfuls of wine caused nausea and unpleasant wooziness. That summer, on Martha's Vineyard, he felt a "numbness, an enervation, but more particularly an odd fragility," as if his body had become hypersensitive and frail. "Nothing felt quite right with my corporeal self; there were twitches and pains, sometimes intermittent, often seemingly constant, that seemed to presage all sorts of dire infirmities." He sought extensive physical workups from specialists and, when the doctors pronounced him fit, he was relieved for one or two days, "until once again began the rhythmic daily erosion of my mood—anxiety, agitation, unfocused dread.... Mysteriously ... and in ways that are totally remote from normal human experience, the gray drizzle of horror induced by depression takes on the quality of physical pain."

Depression can contribute to chronic illness and chronic illness to depression; the two tend to feed on each other. Some illnesses seem to trigger depression biologically, and some medications, like steroids, can lead to depression. Once depression is detected and treated, sick patients often get better. Masked, depression can make illnesses worse. A study of patients with rheumatoid arthritis found that those who reported the greatest pain and had the hardest time sleeping were most likely to be depressed. Patients who experience serious depression following a heart attack are five times more likely to die during the six months after their attack than patients who aren't depressed. In an attempt to shed light on the chicken-egg dilemma of whether depression or physical sickness comes first, researchers at Columbia University evaluated eighteen patients with shingles at the beginning of their illness. (The virus, known as herpes zoster, is characterized by painful blisters that, in a middle-aged person, take six to eight weeks to heal.) The six patients who developed post-herpetic neuralgia, shingles pain lasting more than three months, had higher scores on a variety of psychiatric scales, including depression, anxiety, and hypochondria, than those who didn't develop a chronic problem.

JOHN: A CASE OF MALE MENOPAUSE

Shortly after John, a forty-eight-year-old chemical technician, was laid off from the company where he had spent his career, he developed shingles across his chest and back. Within weeks the blisters healed; but when John's pain failed to abate after several months, a neurologist, believing the complaints were out of whack, referred him to Mack Lipkin, Jr.

"When John came to see me he was quite anxious, and very angry," recalls Dr. Lipkin, an internist affiliated with New York University who specializes in somatoform illnesses. "He kept saying over and over, 'There is something wrong with me and you bastards aren't doing anything.' He believed his pain was symptomatic of cancer or a spinal disease."

Dr. Lipkin initially met with John four times and spoke with John's wife, who was worried about the pressure her husband was putting on himself. He couldn't find another job commensurate with his experience and was ashamed that his wife had to work while he collected unemployment insurance. John also displayed symptoms that included a decreased libido, difficulty maintaining erections, forgetfulness, and bouts of intense irritability in which he'd lash out at his wife and grown children.

The problem, as Dr. Lipkin saw it, appeared to be a classic

case of male menopause. Shingles, like other herpes viruses, tends to break out at times of high stress, when the body is vulnerable. In John's case, the lesions had healed, but the persistent burning and shooting pain, and the fear and anxiety related to it, provided a focus for his emotions. "The neuralgia became a scapegoat for his depression and damaged self-esteem," Dr. Lipkin said.

He spent several months talking with John about feelings related to no longer being the breadwinner and his change in social role. Together they searched for ways he could soothe himself. The most effective turned out to be simply immersing himself in hot baths with a sprinkling of oil, which helped him relax and get to sleep. Slowly, John began to find new interests and expand his life—community volunteer work, playing basketball with friends—and eventually he was able to get part-time work teaching science at several local schools. Within a year, the neuralgia disappeared.

Depression is the most treatable of all the psychiatric illnesses: studies show that 80 percent of depressed people can obtain relief through medication and relatively brief psychotherapy. It's the mood disorder that receives the most publicity. Famous sufferers—Art Buchwald, William Styron, Dick Cavett, Mike Wallace, Patty Duke—who have spoken candidly about their illnesses have helped raise public awareness, as have widely published studies estimating the national tab for depression at anywhere from $27 billion to a whopping $43.7 billion.

If only depression were the entire answer. For years, people, including my therapist, tried to convince me that I was depressed. Sure I was, at times. I had horrible symptoms and fantasies about crippling illness and death which, in my more rational moments, I realized were ludicrous. Who wouldn't be depressed? But depression wasn't my primary trouble. The routine tricyclic antidepressants I tried didn't have an impact on the depression, and the side effects—dry mouth, weight gain, extreme sleepiness—were intolerable. If anything, having an obsessional personality—psychiatrists categorize obsessive-compulsive behavior as an anxiety disorder—was the main culprit, manifesting itself during my teens in the eating disorder anorexia nervosa and later in hypochondria. Depression was merely a by-product.

The clinical picture, again, is confusing, as depression doesn't necessarily occur alone; it may coexist with hypochondria, and any other somatoform condition, and more often than not goes hand in hand with anxiety. The comorbidity puzzle, which supplies endless material for the splitters and the lumpers to debate, is a mystery the psychiatric profession is working hard to unravel. Consider a 1994 program brochure for a meeting of the American Psychiatric Association. Among the seminar topics listed were Mixed Anxiety and Depression: Current Controversies and Treatment Considerations; Panic and Bipolar Disorders: Is There a Link?; Mixed Anxiety/Depression: What It Means for the Clinician; Management of Anxiety/Depressive Syndromes in the Elderly.

ARE YOUR SYMPTOMS RELATED TO ANXIETY?

Millions of Americans, perhaps 10 to 13 percent of the population, suffer from severe anxiety. This is not the occasional worry about a test or job interview or the panic one feels when a child is late coming home. That's garden-variety agitation, generally considered an adaptive mind-body response that alerts us to stressful situations and prepares us to deal with the challenge. Anxiety in this case refers to the unremitting onslaught of dread, uncertainty, and nervousness that comes with a racing heart, sweaty palms, and churning stomach. The symptoms may come upon you suddenly as a rush of overwhelming fear, or you may feel tense and worried all the time. Defining the point at which anxiety outweighs its productive function and becomes excessive is not always easy. At its most severe, it can be a form of torture that prevents a person from carrying on normal day-to-day activities.

Panic attack, that inexplicable ambush of terror which strikes seemingly out of the blue, is probably the best known psychiatric condition after depression. It is certainly the most publicized anxiety disorder, though only one of a group of six anxiety syndromes, and has the greatest link with somatic symptoms and hypochondria. The attacks are accompanied by a multitude of such somatic symptoms as shortness of breath, accelerating heart rate, choking sensations, dizziness, stomach upset, sweating, and trembling; some people fear they are going crazy or dying or that they will lose control. To be diagnosed with panic disorder, a person must have at least four such symptoms that develop abruptly, reach a peak within ten minutes, and are followed by a month of persistent fear. The disorder, estimated to affect 8 percent of primary care patients and twice as many who see cardiologists, is known among clinicians as the great masquerader because it mimics many physical diseases and is difficult to diagnose.

Panic sufferers, who are two to three times as likely to be women, have a tendency toward hypochondria. Experiencing chest discomfort and breathing difficulties, they may rush to emergency rooms, convinced they are having a heart attack. The problem is so common that it has been given a name: cardiophobia. Each year 100,000 people in the United States complain of chest pain, but tests show normal coronary arteries and no heart disease.

Patients with cardiophobia, which involves a complex interplay of chest pain, autonomic arousal, and anxiety, may have panic disorder as their primary problem. Or, if conviction or fear of illness is pervasive and full panic attacks never occur, they may be suffering from hypochondria. Generally, panic sufferers believe that physical harm is imminent—that they are in the midst of a heart attack—while hypochondriacs tend to fear degenerative illnesses with more insidious courses.

Before 1987, patients who had panic attacks were often diagnosed with hypochondria, but in the third revision of DSM panic disorder became clinically distinct. One reason is it's much easier to cure—nine out of ten panic sufferers respond rapidly to early diagnosis and treatment. So now the manual explicitly states that hypochondria should not be diagnosed if the illness fears are primarily triggered by symptoms of panic. Still, even when panic sufferers seek help, they don't always find out what's wrong. Generally, people have seen nine or ten physicians before they receive an accurate diagnosis.

JUDITH: HEART PALPITATIONS

Judith, a thirty-three-year-old graphic designer, began to develop frightening symptoms a year after her mother's sudden death. She could be driving, talking to a friend, or reading at home when an intense, wild fear came over her. "I'd feel dizzy, nauseated, and shaky all over. My heart would begin to race, like it was beating out of my chest. I could barely catch my breath." Sometimes the feelings would last ten minutes, sometimes half an hour, and she thought she was about to die. The first doctor she consulted hinted at an irregular heartbeat and sent Judith to a cardiac specialist. He found nothing wrong with her, but her terror didn't go away. She avoided going places alone, for fear she'd get sick. At work she kept checking her pulse, certain some terrible abnormality would show up. She needed constant reassurance from friends that she was okay. At one point she thought she might have to quit her job. "I couldn't figure out what was happening to me. I was driving myself and my boyfriend crazy. I wasn't sleeping well. I didn't know how to find the healthy person I once knew."

A friend, a nurse who saw a notice advertising a hypochondria study at Columbia Presbyterian Hospital, jokingly suggested that Judith check it out. Judith decided to try it, but didn't tell a soul. She began to meet regularly with a psychiatrist, who diagnosed her with panic disorder, which he believed had triggered a hypochondriacal reaction. He suggested she begin a trial of imipramine, a tricyclic antidepressant effective in stopping panic attacks. But Judith was afraid of side effects, so they opted for a short course of intensive psychotherapy, including cognitive behavioral techniques, which enabled her to recognize signs of an impending attack and rebuff it with relaxation exercises.

What helped most, she believes, were the hours she logged simply talking. "Everything came pouring out," she recalls. "I'd cry for nearly the entire session." After three months of therapy, Judith came to see her attacks and hypochondriacal fears as a manifestation of the conflict over her mother's death. "I *thought* I was mourning my mother and that I had coped with her death fairly well, but emotions ran deeper," she says. They were tied to the fact that her mother had died of a heart attack in her fifties, before Judith could marry or have children. "I was angry and frightened that she left me, and because I had to live with the possibility that she may have passed her condition on to me." Once she drew the connection between her attacks and emotions, the problem began to resolve. Today Judith is productive and happy, and though not entirely free from anxiety, she has not had an attack in two years.

Do Symptoms Signal Obsession?

The most tantalizing research in hypochondria these days involves the exploration of the relationship between hypochondria and obsessive-compulsive disorder. OCD is a psychiatric illness in which a person is besieged by unwanted, disturbing irrational thoughts or sensations. Obsessions typically involve hygiene, violence, or sexual impulses, which compel sufferers to carry out ritualized behavior, such as washing, checking for example, doors, locks, and appliances, touching, hoarding, and counting. For people to be diagnosed with OCD, their thoughts and rituals must recur persistently, last more than an hour a day and cause marked distress or significantly interfere with functioning and interpersonal relationships.

Psychiatrists place OCD on a spectrum with anxiety disorders, the rationale being that obsessives act out their ritualized and aimless behaviors to calm their piercing anxiety that unless they act, something terrible will happen. While there is a slim justification for each obsession, OCD patients often realize that their fears and compulsions are totally senseless. "These people aren't crazy. The thoughts may be silly or crazy, but they can't get them out of their head. They have a hard time getting unstuck," says Eric Hollander, an expert in OCD-related behaviors and vice chairman of the Department of Psychiatry at Mount Sinai School of Medicine.

OCD sufferers can be plagued by nagging anxiety and persistent doubt about their health, but health concerns in OCD are not always hypochondriacal. For example, someone with OCD might obsess about an irregularity on her skin but not fear that it is cancerous. However, for a number of people, OCD and hypochondria do overlap. Dr. Barsky's study of sixty hypochondriacal patients found that about 8 percent also suffered from OCD at some point in their lives. In Dr. Brian Fallon's study of twenty-one hypochondriacal patients, nearly one-third had a lifetime history of OCD.

NANCY: "MOMMY, STOP TOUCHING YOUR BREAST!"

Nancy, a thirty-six-year-old mother of a four-year-old boy, remembers being headstrong and compulsive, even as a kid. "I had to do things a particular way, eating food in the right order, dressing in a certain manner, that kind of thing," she recalls. As she got older, she began to notice a certain inflexibility in her behavior. While entertaining, she'd become transfixed by a spot on the kitchen floor. "I hated to see a speck of dirt. I couldn't wait for the company to leave so I could clean, even though I knew I was being stupid, sabotaging a good time."

Three months into her second pregnancy, Nancy miscarried and became quite depressed. She blamed herself. "I had this sense I was being punished, that something worse was about to occur." Over the next months, she and her husband tried to conceive, but nothing happened. About that time, she thought she felt a lump in her breast. She saw her gynecologist, who told her what she already knew: she had lumpy breasts, the same benign fibrocystic condition her mother and grandmother had. She was in perfect health. When she told her doctor she felt depressed and anxious, he said, "Your feelings are normal. You've suffered a loss. Keep trying to have that baby."

As months went by with no signs of a baby, the worry escalated. Something was wrong, she thought, like ovarian cancer. A few times she had night sweats, which she'd read were a sign of AIDS. She kept checking her throat for thrush. Phobias would come and go, but one thought remained constant: she would soon find a malignancy in her breast. That thought remained even after she consulted an eminent breast surgeon and had a mammogram, which was normal. "I had promised myself if it showed nothing, I'd relax; but three hours later I was obsessing that they'd missed something."

Nancy would never know when the compulsion to check herself would hit: while she was cooking (she once burned dinner); in the car (she almost got into an accident with her son); in bed (during sex she'd ask her husband to reassure her that there was no mass). "I could visualize the doctor giving me the news; the chemotherapy, losing my hair, having to tell my son his mommy was going to die." She went back to her gynecologist, who ordered her to stop checking her body. One day in McDonald's she almost fainted when her son, who had accompanied her on several physician visits, leaned over the table and said: "Mommy, the doctor told you not to touch your breast!"

Embarrassed to tell her friends, Nancy isolated herself. She experienced panic states in which she felt she was going insane. Her husband was at his wit's end. "I'd be hysterical, petrified, constantly crying. My husband would have to take a day off from work to stay home to take care of things." Finally, her father approached her at a family dinner. To her surprise, he told Nancy that for a year he'd been treated at a local clinic for depression. "It's helped like nothing ever has," he said. "I'm not sure what's eating you, but I think it would do you some good." She and her dad hadn't been close. Never a forceful parent, he'd been remote and uninvolved, but about this he was persistent. "He practically took me by the hand."

Nancy was evaluated at that same clinic and initially diagnosed with mixed anxiety and depression. She began a trial on the antidepressant Zoloft and learned behavioral techniques to control the panic and obsessive thinking. Her depression lifted quickly. The impulse to check her breasts continued, but she didn't act on it as often or judge herself so harshly. After six weeks on the drug, however, she got into another state. The compulsion intensified, then came back in full force. All of a sudden, there it was: a real lump, the size of an egg, black and blue and painful. "It was the strangest thing. For the first time I knew that this was real. I had this perverse sense of satisfaction. So *that's* what I've been searching for all these months. It was almost a relief."

An internist at the clinic diagnosed the lump as a hematoma, an enormous swelling filled not with cancerous tissue, but with blood. The irony was that, with all her pushing and prodding, she herself had brought it on! A second opinion confirmed the diagnosis. "You've got to stop touching yourself or you're really going to cause damage," the doctor told her. Nancy's hematoma turned out to be a blessing. With the bandage, she could no longer touch herself. Her physicians decided to stop Zoloft and start her on Anafranil, the preferred medication for OCD. They explained that her depression had hidden the more

primary problem of OCD, which coexisted with, or had mani-
fested itself in, hypochondria.

Since starting Anafranil, Nancy has enjoyed great success and
gets much more out of behavioral therapy, which she began
while on Zoloft. She's joined an OCD support group and is
pleased to have found a name for her problem. It's not that the
intrusive thoughts don't come, but now she can say stop. She's
learned how to get unstuck. "No one can guarantee me that I'll
feel this good a month from now, but today I'm happy, and I'm
determined to fight this." The next challenge will be going off
the drug to get pregnant, something she's looking forward to. "I
think I can do it, knowing that if things get bad, I can go back on."

COULD SYMPTOMS POINT
TO POST-TRAUMATIC STRESS?

Nightmares, flashbacks, and extreme agitation years after a
traumatic event have been well described in Vietnam veterans.
Once called combat fatigue or shell shock, it is now known that
post-traumatic stress disorder (PTSD) can strike anyone who
has suffered a trauma. The symptoms, which tend to come in
waves, include night terrors, impulsive or avoidant behavior,
irritability, intense anxiety, emotional numbness, fears of illness
or death, and bodily aches and pains. PTSD isn't diagnosed unless the symptoms are clearly related to "an event outside the
range of usual human experience," such as rape, torture, accident, or assault.

By definition, a trauma is something we cannot easily inte-
grate into the conception of who we are. "When an event is so
overwhelming that we have no means to express or resolve it,
pieces of it may get tucked away in the unconscious as a protection against psychic pain," explains Debra Neumann, a clinical
psychologist at the Traumatic Stress Institute in South Windsor,
Connecticut. Sometimes a trigger, like therapy or the birth of a

child, can rekindle these "body memories" and bring them to the surface. The knowledge may first appear as physical symptoms, then filter into the emotional realm, and, with therapeutic assistance, finally emerge in mental consciousness as memory.

There has been a great deal of controversy about cases in which victims of sexual abuse have claimed to uncover memories of early sexual trauma years, even decades, after the event. Priests, parents, and other relatives, accused by adult children of sexual molestation, have been convicted on the strength of recovered memory. Some cases have yielded multimillion-dollar verdicts for the victims; a few adult children have sent parents to prison; others have recanted and with their families sued former therapists for contributing to the confabulation of childhood incidents they come to believe never occurred.

The issue of recovered memory is highly charged, and so far the theory has not been substantiated by research. In fact, initial studies have found the accuracy of repressed memory to be questionable—scientists agree that neurological and cognitive mechanisms can, indeed, foster false memory—and an American Medical Association task force is continuing to investigate the matter. Despite the uncertainties, some highly regarded psychologists and psychiatrists support the principle, believing repression is one of the few mechanisms with which young children can attempt to cope with the trauma of incest.

A. G. Britton, an incest survivor, wrote of her struggles with hypochondria and somatic symptoms during the painful process in which she uncovered memories of being forced as a child to have oral sex with her father. The resurrection of her ordeal began with uncontrollable bouts of anxiety and fear and numbness in her arms and legs during her second pregnancy. The truth began to emerge in psychotherapy and through her dreams. She relived the experience as a child would, "in symbols, body problems, and emotions that seemed to come out of nowhere." Britton had one dream about a little girl, "naked, unconscious, and strapped down with her legs apart." At the end of the bed was a man holding surgical instruments in his hands. She heard him say, "I've penetrated too far."

"Incest survivors repeat the trauma that was done to their bodies in order to regain some sense of control," Britton explains. Many find themselves fantasizing about self-mutilation and physical violence and are plagued by bizarre, irrational fears. Britton herself was tortured by disturbing visions: of dropping her baby and smashing his head on the floor, of burning or cutting a child while she was cooking, of biting her son's head. Attempting to squelch memories, survivors may harm themselves. "My trauma was stored in my upper left leg and left arm, producing numbness in those areas whenever my mind threatened to remember," she says. "Ten years before my memories emerged, I carved up those spots on my body. It clearly wasn't an attempt at suicide; I just had a vague feeling that something had to be released. I never felt well physically. And being sick panicked me. Every time I had a fever, or even a toothache, I thought I was going to die."

CHAPTER FOUR

Are Hypochondriacs Born or Made?

The Nature-Nurture Debate

How shall a man escape from his ancestors, or draw off from
his veins the black drop which he drew from his father's or his
mother's life?

— Ralph Waldo Emerson, *Conduct of Life*

THIRTY YEARS AGO, when Nora was in her twenties, she had
what doctors termed a nervous breakdown, the catch-all diagnosis back then for most mental problems. It began with cloudy
vision, insomnia, and a sudden loss of twenty pounds. Nora
sought answers from medical specialists all over the country, a
quest that ended with her committal to a psychiatric hospital.
There she was "drugged up like a zombie," unable to see her
two small children for two months.

As mysteriously as she got sick, she got better. For years,
Nora had no major psychiatric troubles, though her family, especially her physician-husband, thought her a hypochondriac.
She had a phobia about her blood pressure: it shot up whenever
she was tested in a doctor's office. (Her husband had managed
to get normal readings at home.) The problem, a phenomenon
known as white-coat hypertension, stemmed from the time her
mother, then in her fifties, died from a stroke and Nora has
worked hard to overcome it in therapy.

Two years ago, when her teenage son, always a bit mercurial, began exhibiting symptoms of depression after a romance broke up—headaches, fatigue, weight loss, blue mood—Nora, with her history, wasn't surprised. But when he announced that what was really wrong was chronic fatigue syndrome—no doctor had made that determination—and for months pursued tests and treatments, she and her husband were caught off guard. Last year the couple's twenty-two-year-old daughter was diagnosed with an atypical form of manic depression. She quit her job and has been through four psychiatrists. "Where did we go wrong?" Nora asks. "All my daughter talks about these days is whether she's bipolar one or two, if she has attention deficit disorder, or what new medication she's going to try. Our son isn't back on his feet either. Did I mess them up when they were little? Or is it something in our genes?"

Throughout the ages, those in the throes of emotional turmoil have examined family trees, trying to locate the origins of their pain. The Victorian poet, Alfred, Lord Tennyson, afflicted with hypochondria, depression, and fear of going mad, referred to his torment as a taint of "black blood"; five brothers and two sisters suffered from depressive disorders, and his father, grandfather, and two great-grandfathers were similarly plagued. In the eighteenth and nineteenth centuries, physicians suspected that hypochondria, which tends to run in families, was a heritable condition that could be passed from generation to generation. Early biological theories attributed the problem to constitutional inadequacies, inborn and ineradicable.

Then, in the first half of the twentieth century with the rise of psychoanalysis, hypochondria increasingly became regarded as a malfunction of the psyche, its symptoms put down to bad mothering, unhealthy social influences, and other environmental factors. The key to the disorder was sought among unhappy childhood experiences and early psychological trauma. Change was presumed possible but difficult. Only by cleansing the psyche of repressed, neurotic conflict could one hope to overcome hypochondria and heal the emotional wounds of the past.

Today, with the revolution of molecular genetics and discoveries of neurotransmitters and psychoactive medications that can change brain circuitry, even transform personality, biological theories are once again in fashion. Psychiatry has been "remedicalized" while psychology, perceived as lacking academic rigor, is feverishly working to adopt the quantitative methods of the hard sciences. According to Alfie Kohn, author of *The Brighter Side of Human Nature; Altruism and Empathy in Everyday Life*, the nature–nurture debate has come full circle. "On just about any given psychological issue, genetic factors get more attention than cultural factors do; emotional problems are more likely to be investigated by looking at brains than at families," Kohn says. "Nurture receives lip service while nature receives enormous grants."

What Causes Hypochondria?

Understandably, one of the first questions individuals and family members touched by mental illness ask is Why? What went wrong? Is the problem caused by a biological glitch in the brain? Is it due to heredity? Faulty thinking? An unhappy childhood? What creates this subversive pact between body and brain? Anxiety and depression can shed some light on the mystery, but not much. After all, what causes someone to become depressed and anxious? Additionally, not everyone with health worries suffers from depression or anxiety. Research tells us that at least a fifth, or perhaps more, of those who score high on tests for hypochondria don't have any other psychiatric diagnosis. "Pure" sufferers tend to be harder to cure than hypochondriacs with underlying psychiatric conditions. They have a longer history of the problem, their health fears are more entrenched, and while they have a greater distrust of physicians, they seek the most medical help.

If for no other reason than to determine what type of assistance to seek, it makes sense to try to figure out the underlying cause of any behavior that makes one unhappy. (For a detailed discussion of various therapeutic approaches, see Chapter 10.) But there are limitations: why people feel and act the way they do is an intricate puzzle, the pieces scattered across psychology, biology, and culture. No matter how deeply you dig, it's unlikely you'll uncover one specific "first" cause of your problem, be it hypochondria, anxiety, depression, or any combination of such disorders. After all his introspection, William Styron was resigned to never learning what caused his depression: "To be able to do so will likely forever prove to be an impossibility, so complex are the intermingled factors of abnormal chemistry, behavior, and genetics."

Nonetheless, it may be instructive to examine the forces that together shape human behavior and personality, even physical traits. Although the question isn't simply whether hypochondria is driven by a genetically predisposed constitution or socially conditioned mind, both play a part in influencing how different individuals respond to symptoms and stress. What we seek to know is how genes and culture interact to make us vulnerable to the syndromes society chooses to label abnormal, how nature and nurture conspire to make us who we are.

The following provides an overview of three important theories of human functioning—psychodynamic, cognitive-behavioral, and biological—and explains how each regards hypochondria. Later in the book you will learn about specific therapies derived from these philosophies, treatments that have been found helpful in ameliorating hypochondria.

THE PSYCHODYNAMIC VIEW

This approach, derived from the Greek words for mind and power, is based on the principles of psychoanalysis, which seeks to resolve intrapsychic conflicts that originate in childhood and are repeated in adult life. Traditional psychodynamic theory

presumes that by understanding one's unconscious conflicts—
the neuroses that represent the ongoing battle between repressed
drives and unconscious defenses—these hidden urges and terrors lose their power over us.

Freud's initial view of hypochondria was as a neurosis with a
biological basis, the consequence of a damming up of sexual energy displaced onto bodily organs. His earliest writings about
the disorder revealed a strong belief in the coexistence of physical and mental processes. But as Freud became increasingly involved in working with hysterics, his notion of undischarged
sexual desire became more symbolic than biological. Hysteria
was irresistible as a classic psychoanalytic problem, its pseudo-
symptoms tantalizing material for exploration and interpretation,
and hysterics were prime candidates for the psychotherapeutic
relationship. The more somatic riddle of hypochondria Freud
left to his followers, saying, "It is not within the scope of purely
psychological inquiry to penetrate so far behind the frontiers of
physiological research."

Many years later, Freud's own followers chastised him for
having dismissed physical symptoms as little more than mastur-
batory equivalents. These disciples took the psychoanalytic doctrine a step further, placing hypochondria within the framework
of dependency issues and low self-esteem. One popular analytic
interpretation has been that hypochondria develops as a narcissistic response to loss. A child who has difficulty separating
from a parent fails to acquire a strong sense of self. She becomes
confused about the boundaries of her own thoughts and physical feelings and has little confidence that the world can gratify
her overwhelming needs. Symptoms are an attempt to soothe
herself and survive on her own.

Complaining of physical symptoms, then, becomes an indi-
rect method of communicating with others, an unconscious way
of eliciting support and encouragement, hearing and attention.
Hypochondriacs learn that pain brings love, but the behavior is
also an aggressive means of punishment. Hypochondria, in a

psychoanalytic context, is a way of displacing anger against the parent onto a more acceptable target, oneself, or more precisely, the part of oneself that identifies with the parent.

George A. Ladee, a Dutch doctor who wrote one of the first modern books on hypochondria, theorizes that it may serve as a safe way of letting conflict partially express itself, certainly in a less threatening and destructive manner than such other behaviors as violence or alcoholism. Physical complaints become a sponge for soaking up the anxiety and confusion that stem from the hypochondriac's complicated feelings of dependence, hostility, and guilt, thus allowing him to be loved and to suffer at the same time.

Another psychoanalytic explanation centers on low self-esteem, the belief that one is a failure and no matter what one does it is never good enough. Being sick can hide deep feelings of inadequacy and "interesting" symptoms can compensate for a lack of self-worth. Hypochondriacs are often accused of being narcissistic, which has the negative connotation of being in love with oneself. (In the movie *Manhattan*, the Woody Allen character is briefly married to a woman, played by Meryl Streep, who leaves him for a female lover. She writes a book in which she describes her hypochondriacal husband as having "a fear of death which he elevated to tragic heights, which, in fact, was mere narcissism.") No question, dwelling on sickness can make people self-absorbed, and poor self-esteem often goes hand in hand with narcissism. As Susan Baur puts it: the hypochondriac "substitutes illness, a blameless form of failure, for his sense of general worthlessness." To make himself feel better, "he desperately maintains his belief that he would be strong, independent, and lovable if only he were not sick."

Psychoanalytic doctrine implies that the hypochondriac doesn't want to get rid of symptoms or that he can't; they are essential to his identity. Hypochondria can protect people against "an overwhelming sense of annihilation," says Harvard professor Donald R. Lipsitt. Or in the words of Ladee, the disorder is

"capable of safeguarding a person from psychotic disintegra-
tion." That may partly explain the "help-seeking, help-rejecting"
behavior of hypochondriacs, who "parade their suffering, then
thwart efforts to make it better," Dr. Lipsitt says. The dynamic,
which exists within family life as well as in the physician–patient
relationship, allows people to remain helpless and in control at
the same time. In a sense, he says, the physician becomes the
idealized, and ambivalently held, parent, and the patient the
dependent child. Dr. Lipsitt believes that if physicians better
understood the psychodynamics underlying hypochondria, they
might find hypochondriacal patients a therapeutic challenge,
more interesting than vexing. In his experience, "when doctors
are tolerant and informed, patients feel connected, and physical
complaints begin to melt away."

The value of insight when applied to illness dynamics, a de-
ceivingly simple yet crucial ingredient of good medicine, may
have fallen victim to the current disdain for anything that
smacks of psychoanalytic doctrine. Certainly classical psychoanalysis, harshly criticized for its tendency to boil human behavior down to defense mechanisms and reaction formations,
does have its shortcomings. For one, the psychogenic tradition
grants too much power to the workings of the human mind and
fails to acknowledge the biologic and genetic basis for mental
illness. The legacy of such thinking is that hypochondria continues to be regarded as a sign of weakness. Second, psychodynamic theories, critics say, fail to place enough emphasis on
cultural factors—patterns of family life, ethnicity, class, gender,
the influence of the medical community and the media—all of
which contribute to how people interpret and act upon symptoms. A third difficulty with the approach is that, while anecdo-
tally fascinating, its efficacy is nearly impossible to demonstrate.
You can't isolate an id in the laboratory, which has led to a
dearth of empirical research and the perception of psychology as
a soft, inexact science. Last, psychoanalytic process is a terribly
slow cure, and many who've used the tools of free association

and dream interpretation to gain intellectual insight have found themselves, despite all the work, unable to change. As the poet Edna St. Vincent Millay wrote:

> Pity me that the heart is so slow to learn
> What the swift mind beholds at every turn.

COGNITIVE-BEHAVIORAL VIEW

From a cognitive-behavioral perspective, whether hypochondriacal symptoms come from nature or nurture doesn't matter. What's important is doing something in the here and now to get rid of them. The cognitive approach, developed in the 1960s by Aaron Beck, a Philadelphia psychiatrist, is based on the principle that negative moods are a result of negative thinking and distorted perceptions. From a cognitive perspective, then, hypochondria is a learned response, more like a bad habit than a neurosis. We think our way into trouble, and we can learn our way out by replacing maladaptive thought patterns with healthier ones. Behavioral and cognitive theorists hold a similar belief that bad habits are rooted in one's upbringing. But rather than changing the way we think, as cognitivists recommend, behaviorists emphasize modifying specific behaviors by stopping what have been reinforcing patterns, such as avoidance or seeking reassurance, and encouraging more desirable responses, for example, exposure to the feared situation.

Psychiatrists and psychologists, particularly in England, have been successful in applying cognitive and behavioral techniques in the treatment of hypochondria as well as of panic attacks. From a cognitive-behaviorist viewpoint, the cause of health anxiety in both disorders is presumed to be catastrophic misinterpretation; physical sensations are perceived as more dangerous, and illnesses more probable, than they actually are. Such heightened vulnerability seems to be exacerbated by a growing societal preoccupation with health and disease, particularly the AIDS epidemic, a threat that is rooted in reality to a degree but is also blown out of proportion by the media. In a study at Temple University School of Medicine of 176 heterosexual students with no known risk factors for HIV, 15 percent reported that they thought about the possibility of getting AIDS almost daily or even more frequently, and 17 percent had consulted a physician because of AIDS fears.

At Boston's Brigham and Women's Hospital, Arthur Barsky conducts cognitive-educational seminars in which patients with distressing physical complaints and health concerns are taught new ways to cope with symptoms and fears, a sort of reality-checking therapy. In Dr. Barsky's view, hypochondria is primarily a problem of cognitive and perceptual distortion, set in motion by a process he calls amplification. People who are amplifiers, he says, are more sensitive to minor physical sensations and have a greater awareness than others of the grumblings, twitches, and creaks of the body. They're bothered by sensations not generally connected with illness — dry ears, tired hands, weak ankles — and feel them acutely. Their discomfort frightens them and they become anxious, which in turn produces more symptoms. "The emotional and bodily distress become a loop in which each form of suffering perpetuates and intensifies the other," Dr. Barsky says.

Dr. Barsky's research indicates a robust connection between hypochondria and those scoring high on amplification scales. Overestimating the significance of symptoms and the degree of harm they can cause is what puts hypochondria's vicious cycle in motion: catastrophic thinking leads to hypervigilance and repetitive checking behavior, as well as a need for reassurance, which the hypochondriac rejects because it doesn't confirm his belief that he's sick. One person in Barsky's study couldn't go into shopping malls because the bright colors gave her nausea; another called to cancel an appointment because of a hunch that his cholesterol might be high that day.

Many illness phobics can relate to this heightened sense of alarm and vulnerability. One man I interviewed recounted an anecdote about a fear that crossed his mind in a movie theater, then haunted him for a year. The man couldn't understand why he always had to urinate when most people made it through a two-hour film without difficulty. An urgent and frequent need to relieve himself had been present most of his adult life, but in middle age it suddenly became significant. He consulted several physicians. Tests for prostate and kidney problems, as well as for diabetes, came up negative. Still, he obsessed. When doctors would say nothing was wrong, it worried him more. If I'm okay, why is the problem still there? he wondered. One urologist finally hit on an answer he could live with: a nervous bladder. "You're a high-strung, anxious person with a hair-trigger central nervous system that's exquisitely sensitive to discomfort," the doctor told him. "Sure, others wait five hours until their bladder hits 500 cc's. You want to pee at 250 cc's. It's not that you *can't* hold your urine, you don't want to."

Another person told me of the horror of glancing down at her foot one day and seeing a black line across the back of her heel. "I had an immediate sense of doom. The old panic siren went off. That's it, it's over, I'm gone." As she dashed through the kitchen to show her husband the latest abnormality, a jar of shoe polish on the counter caught her eye: she had polished her black shoes that morning while they were still on her feet. So much for the black plague.

In *Worried Sick*, Barsky outlines four factors that play a role in amplification:

Attention. The more attention you pay to a symptom, the more discomfiting it becomes. Distractions, on the other hand, help minimize physical woes. For example, in a study of patients undergoing dental extractions, two groups of subjects were asked to report periodically on how much pain they were experiencing from the procedure. Over a two-hour span, one group reported their pain every twenty minutes, the other group only once. Not surprisingly, the patients who monitored their misery more frequently complained of greater pain.

In another study, James W. Pennebaker, a psychology professor at Southern Methodist University in Dallas, observed college students while they worked out on treadmills. Wearing headsets, half the subjects listened to music and street noises; the other half were treated to sounds of their own breathing and heart rate. The subjects who focused on their bodies complained of being more winded and had far greater physical discomfort than those who were provided with distraction.

Circumstances. How a person experiences sensation and whether he or she perceives it at all depend on its context. A backache is worse when you're facing onerous household chores than when you're relaxing on the beach under sunny skies. A child ordered to come in from playing outdoors to do homework becomes aware of the stomachache that hadn't bothered him outside. Soldiers during battle can sustain a high level of pain, even be oblivious to severe wounds that might be unbearable under other circumstances.

Expectations play a role in shaping what people feel. When relief is anticipated and doesn't come, symptoms become worse. Conversely, curable pain is bearable. Take childbirth. For most women the agony of labor is mitigated by what they know: that relatively safe anesthesia is available and can be provided if necessary; that the severe pain of contractions is generally of short duration; and that after it's over, there's a wonderful reward!

Mood. Mental discomfort increases any ache, pain, or minor physical annoyance. Anxiety and depression are major amplifiers. Stressful events—arguments, rejections, defeats—tend to make symptoms worse, while triumphs and happy occurrences can act as what Barsky calls symptom reducers. When you're about to cross the finish line in a marathon, you aren't likely to notice the degree of pain you felt at mile 13!

Beliefs. When people suspect that the cause of physical discomfort is serious, the symptoms become more acute. For instance, if you attribute a headache to eyestrain from reading, the pain is profoundly more tolerable than if you believe it is caused by a brain tumor. The problems of hypochondriacs arise in part from mistaken beliefs—for instance, "I should always be able to find an explanation for my symptoms"—which cause them to interpret whatever routine physical symptom they experience as a significant event. Says Barsky, "Hypochondriacs tend to have an unrealistic notion of what it means to be healthy. One reason they have so many complaints is they think they're not supposed to have any."

The Biological View. With the growth of biomedicine, neurobiology has become the hot ticket in mental health research. Scientists in pursuit of innate mechanisms to explain mental illness are discovering biochemical underpinnings for just about every type of human behavior—depression, eating disorders, violence, premenstrual syndrome, alcohol and drug addiction, to name but a few. Effective chemical treatments have shown a biological basis for mental disorders that have baffled psychiatrists for decades. Who would have thought ten years ago that technical terms like "neurotransmitter" and "serotonin" would become practically colloquial and, within some families, household words? Mental illness has become something tangible—it's in our cells, our genes, our brains. The problems aren't our fault, maybe not even our parents'. We're hypochondriacs because we have biochemical imbalances, neurodeficient circuits, trouble quieting some regulatory system in our brains.

There's some evidence to support the notion that hypochondria may be at least somewhat biologically driven. Most biologic theories of illness phobia center on the dysregulation of the serotonin system, the network of neurotransmitters that shuttles messages between brain cells. Serotonin, especially plentiful in the limbic region of the brain, which regulates emotion, seems to influence a number of bodily and mental processes, such as mood, appetite, pain transmission, sexual behavior, and sleep. At appropriate levels, the chemical promotes a sense of equanimity, helping to keep emotions like anger and worry in check; depleted or in excess, it can trigger chronic disturbances in mood, behavior, and thought. Scientists believe that a metabolic flaw in neural pathways that connect via serotonin may be the culprit in a variety of psychiatric problems: compulsive behavior, such as that seen in obsessive-compulsive disorder (OCD), eating disorders, and hypochondria, as well as in impulsive behavior, such as violence and suicide, though the mechanism by which serotonin-secreting cells misfire is still unknown.

The implication of neurotransmitters in obsessive thinking appears so strong that some bioresearchers suggest that the disorders characterized by compulsive and impulsive behavior, rather than being discrete diagnostic entities, are a related constellation of conduct that reflects a single organic disturbance or physiological state. Hypochondria, according to the theory, would be only one of a number of neurologically linked conditions that exist along a continuum of psychiatric illness; they are classified under the umbrella term "obsessive spectrum" disorders, according to Eric Hollander, one of the primary advocates of the theory.

Dr. Hollander, who is the director of both Clinical Psychopharmacology at New York's Mount Sinai Medical Center and the Anxiety, Compulsive, Impulsive and Dissociative Disorders program, explains that obsessive-compulsive-type illnesses are connected by common neurological markers and core symptoms. At one end are compulsive-style, or risk-aversive, disorders, characterized by ruminative thoughts or bodily preoccupations. For example, those with body dysmorphic disorder focus on body appearance, with anorexia nervosa on body weight, and with hypochondria on body illness. At the other end are impulsive-style, or risk-seeking, disorders marked by ritualistic, driven behaviors, such as the tics of Tourette's syndrome, the hair pulling of trichotillomania, or explosive sexual or aggressive urges.

The OCD-related disorders share other features: the onset of illness in adolescence or early adulthood, a clinical course in which symptoms wax and wane, and a tendency to be passed from one generation to another. Compulsive and impulsive symptomatology tends to overlap in families as well as individuals. It's not unusual to see the behaviors come in clusters, with different symptoms emerging at different times. But the traits seem to stick to their own camps: impulsives stay risk seeking and compulsives stay rigid.

A typical case might be a highly strung college student away from home for the first time. She feels insecure academically and socially and develops a fear of gaining weight. She soon becomes anxious about food, obsessed with exercise, and begins to starve and binge. The young woman is able to resist the preoccupation enough so that it doesn't reach full-blown anorexia nervosa or bulimia. But she begins to think that something doesn't look right with her nose. Later she worries that she has AIDS.

Although research on the connection between hypochondria and OCD is still in its early stages, more thorough data exist on the OCD-anorexia link. One controlled study found that half of anorectic patients would qualify for a diagnosis of OCD even after excluding food and body-related obsessions. Another study evaluated nineteen anorectic patients, finding that all had OCD types of symptoms beyond body image, exercise, and eating obsessions: 18 percent worried about loved ones getting ill; 23 percent had somatic preoccupations and body-checking rituals; 55 percent feared something terrible was about to occur.

Those with anorexia nervosa, hypochondria, and other compulsive behaviors share common characteristics: they exaggerate the possibility of harm associated with actions or thoughts; they're hypervigilant, sensitive to subtle changes in sensory information. "They seem to have an internal alarm, a very primitive kind of biological mechanism, that goes off when something doesn't feel right, look right, or fit right. It's kind of a mismatch detector," Dr. Hollander says. The mismatch hypothesis, isn't so different from the cognitive notion of amplification; but rather than blame bad habits or faulty learning, neurobiologists would attribute the problem to a brain abnormality that causes people to scan their environment with undue hypersensitivity.

Research supports the idea that a specific brain circuit may indeed be responsible for the bizarre urges and distinctive conduct of obsessive-compulsives: the brains of OCD sufferers look different from other people's. Sophisticated brain-mapping techniques show increased activation of the orbital region of the frontal cortex, just above the eyes, when compulsions are being acted out. Impulsive conduct seems to have the opposite effect, reducing frontal lobe activity. Additionally, compulsivity is associated with increased sensitivity to serotonin, and aggressive or impulsive behavior with reduced serotogenic function. That may be one explanation why Anafranil and Prozac, which initially raise serotonin levels, then reduce brain receptivity to the chemical, have been so successful in diminishing obsessions and compulsions in OCD, anorexia, and hypochondria, while the impact of these medicines on suicidal and violent behavior is less clear.

THE HEREDITY LINK

Should neuroanatomical theories prove correct and it turns out that depression, OCD, and hypochondria are hardwired into neurochemical circuits, a puzzle would remain: Are these illnesses genetic, imprinted in us from birth like the color of our eyes, the size of our feet? Or does something in our environment provoke biology? Most important, can we change brain circuitry once the damage is done? One of the best methods science has of distinguishing nature and nurture are studies of identical twins. The idea, of course, is that if a disorder is genetic, there is a high possibility that both twins will have or will develop the disorder. Studies of adopted children removed from their birth families also help researchers distinguish hereditary effects from environmental ones.

Enormous efforts have been made to study twins and adopted

children with all kinds of genetic disease. Thanks to advances in genetic technology, scientists are isolating human genes, the discrete segments of DNA that are the units of heredity, at the rate of more than one a day. They've come a long way in pinpointing genetic markers that cause or trigger some forms of heart disease and cancer. More recently, researchers have located genes that play a role in Huntington's disease, Lou Gehrig's disease, ataxia, the disease featured in the film *Lorenzo's Oil*, as well as genes linked to a common form of colon cancer and a hereditary breast cancer that strikes women at an unusually early age.

Scientists have achieved less success, however, in unmasking genetic flaws that lead to mental illness. There is little dispute that psychiatric illness runs in families, but questions remain as to whether specific genes play a role in who suffers these disorders. It is more likely that traits carried by several genes predispose a person to develop certain psychiatric conditions, which surface only if the right—or wrong—environmental buttons are pushed. One complication is that even if psychiatric disorders do involve the interaction of multiple genes, scientists don't know how many there are, where they lie, or what they do.

Aubrey Milunksy, a leading medical geneticist at the Boston University School of Medicine, has found little evidence to confirm genetic theories in the vast majority of mental disturbances. The exceptions are schizophrenia, manic depression, and possibly severe depression, which appear to be strongly influenced by hereditary factors alone. For instance, twin studies of schizophrenia, a psychotic disorder characterized by hallucinations, paranoia, and loss of contact with reality, have shown that both identical twins develop the disorder in one third to one half of all cases. (By comparison, the occurrence rate in pairs of non-identical twins is 10 to 12 percent.) As for the heritability of common neuroses such as mild depression, the data aren't persuasive. "There is no evidence that neuroses have a genetic basis," Dr. Milunsky says. "Through a shared environment, it could be anticipated that severely neurotic parents will have neurotic children."

A hereditary basis for hypochondria is on even shakier ground. Partly because of its muddled definition, few family studies on hypochondria have been conducted, and the limited attempts to find genetic links have yielded contradictory results. One study of twenty-four pairs of identical twins and twenty-four pairs of nonidentical twins, ages fourteen to eighteen, determined that "neuroses with hypochondriacal and hysterical elements have no, or low, genetic component." In the same study, depression and schizophrenia were found to have a substantial genetic basis. Another study of forty-four pairs of identical twins reared apart for most or a period of their childhood found a high degree of either somatic symptoms or hypochondriacal traits in four of the pairs. One of them, thirty-nine-year-old Olga and Viola, had been separated from birth until age eleven, then again at sixteen, with minimal contact during adult life. At twenty-five, Olga had a sudden panic attack in which she developed the idea that she was going to choke and became afraid to swallow her own saliva. Viola, who knew nothing of her sister's problem, developed similar symptoms and for several years would not eat any solid food.

The search for hereditary links is intriguing, but coincidences of this sort may be just that, no more than a biological accident. In fact, every time researchers think they've unmasked a genetic abnormality to explain a mental disorder like manic depression or alcoholism, the finding disintegrates on closer inspection or is cast into doubt. Those in the behavioral sciences say that investigators in eager pursuit of biological solutions may overlook environmental factors that may be better predictors of mental function and dysfunction, for example, twins' ages when adopted or the backgrounds of their adoptive parents.

The ascendance of biopsychiatry has hit a raw nerve among many mental health practitioners who believe its power is being oversold. Keith Russell Ablow, a psychiatrist who writes for

The Washington Post, is disturbed by the false public impression, which, he says, some biopsychiatrists have helped create, that biochemical causes of mental disorders are rapidly being uncovered and that pharmacological "cures" are at hand. "The truth is that no one knows how abnormalities in the brain cause psychiatric illnesses," he writes. "The medicine used to change brain chemistry offers symptomatic relief, not cures." That disturbed neurotransmitters appear to play a role in psychiatric disorders shouldn't diminish the importance of self-understanding and insight: disordered biology, says Dr. Ablow, can be rooted in traumatic experience.

Martin Seligman, a professor of psychology at the University of Pennsylvania, also campaigns against constraints he contends biological and pharmacological models have placed on the humanistic concept of self. The premise of his book *What You Can Change and What You Can't*, put simply, is that some traits are malleable and some aren't. Most important, a great deal of our genetic inheritance can be overridden or deeply modified through learning or life experience. The view that all is genetic and biochemical and therefore is often wrong, he says. "Many people surpass their IQs, fail to 'respond' to drugs, make sweeping changes in their lives, live on when their cancer is 'terminal,' or defy the hormones and brain circuitry that 'dictate' lust, femininity, or memory loss."

No matter to what side one leans in the nature–nurture debate, few scientists today posit that biology is destiny. Not even the strictest biological determinist would insist that having the gene or group of genes for schizophrenia—or hypochondria, for that matter—automatically means you'll develop the illness regardless of the hand life deals you. Most mental and many physical illnesses are multifactorial; you need two hits: biology and environment. "People are born with a genetic predisposition to develop certain psychiatric disorders," Dr. Milunsky says, "but a number of things can happen in life to trigger the onset of the illness or make it more likely."

The kinds of stressors thought to play a role in hypochondria aren't exactly surprising. At the top of the list is experience with illness, especially when young. A number of adult sufferers of hypochondria, as children, were either sickly themselves or witnessed a critical illness of a parent, sibling, relative, or close family friend.

Jim, an actor in his fifties, links his overconcern with physical well-being directly to childhood. During World War II, when he was a baby, his uncle was lost at sea. Both grandparents died shortly afterward "from grief." At ten, Jim's younger brother was stricken with what was thought to be leukemia but turned out to be infectious mononucleosis. Though the brother, at forty-three, is healthy, his mother never quite believed the doctors and, Jim says, "she's still waiting for the other shoe to drop." As a child Jim himself was troubled by asthma, eczema, and constant stomachaches. The maladies didn't worry him then, but he felt emotionally isolated without them. "I had it figured out—*I* knew what got attention in my family," he says.

His phobia about illness didn't set in until college, when a close friend's mother was diagnosed with colon cancer. "I knew the woman well and though my friend begged me to see her, I couldn't," Jim recalls. On some level, he believes, he must have connected his stomach trouble to the cancer, because ever since then he has struggled with fears of intestinal and colon cancer. Another contributor to Jim's hypochondria was that his mother always "bought into" his health concerns. Even at age seventy-five, she treats her two sons like patients, querying them about their diets, weight, even bowel movements, and inquiring about doctor visits and test results.

Parental cues are significant in the making of a hypochondriac. Children tend to mimic hypochondriacal behavior they observe in a parent, either becoming hypochondriacs themselves or repeating the pattern with their own children. Overprotected children whose parents were anxious about health often exhibit this vigilance in adulthood. "Quite often, a hypochondriac had parents who analyzed every sneeze, took them around to doctors, and left them feeling vulnerable and insecure about their bodies," says Laurence Kirmayer, a psychiatrist at McGill University. Impressive data are also emerging about the relationship of childhood trauma to hypochondria, the studies revealing a high correlation of the disorder with physical abuse in childhood as well as early loss.

One twenty-eight-year-old woman, a patient of Dr. Hollander's with both hypochondriacal and OCD symptoms, bore the terrible trauma of her mother's having died while giving birth to her. As an adult, the woman felt a perpetual sense of doom, believing not only that some mishap, such as early death or disease, would befall her but that she might cause harm to other people. At one point this obsession turned into a paralyzing panic. She'd be walking down the street and suddenly an intense fear would creep over her: if she kept going, she might be responsible for killing somebody. Dr. Hollander describes what happened next: "The patient, call her Susie, would come to a complete stop, unable to go backward or forward, because she believed she might knock somebody off the sidewalk or a car might come by and run a person over. When she finally could move, she'd go to a telephone booth to call her husband, asking him to contact the police precincts to see if there had been a pedestrian accident."

The woman, a television production assistant, would be unable to return to her office. "Her preoccupations were interfering with her job and marriage," Dr. Hollander says. "She was so bright, yet she was barely functioning, unable to move forward in her life." Eventually she sought treatment and was helped by a combination of talk therapy and one of the serotonin reuptake blockers; but once off medication, she relapsed. Insight alone wasn't enough to curb her self-destructive tendencies. "Anyone who loses a mother in this terrible way is bound to be profoundly affected, but not everyone goes on to develop a pathological sense of responsibility," Dr. Hollander says. In this case, he believes, a clear biological substrate underlay the patient's behavior, which included a family history of eating disorders, OCD, and other related problems.

Ironically, biological theories may end up reviving scientific interest in Freudian principles, generally out of favor with today's neuroscientists. Modern theory of obsessive behavior echoes much of what Freud had to say about intrapsychic conflict: that in OCD, the "automatic gatekeeper" in the brain which filters out impulses associated with "primitive" drives, related to sex, aggression, appetite, is weak, giving rise to repetitive thoughts and rituals. Freud believed that compulsions reflected a need to silence unacceptable urges and unconscious fears, and his initial theories connected compulsivity, sometimes referred to as anal behavior, with the toilet-training phase. For example: a toddler holds back feces to control harsh, demanding parents and ends up rigidly perfectionistic, a tempting hypothesis that hasn't been borne out by research. Freud himself was never certain that early trauma alone was responsible for obsessional or hypochondriacal neuroses, and his writings included speculation about genetics and other biological influences. In fact, he predicted that someday science would discover a mechanism to explain the enigmatic leap between mind and body that mystified him in these disorders. "In view of the intimate connection between things physical and mental," Freud wrote, "we may soon look forward to a day when paths of knowledge will be opened up leading from organic biology and chemistry to the field of neurotic phenomena."

CULTURE: THE MISSING LINK

We've come a long way since Freud in unraveling the mind-body connection, yet the picture of hypochondria remains incomplete. Social scientists would argue that the experience of health and sickness, which goes beyond even psyche and soma, must be examined within a third context: the time and culture in which we live. Those considered hypochondriacs live in a society that dictates whose ailments are legitimate, which symptoms are acceptable, and how sick people should behave. "Symptoms have a social as much as an individual stamp," writes Edward Shorter in his most recent book, *From the Mind into the Body: The Cultural Origins of Psychosomatic Symptoms*.

Unconsciously one may choose to express emotions in the physical language of the body, but there is also an external pathology that drives and maintains somatic distress. Genetics may influence the manner in which people interpret physiological signals. Trauma can increase the likelihood that the delicate balance of thoughts, emotions, and physical processes may fall out of sync. Yet, as Shorter notes, disruptions in neurochemistry and personal equanimity "don't account for the choice of symptom, or the timing and the duration of the illness." It is something outside of self, be it national character, ethnic group mores, marital dynamics, or the medical dictates of the day, that directs behavior for dealing with emotions and being ill.

Talk to cultural anthropologists and sociologists about hypochondria, and the picture that emerges is one less of individual behavior or biochemistry than deprived social conditions. People who don't have a sense of mastery of their environment, or are bored and lonely, tend to turn inward and focus on their bodies. They may look toward the health care system for social support and validation of their lives. When social workers encounter bodily preoccupation among the poor, who are collectively at higher risk for both mental and physical illness, according to Susan Baur, they construe it as a defense against powerlessness and vulnerability, a response to social stress. The therapy of choice, Baur says, becomes "employment, good housing, a sense of community, and other external signs of security and self-esteem" that community mental health advocates maintain can empower individuals and help "prevent the common retreat into hypochondria."

If hypochondria represents, for many, an unconscious escape

from difficult life predicaments, is there a general profile of someone apt to take refuge in illness? Not really. Hypochondriacal
and somatic behavior cross sex, age, race, and ethnic and socioeconomic boundaries. Are some groups more prone to communicate psychosocial distress through physical complaints than
others? The answer is a qualified yes. A young black or Hispanic woman who is separated and has experienced physical or
sexual abuse is at far greater risk for somatic complaints than a
middle-aged, white Anglo-Saxon male who has been happily
married for twenty-five years.

Here's some of what we know about the social dimension of
symptoms from a handful of research findings in this area.

• Jews and Italians are more apt to fixate on their bodies and
complain about pain than Anglo-Saxons or Irish-Catholics.

• Those with less education and of lower socioeconomic status suffer more unexplained medical symptoms than the well-
to-do, but disease phobia is equally common among middle and
upper classes.

• Single people—the separated, divorced, and widowed—
are at greater risk for disease and physical symptoms than married people.

• Older people suffer a great deal of organic disease—75
percent of those over sixty-five have some form of chronic illness—yet, surprisingly, are less prone to hypochondriacal fears
than younger folk.

• Women suffer from more vague physical ailments for which
they seek medical attention than men, but both sexes appear
equally affected by hypochondria.

Since hysteria's heyday, the culture has borrowed ideas from
medical sciences to explain the human condition. Once histrionic behavior no longer was attributed to the female reproductive system, hysteria became not a symptom of a disturbed
psyche but, in the eyes of some historians, a feminist reaction to
a male-dominated social order. This was the mid-nineteenth
century, when feminist voices, like Mary Wollstonecraft, began

speaking out, and oppressed Victorian women caught a glimpse of the freedom that the culture remained largely unwilling to grant. "Hysterical pain and numbness served as ballots cast secretly in an election from which women were still legally excluded," David Morris writes in *The Culture of Pain*. The "rest cure," made famous by S. Weir Mitchell, a nineteenth-century physician, became the prescription of choice to quiet the symptoms of nervous, emotional women. Dr. Mitchell's advice to one "hysterical" writer of the period: "Live as domestic a life as possible. Have your child with you all the time . . . Have but two hours' intellectual life a day. And never touch pen, brush, or pencil as long as you live."

By World War I, neurasthenia, a condition with a multitude of poorly defined symptoms that plagued America's intellectual and economic elite, had replaced hysteria as the disease de rigueur. In *American Nervousness, 1903*, sociologist Tom Lutz maintains that the illness helped the American upper class come to terms with the pressures of industrial modernization—labor unrest, a massive influx of immigrants, the addition of women in the workforce, and innumerable technological advances. Neurasthenia, which unlike hysteria affected both sexes, was understood to be a form of nervous exhaustion. Among the famous afflicted were Henry James, Charles Darwin, Teddy Roosevelt, Edith Wharton, and Emma Goldman. The medical advice dispensed to men and women differed completely: women were prescribed rest and quiet, men vigorous muscle building and exercise cures. The remedies, which Lutz says symbolized "a return to traditional values of passive femininity and masculine activity," nonetheless couldn't stem the march of culture: Edith Wharton, for instance, made the best of her neurasthenic career by writing in bed.

The rise of psychiatry stripped neurasthenia of its power, and today the diagnosis has virtually disappeared in North America, though some claim that the "disease" has simply acquired new names. According to Charles Ford, the University of

Alabama psychiatrist, every generation has its own brand of vague, neurasthenic–type complaints for which "fashionable" diagnoses periodically emerge. Even if a genuine organic basis exists for some, such fad or marginal diagnoses—which often represent an unconsciously motivated collusion between doctor and patient—generally lead to overdiagnosis in the population at large. Twenty-five years ago hypoglycemia, a low blood sugar condition rarely mentioned these days, was used to explain a myriad of ambiguous symptoms. Back then "physicians were far more comfortable in making the hypoglycemia diagnosis and prescribing treatment for it than they were diagnosing anxiety or depression," Dr. Ford opined. Some would claim that the same holds true for today's chronic fatigue syndrome complaint. In fact, the debate in medical circles over the chronic fatigue epidemic is not unlike the controversy that swirled around neurasthenia earlier in this century.

A diagnostic label that helps symptoms qualify as a disease isn't altogether bad. For some, having a name for pain and discontent provides positive illusion, a crutch for coping with uncertainty and emotional distress. For others, a fad diagnosis can contribute to lifelong hypochondria, both costly and destructive. Cultural explanations of hypochondria, however, contain a message of hope. For as difficult as it is to change one's psychology or biology, as Shorter points out, "understanding the way in which others make us sick is within reach of us all."

....

CHAPTER FIVE

Healthism: A Symptom of Our Time

For each disorder that doctors cure with drugs . . . they produce ten others in healthy subjects by inoculating them with that pathogenic agent a thousand times more virulent than all the microbes in the world, the idea that one is ill.

— Marcel Proust, *The Guermantes Way*

THE FACES STARE mournfully from the cover of the magazine: mother and son wrapped in a blue blanket, looking stricken and petrified as if nuclear war has broken out. The headline screams, IS MY ELECTRIC BLANKET KILLING ME? This oversize photograph, which promotes an article about the health risks of electromagnetic fields, was journalistically conceived after Colleen Drischler, beside herself because she had slept under an electric blanket during pregnancy, wrote a letter to *USA Weekend*. She was worried that her five-year-old would develop leukemia and was embarrassed to bring up her fears to her pediatrician — but apparently not to reveal them to 33.5 million subscribers.

Not until well into the magazine could readers discover that Ms. Drischler needn't have looked so glum. There is no scientific proof linking electric blankets to cancer, they learned, although one study of their use during pregnancy found the rate of childhood leukemia to increase from one in twenty thousand to two in twenty thousand. So the editor told Ms. Drischler, "As you can see, the chances your son will develop leukemia are small," a text message quite different from the visual one.

BLURRING THE LINE BETWEEN
HEALTH AND HYPOCHONDRIA

Never mind extraordinary progress in health and medicine— preventive vaccines that have eradicated deadly diseases, advances in antibiotic therapy, the rise in life expectancy. The gulf between people's objective health and their perception of it has clearly grown. Middle-aged baby boomers consider themselves "sicker" than their counterparts did fifty years ago. Our generation spends a greater number of days in bed for acute and chronic illnesses than our grandparents', and a higher proportion of our population is on permanent disability. In the course of a given year, a typical forty-five-year-old consults a physician three times, in contrast to the 1920s, when the average person saw a doctor less than once a year.

It's hardly a coincidence that society's definition of who is sick has expanded as the threshold for what's considered worthy of medical attention has declined. Books, magazines, newsletters, television programs, and medical hot lines promoting health awareness add to the flood of knowledge demanded by a seemingly insatiable public seeking to strengthen their minds and bodies and ward off all manner of illnesses. Some suggest that in the rush to embrace wellness, our generation has become increasingly intimidated by disease. We seek relief for every discomfort. We research symptoms in libraries and on computer databases. Our expectations for diagnosis and treatment are high. As the late magazine editor Norman Cousins said, "We fear the worst, we expect the worst, and the result is that we are becoming a nation of weaklings and hypochondriacs, a self-medicating society incapable of distinguishing between casual, everyday symptoms and those that require professional attention."

This hypochondriacal mind-set is further fed by our disease-defining health care system. Symptoms once considered inexplicable, benign, or trivial are now attributed to popular, nonscientifically documented disorders. Feeling well is no longer a good enough reason to put ideas about illness out of mind. If you don't have a detectable disease, you have hidden risk factors. Commonplace conditions—menopause, childbirth, hair loss, even shortness—have increasingly become medical concerns, while conduct once considered within the range of normal behavior, like having a short attention span or being crabby before your period, is relegated to the pathological.

Donna Stewart, a professor of psychiatry, obstetrics, and gynecology at the University of Toronto, has made a career of studying "disease of the month" syndromes, illnesses she believes are driven by the media. She includes in the fad diagnostic category such conditions as fibromyalgia, chronic fatigue syndrome, temporomandibular joint syndrome, environmental hypersensitivity syndrome, also called total allergy syndrome, and candidiasis sensitivity, in which sufferers attribute disabling health problems to common yeast. In Stewart's opinion, if these so-called illnesses exist at all—and despite extensive research efforts into these disorders, no virus or pathogen has yet been identified—they are overdiagnosed in the population at large. "My clinical impression is that chronic somatizers are especially prone to elaborate on nonspecific symptoms and tend to embrace each newly described disease of fashion as the answer to long-standing multiple, undiagnosed complaints," Stewart writes. In her study of fifty sufferers of environmental hypersensitivity syndrome, which reputedly triggers immune dysfunction in people allergic to chemicals and pollutants in food, air, and water, Stewart discovered that 90 percent of those afflicted had previously incurred at least one other media-popularized disorder.

The "diseasing" of risk factors, life events, and relatively benign symptoms means people increasingly carry around labels that may create more problems than they solve. On the one hand, labeling symptoms as a disease can bring long-standing suffering out of the closet. Medical acronyms, like PMS, for premenstrual syndrome, promote openness and increase public awareness of hidden problems. For many people, just naming a distress can have a placebolike effect, encouraging self-acceptance as well as positive lifestyle changes. Parents whose children display behavioral difficulties may feel relieved when a doctor labels the problem ADD, attention deficit disorder. Employees disabled by job-related aches and pains are increasingly suing employers, claiming RSI, repetitive strain injury. And those who suffer from extreme winter doldrums can hang their troubles on SAD, seasonal affective disorder, a bona fide disorder that responds well to antidepressants — and is less stigmatizing than major depression.

On the negative side, disease labels like these can exacerbate symptoms and deepen an illness. They may catapult a disorder into public consciousness, triggering a new epidemic and causing relatively healthy people to build their lives around a given diagnosis. People who feel sick and don't know why often embark on a torturous odyssey in the mistaken belief that diagnosis means cure. The search for a "mystery" illness can be counterproductive. Doctors and patients become caught up in a fishing expedition, ignoring deeper troubles and more crucial aspects of the doctor-patient relationship. Worst of all, high-tech treatment for common physical and psychological conditions is costly and potentially harmful. Warns Clifton K. Meador, an endocrinologist and director of medical affairs at St. Thomas Hospital in Nashville, writing in the *New England Journal of Medicine*, "A public in dogged pursuit of the unobtainable, combined with clinicians whose tools are powerful enough to find very small lesions, is a setup for diagnostic excess."

The irony is that most people don't get sick because of carelessness about health or a failure of vigilance. As the author and physician Lewis Thomas wrote, "Most illnesses, especially the major ones, are blind accidents that we have no idea how to prevent." Nevertheless, that doesn't stop the hypochondriac from being on red alert, just in case, or from being taken advantage of.

ARE THE MEDIA TO BLAME?

Of course, hypochondria isn't just a condition of modern-day America or its reading public. The malady has been around since the dawn of medicine and occurs in other cultures. The difference is that never before has our collective vulnerability been seen as such a goldmine. Medical expenditures have risen to more than 13 percent of the U.S. economy, nearly double what it was twenty years ago. Americans spend about $60 billion on prescription drugs and $25 billion on over-the-counter medications—in 1960 the figures were, respectively, 4.2 and 1.6 billion; $33 billion on diets and diet-related services; $4 billion on cosmetic surgery; and $3.5 billion on vitamins. The home diagnostic test industry, which took in $780 million in sales in 1993, is growing 20 percent annually.

Drug companies, hospitals, diagnostic centers, publishers, and doctors, chasing after a larger market for their products and services, spend a great deal of effort to tap into the national vein of hypochondria. "You'll feel better knowing," claims a magazine ad for Medical Information Line, an encyclopedia of health information for which callers pay $1.95 a minute to listen to one of three hundred recorded selections on topics from brain tumors and herpes to premature ejaculation and PMS. Just take a ride on the New York subways. The posters in one car alone, hawking everything from designer braces to abortions, screech, "Is It a Mole or Melanoma?" "Get Ahead of Lead, Have Your Child Tested," and in case you didn't have enough on your mind, alert you to "The Itch to Worry About." Promotional gimmickry such as this certainly causes people to pay more attention, even if only subliminally, to symptoms and appearance and may pressure them to take unnecessary or ineffective actions.

That's why it's essential that the media, in their dual role as neutral mirror and influential shaper of human behavior, get it right. The way journalists report medical news is reflected in the way the public makes decisions about health. Much of what's out there serves people well. Media can educate us about our bodies, draw attention to health hazards, inform us of precautionary measures and treatments that may delay or prevent disease. Good medical journalism can offer sound advice and help us determine when to call, and not to call, a doctor. Think of how the common-sense wisdom of Dr. Benjamin Spock guided two generations of parents in managing the illnesses, as well as the psychological development, of their children.

Media can also serve as a watchdog to keep the public aware that medicine is often more art than science, and that physicians vary in their approaches and treatments. If a woman is told she needed to have her uterus removed, might she find it helpful to know that 25 to 50 percent of hysterectomies are deemed unnecessary? Similarly, a man diagnosed with early prostate cancer, facing the decision whether to undergo or forgo treatment, might want to consider that the outcome of "watchful waiting" has been found to be as effective as radiation or surgery, procedures that can bring on serious side effects.

Perhaps a *little* media-generated hypochondria isn't such a bad thing. On the whole, our health as a nation has never been better. Thanks in part to public education campaigns, millions of us realize that several of the biggest killers, such as cancer and heart disease, are associated with lifestyle factors within our control. Death rates from coronary disease have dropped 20 percent in the past two decades. Life expectancy is at its highest ever, with the average American looking forward to 76 years of life, the high being 78.7 for white women and the low 64.6 for black males. In 1900, few could expect to make it past 50. We're smoking less, drinking less hard liquor, eating more nutritiously, examining our breasts, and wearing seat belts.

Nevertheless, there's a downside to all this vigilance. Just because a little prevention is good doesn't mean a lot is better. We live in an era of activist medicine when doctors are eager to test, prescribe, and operate to make sure problems are detected early and treated vigorously. The public has been made so hungry for "magic bullets" that there's a tendency to oversell, if not downright misrepresent, solutions and cures. Lynn Payer, a medical journalist, calls this aggressive marketing practice disease mongering—convincing the healthy that they are sick, or the slightly sick that they are very ill—and, she says, it's big business in America. In *Disease Mongers*, Payer explains how pharmaceutical companies, insurers, and health care providers methodically exploit the "worried well" by taking the symptoms of daily living and converting them into diseases requiring medical attention. Payer writes, "To tell us about a disease, then imply we have it—either by citing the huge number of Americans who do or by listing symptoms that are universal, such as fatigue—is to gnaw away at our self-confidence, not to mention our wallets."

THE PITFALLS OF HEALTH PURSUIT

The impact of disease mongering came home to me at a gathering of friends for a backyard barbecue. Of eight men and women in their thirties and forties, just about everybody had a medical condition that caused some degree of angst. Two people were being monitored for high cholesterol, three had a prescription for Prozac, another was lactose intolerant and suffered from bouts of PMS, and one couple worried that their rambunctious three-year-old exhibited signs of attention deficit disorder. Most in the crowd were fanatical about exercise. Four were vegetarians; another couple was concerned enough about diet to consult a nutritionist and consume large quantities of vitamin supplements.

Unfortunately, amid the welter of health studies, health news, health tips, and health warnings, medical consumers are exposed to much that is confusing and contradictory. They don't know what to make of precautionary advice or whether the risks are real or perceived. Nor are they clear about what actions to take. In an experiment in which fifty-three women were shown an article from *The New York Times* headlined "A Clear Link Between Dietary Fat and Breast Cancer Eludes Study," more than half said the headline indicated that there was a link, a third said there was no link, and the rest weren't sure.

The coverage of medical issues often involves complicated, unresolved debates on science and policy. Faculty academics, facing the publish-or-perish syndrome, churn out a constant array of research papers. One study finds that vitamins boost the immune system, another doesn't. For years women were warned that coloring their hair put them at risk for cancer; now they are told that the danger is minimal and exists only for black dye. Health-conscious consumers switch from butter to margarine and give up burgers for fish only to read that these "heart healthy" foods may drive up cholesterol, too.

The public fixates on endless reports of what to do and avoid, unaware that a single study is usually just a piece of a puzzle and not definitive. It can take years of investigation to convert promising theory into scientific truth — and the theory may still turn out to be a bust. But readers and listeners want to know: What does this discovery mean for me? Does exposure actually cause disease? To satisfy the public's quest for answers and avoid reporting dry, scientific findings, which can hurt ratings, the media tend to hype and oversimplify. Remember the flesh-eating bacteria surging across the country? That made for great sound bites and electrifying photos. For two days television audiences watched as an unfortunate stricken man had his arm gobbled up by the bacteria. The clarification that infection from this strain of group A streptococci was rare and likely to remain so came days after the story broke.

For those prone to hypochondria, such sensationalized medical stories can cause unwarranted panic and create lingering fears that are hard to erase. The result of headline hysteria and hit-and-miss coverage is that those who think they are warding off disaster may actually be courting it.

Here are some of the potential dangers.

Overtesting. Each year Americans submit to close to $10 billion's worth of medical tests among a bewildering array of fifteen hundred. Some of these diagnostic inquiries may be life-saving, revealing hidden tumors or abnormalities before diseases take hold. Others can lead to false positives, exposing patients to unnecessary and possibly risky procedures. After Gilda Radner's death from ovarian cancer, a surge of fearful women demanded tests for the disease. A subsequent investigation found that routine blood and ultrasound examinations did not save lives but instead resulted in unneeded surgery. An advisory panel later recommended that only women at very high risk for ovarian cancer, for example, those whose mother or sister had the disease, undergo screenings.

Another example of testing excess, at least among the young and healthy, is mammography. How often have you heard the statistic that one woman in eight stands a chance of getting breast cancer? But that's if she lives to ninety! The risk of women in their thirties is more like one in six hundred. Yet they're the ones having mammograms, even though the benefits of the test for that age group are questionable, while older women, whose odds at age sixty are one in twenty-four, are more likely to skip them.

Even testing for cholesterol levels or high blood pressure can be risky. With the almost solipsistic interest people have in their cholesterol these days, learning they have a reading outside the normal range can have a tremendous effect on their lives. As a result of a single test, which is notoriously inaccurate because readings vary over time, people have been known to consume vast quantities of the B vitamin niacin, cheap and available in drug and health food stores, which in large doses can cause jaundice and liver failure. Studies of asymptomatic people who learn they have high blood pressure have suggested that the diagnosis results in more absenteeism from work and a greater dissatisfaction with marriage and home life.

The majority of medical tests are designed to detect pathology, not health, and diagnostic processes as well as results are almost always imperfect. This perpetuates what psychologist Delia Cioffi, describes as the "ambiguity of uncertain wellness," which plays a role in maintaining hypochondriacal concerns. For example, many women who examine their breasts feel doubtful about giving themselves a clean bill of health. Here's one woman's description of her monthly "cancer-detecting" exam: "It's a no-win situation. I don't feel reassured after doing the self-examination, mainly because I'm never really sure I didn't find anything. It's funny; I'm pretty sure I would find a lump if I had one, but I'm not really sure about finding nothing!" Such ambiguity doesn't mean diagnostic testing should never be done but, as Dr. Cioffi points out, it should make practitioners think twice about whether the tests are necessary.

Overtreatment. Much has been said of the danger of overprescribing antibiotics, the lifesaving drugs that fight infections. Nevertheless, some physicians say they find themselves prescribing antibiotics for viral infections, for which they are useless, simply because patients expect to be given them. When antibiotics are inappropriately used, drug-resistant disease strains can arise, increasing the likelihood that the medication won't do what it's supposed to do when it's needed. Overuse of ibuprofen, the main ingredient in many nonprescription pain medications, can have serious consequences. Since ibuprofen products went over the counter a decade ago, sales have tripled, and today people think nothing of popping an Advil or Nuprin to relieve any minor discomfort. Yet the medication can cause such complications as stomach upset or gastrointestinal bleeding. Worse, it can cover symptoms and delay treatment of more severe illness. Even the widely used painkiller Tylenol isn't risk free: over years of steady use the medication can damage the kidneys or liver, particularly in people who consume three or more alcoholic drinks a day.

Unnecessary surgery. Surgical procedures are always risky, especially when anesthesia is involved—the risk of death or brain damage related to anesthesia is about one in 200,000. Occasionally certain operations have become trendy, even before they're proven safe. The silicone-gel breast implant disaster is probably the best example of biotechnological engineering gone awry. More recently, synthetic jaw implants for temporomandibular joint syndrome have left thousands of patients unable to eat and speak normally. The surgical implants, which were pulled off the market in 1988, were found to break into microscopic pieces, causing a biochemical reaction that erodes the jawbone.

Unblinking zeal to promote healthy behaviors. Misguided good intentions about what is best can occasionally lead to tragedy. Unproven health claims are rampant these days, and the dispensing of questionable advice isn't usually halted until someone is hurt. Consider tryptophan, an amino acid purported to have a sedative effect. In 1989, fifteen hundred people became ill and thirty-eight died of a rare muscle disease from taking the dietary supplement, which was readily available in health food stores. Though a chemical contaminant in one brand appeared to be at fault, the Food and Drug Administration took no chances and banned over-the-counter sales of tryptophan.

Even something as wholesome as mother's milk can be lethal when health fads cause people to abandon common sense. For the past decade, medical experts and the news media have touted the wonders of breast milk so strongly that nonnursing mothers have felt ashamed and guilty for using formula. While most studies show that breast-fed babies are less prone to diarrhea and allergies, what is seldom mentioned is that they're also in danger of not getting enough milk. Babies have been returned to hospitals dehydrated and starving, suffering from insufficient milk syndrome, a problem for about 5 percent of women who breast-feed. One nursing mother who kept telephoning her pediatrician saying her days-old baby wasn't getting enough milk was told to keep trying. The result: today her son suffers from irreversible, dehydration-induced brain damage.

The Quest for Perfection

There is another injurious dimension to the national health obsession, perhaps less threatening to physical well-being than to the psychological and spiritual aspects of our lives. That is, in our quest for bodily perfection, we're finding ourselves less capable of taking satisfaction in who we are. Remember the Billy Crystal character on *Saturday Night Live*, the Ricardo Montalban look-alike whose distinguishing line was "You look maahvelous"? The sketch satirized the look good–feel better philosophy that since the 1960s has become more and more pervasive. Our culture prizes whatever society happens to define as desirable at the moment, setting up the parameters of the normal and acceptable, only occasionally making quirky allowances, like Lauren Hutton's front tooth gap or Cindy Crawford's mole. The result is intolerance of anything deemed unbecoming or odd: breasts too large or small, noses too big or pug, crooked teeth, pimply skin, too-tall women, and too-short men. And though we hate to admit it, the list includes even larger transgressions against the norm, like obesity, dark skin color, terminal sickness, physical deformity. Those with characteristics that deviate from this so-called norm may even require laws to protect them.

The society that defines such values is also fickle, requalifying its ideal just enough to keep attainment out of reach for most

Judging the Medical News

These are a few suggestions on being "healthily skeptical" in in-terpreting research and evaluating the health benefits and risks of any study.

Consider the source. Scientists usually avoid words like "break-through" and "ground-breaking" when describing their research, but such adjectives are a journalistic staple. The popular media, to varying degrees, tend to overstate to give a study a more news-worthy spin. Look for research that first appeared in reputable sci-entific publications like the *Journal of the American Medical Association* or the *New England Journal of Medicine* for which submissions must undergo rigorous peer review. Then, if you want to know more, obtain the journal in a library or an on-line service and read the original.

Watch for what a report does not say. Most scientists list a study's limitations in a discussion section at the end of a journal paper, for example, lack of a control group, too small a sample. These caveats, however, seldom find their way into institutional releases or the media. Take note of or find out who is funding the study. A growing amount of research is financed by industry, particularly pharmaceutical firms, and if a study supports a company's bottom line, the company does all it can to seek publicity. If a report states a health risk, how meaningful is that risk? Mere association does not prove causation. The results should be "statistically significant" — less than a 5 percent chance that the same results would have oc-curred randomly. Be aware of the difference between **relative** and **actual** risk. For example, one study found that the relative risk of breast cancer in women before age thirty-five was 40 percent higher in those who had used oral contraceptives than among those who had not. However, the actual, or absolute, risk was quite small: 11.9 per 100,000 women who used contraceptives had been diagnosed with breast cancer versus 8.5 per 100,000 women who had not.

Evaluate the quality of a study. Medical studies must be wide enough to spot real trends; narrow ones are easily swayed by chance or bias. Data produced in the course of a study at several large medical institutions are more likely to be meaningful than those generated by a small experiment at a single institution.

A controlled, double-blind study is the gold standard. Because patients often improve on their own, it is best if a study compares the use of a drug or new therapy with a control group in which half get a placebo and half get nothing at all. Tests should be double blind so that neither doctor nor patients know who's getting what, to guard against researcher bias.

Other questions you might ask: What was the study population? How many people were included? How was the information gathered? Did other studies precede this one, and are findings consistent? What sorts of studies were they?

Epidemiologic studies of large samples of people in a community measure the relationship between a given exposure, for example, use of a drug, and the risk of developing a disease. They are good at alerting scientists to practices that may cause or prevent disease but, without controls, fall short of establishing cause-and-effect relationships.

Interventional studies provide more conclusive evidence because they test the effects of treatments on groups of people who have similar physical characteristics and habits. Thus, if one group does better than another, the effect is probably attributable to the treatment rather than a variation in genetic endowment or lifestyle.

Another issue to examine is whether a study involved animal or human subjects. Laboratory discoveries often lead to cures for human ailments, but what works well in the lab can turn out to be disappointing, even hazardous, in human trials. It's worth considering how long the treatment has been under study; it can take years of follow-up to determine risks and benefits after the first human experiments begin.

Solicit your doctor's opinion. If you are thinking of making a change in living habits on the basis of a news item, talk to your doctor. Ask how the research and results fit into the larger picture. You might also want to discuss how the information or advice relates specifically to you as an individual. Your doctor should be able to help you weigh the evidence and analyze the risks and benefits of any lifestyle change.

people. Impossible standards serve to keep self-esteem low and self-absorption high. As Patricia Volk, writing in the *New York Times Magazine*, aptly put it, "Beauty's shelf life lasts as long as a tweeze." During the Twiggy years, for instance, with Marilyn Monroe's zaftig, hourglass figure temporarily out of fashion, it was body weight, or rather lack of it, that counted. Twiggy's legacy still lives—a Finnish study found that department store mannequins, if brought to life, would be too thin to menstruate. Nevertheless, the health consciousness of the 1990s may present an even more arduous physical and emotional challenge. Twiggy was famous for her boyish waifishness. Today we would think, Ugh! No abs, no pecs, no chest. Thirty years later, yes, we've permitted ourselves to weigh a little more, but heaven help us if that extra flesh isn't taut, toned, and muscular.

Historically speaking, this isn't the first time Americans have become slightly health crazed, but the 1990s has the distinction of being the decade of fitness excess. For many of us exercise has become a duty, a means of escaping our deeper selves. Witness the phenomenon of celebrities who work out more than once a day. Oprah Winfrey, whose weight we've watched fluctuate over a decade, is said to run four miles at five A.M. and four more at five P.M., in between squeezing in the Stairmaster and 350 sit-ups. Demi Moore, who took a twenty-four-mile bike ride the day her water broke with her second child, reportedly spends four to five hours exercising each day. Even us regular folks, who don't *have* to look good for a living, have become fitness obsessed. My forty-something friends run, swim, bike, Rollerblade, sweat buckets on Stairmasters and NordicTracks, and dutifully sign up for step and aerobic classes, gladly sacrificing lunch hours.

Much of this is positive—a moderate training program can boost immunity, promote better eating habits, and bolster self-esteem—but God forbid we miss a workout! We feel depressed and guilty, rotten about our bodies and ourselves. Even with all this toning and conditioning, few of us, it seems, are fond of our appearance; according to one study, 85 percent of women and 72 percent of men are unhappy with the way they look.

No wonder plastic surgery has become one of the fastest growing medical specialties. Each year approximately 2.5 million Americans opt for cosmetic makeovers—in 1994, 85,000 people got nose jobs, 210,000 hair transplants, 55,000 face-lifts, and as many as 225,000 underwent liposuction, a procedure in which fat is surgically "sucked" away from the body. The American Academy of Cosmetic Surgery reports that men now account for 25 percent of cosmetic surgery patients, up from 10 percent a decade ago. The most common procedures are hair restoration, liposuction, nose jobs, and eyelid tucks, but also gaining popularity are pectoral and buttock implants, calf augmentation, nipple reduction, and phalloplasty, which entails an injection of fat to increase the girth of the penis.

What does all this have to do with hypochondria? Plenty. Preoccupation with our physical selves implies that something is wrong with us, something we must fix. This pervasive "take charge" attitude is based on an unrealistic notion that all of life's infirmities are preventable or medically treatable and that we should be in top form every day. Health has become our prized possession, our bodies the enemy. We polish, tone, and war against their fragility, fighting flab, "bad" cholesterol, and osteoporosis, hoping to outsmart fate. In "The Morality of Muscle Tone," the writer-philosopher Barbara Ehrenreich contends that in pursuing strength, not as a means to any noble purpose but as an end in itself, we've redefined virtue as health, confusing the moral with the physical. "There's a difference between health and healthism, between health as a reasonable goal and health as a transcendent value." Bodily preoccupation, warns Ehrenreich, leads us to avoid examining our spiritual selves and addressing social and political concerns. With virtue "drained out of our public lives," she goes on, "it's reappeared in our cereal bowls . . . and our exercise regimens . . . and our militant responses to cigarette smoke, strong drink, and greasy food."

Spiritual impoverishment, however, isn't the only moral consequence of a body-centered philosophy. As Ehrenreich points out, in attaching so much credit to people for taking charge of their bodies, we're bound to hold them accountable when something goes wrong. The dismal corollary to healthism, she says, is blaming the victim. By equating healthy with good "we've gotten . . . less tolerant and ultimately less capable of controlling the sources of disease that do not lie within our individual control."

GETTING SICK, BLAMING YOURSELF

As far back as the 1970s, Susan Sontag spoke out passionately against victim-blaming, in describing the "sentimental fantasies" and "stereotypes of national character" that surround tuberculosis and cancer. Sontag, who herself had cancer, criticizes the public, in *Illness as Metaphor*, for the special myth it has constructed around cancer, giving credence to the speculative notion that disease reflects some unresolved psychological problem in a sick person's past—lack of parental love, suppressed anger, a profound hopelessness.

Psychologizing cancer may provide a convenient mechanism for distancing oneself from disease—the myth sustains the illusion that we have some control over getting it—but the result is that desperately ill people are made to feel ashamed and guilty, that somehow sickness reflects their personal and emotional failings. Maybe they didn't exercise enough, eat the right food, or think the right thoughts. That's the message underlying the Type C personality theory espoused today in a number of New Age self-healing books. This controversial hypothesis posits that people who repress negative feelings such as anger, fear, and sadness, and constantly put other people's needs ahead of their own, are especially vulnerable to cancer.

In *The Breast Cancer Companion*, Kathy LaTour describes

how, very shortly after her diagnosis, well-meaning friends began dropping off books attributing cancer to unresolved issues and high-fat food. "It's a depressing reality that there are many people out there who believe that people who get cancer somehow caused it—and therefore deserve it," writes LaTour, who for the book interviewed dozens of women about their physical and emotional battle with the disease. One of them, Dottie, describes her feelings after hearing the C-word applied to her for the first time. "But I don't have a cancer personality," she recalled saying as she sat in a surgeon's office blinking back tears. "I'm an artist and I enjoy expressing and creating. How could I develop a terminal illness?"

Many researchers and physicians are deeply troubled by the public's endorsement of unproven cancer-link theories, which, they say, come closer to folklore than science. Not only do such notions attach unfair blame and stigmatize people who experience their illnesses as "happening to them," they also offer false hope: "If I caused my cancer, I should be able to reverse it." Though studies have shown that patients who share fears and emotions are better at dealing with their illnesses, and may live longer than those who are socially isolated, the reasons for this aren't clear. It may be because of what psychiatrist David Spiegel—whose now classic study of women with advanced breast cancer found that those who took part in support groups survived twice as long as those who did not—calls the grandmother effect. It is possible that people who feel cared about are more likely than others to eat sensibly, sleep well, and stick with their medical treatments. They may also have a model for human relationships that enables them to forge more positive bonds with their doctors.

Why some people stay healthy and others get sick is, indeed, a fascinating and important topic. The well-known Grant study, which has been following Harvard graduates for fifty years, has identified some powerful connections between successful aging and traits in earlier life. One finding was that good health at sixty appeared strongly linked to optimism at twenty-five: optimists were at far less risk for poor health in middle age and late adulthood than pessimists. And if along with having a sunny disposition one feels in control over life, physical and emotional health may benefit even more. In a landmark study of nursing home residents, two Yale psychologists found that when people were given simple choices, like making their own breakfast or choosing plants, privileges that were previously denied, they were more alert and happier than those who were told what to do. They also lived twice as long.

It doesn't take a scientist to know that disease cannot be separated from the body in which it grows, and that the mind and spirit shouldn't be ignored in the healing process. That there is a mind-body connection is true beyond a doubt. What is unclear and still unknown is how the physiology of this connection affects physical health and disease. Many popular claims for the mind's power to heal or hurt the body are distorted or inflated, going far beyond what science has established. As yet, there is no conclusive proof that an optimistic outlook can rev up the immune system. The belief that positive emotions can mobilize a compromised immune system, and that we can will ourselves well, amounts to little more than wishful thinking. Unhappy mental states can lead to changes in that system, but it is not known whether the changes, which are small, affect health. Unlike the well-tested theories that tension and hostility can influence the course of heart disease, an ample body of research to detect whether emotional states cause cancer, infections, and other illnesses that involve the immune system is still lacking.

Ground-breaking research in the field of psychoneuroimmunology (PNI), which brings together psychiatrists, psychologists, neurologists, and immunologists, is beginning to reveal how biochemical processes factor into the mind-body equation and the mechanisms that seem to allow the brain and nervous system to affect hormonal and immune responses. Someday, PNI researchers may be able to tell us the degree to which thoughts and feelings influence — or do not influence — physical health, how emotions are translated into chemicals in the body, and how we might best cooperate with our bodies to resist disease and promote recovery.

In the meantime, until disease mechanisms are better understood, it's important that those of us who worry most about our health, and are most likely to gravitate to sensationalistic news stories, dubious self-healing books, and unsubstantiated alternative medical theories, not be swayed by misleading or fraudulent health claims. As most hypochondriacs know, guilt—the myriad sins and infractions for which one will be stricken down or punished—plays a big role in preoccupation with health. There's enough real stuff out there to terrorize us without our believing that bad thoughts will make us sick.

....

CHAPTER SIX

It's Never All in Your Head

"Words cannot express what I have to say. I came to you sick, sick and scared, and you dismissed me. You didn't have the answer, and instead of saying 'I'm sorry, I don't know what's wrong with you,' you made me feel like a child, a fool, a neurotic who was wasting your precious time."

— Dorothy, in *Golden Girls*

ONE OF MY MOST STRIKING experiences in writing this book was a conversation with Melissa, a freelance typist I had hired, through an agency, to transcribe my interviews with patients and physicians. After completing one cassette, Melissa telephoned, introducing herself breathlessly. She told me she'd been typing, listening to the tape with keen interest, when suddenly it dawned on her: "The person speaking could have been me!" She asked whether we could get together and talk.

Melissa, forty-one, married, and the mother of a teenager, since her early twenties had suffered from a gamut of physical and emotional problems that frightened and preoccupied her. She struggled with depression and anxiety, a result, she believed, of her disabling maladies: migraine headaches, jaw pain, stomach cramps, diarrhea, joint tenderness, and backaches, for which she had consulted a host of specialists, including a psychiatrist. She carried a variety of disease labels, some self-diagnosed, others applied by physicians. These included PMS (premenstrual syndrome), TMJ (temporomandibular joint syndrome), IBS (irritable bowel syndrome), lactose intolerance, and yeast allergies. PMS, on which she'd become quite an expert, was by far the most troubling. "For at least half of each month I feel uncomfortable in my own skin," Melissa explained. "Two weeks before my period, any shred of stability goes out the window. I become irritable, tense, and lethargic. My breasts hurt. My face breaks out. I get stomach- and backaches and an intense pressure over my eyes and at my temples. It's as if a meteor has smashed into my brain."

At times the symptoms made her feel suicidal, the pain intensified by shame that her ambiguous ailments weren't genuine. CAT scans and blood tests inevitably came back negative. "If only the tests would reveal something definitive!" she lamented. Though she continued to cling to her own diagnoses — "They're all I have between me and the loony bin" — Melissa had begun to hide her misery from family and friends and temporarily given up on doctors who, she felt, patronized her. Her modus vivendi was to "dress neatly and smile pleasantly" so that no one could guess how she felt inside. "When I talk about my problems I get these weird stares. People think I'm nuts," she said, fighting back tears. "Maybe I really am a hypochondriac, imagining or exaggerating these symptoms. Maybe all of this is just in my head."

There it was, that nasty, fallacious "all in the head" reasoning with its damaging implication that symptoms which smack of psychic or emotional conflict aren't as real or acceptable as those deemed truly organic. Here was another sensitive, attractive person who had come to loathe herself as that most pathetic of beings, a hypochondriac. Her life story, too, had a familiar ring. She had experienced trauma during her teen and early adult years. Raised in a strict Catholic family, she had "gone a bit wild" during college, experimenting with drugs, alcohol, and promiscuity. In her junior year, a close friend died after overdosing on Quaaludes and vodka. This loss precipitated a period of crisis for Melissa: she started feeling intensely anxious. When reports of a herpes epidemic began to appear, she became petrified that she would contract the virus. The phobia followed her throughout her twenties as a secretary in New York, later transmogrifying into a fear of AIDS.

During that period she also lived through stressful familial illnesses. Her father, who died the year before I met Melissa, had been diagnosed in his forties with lymphoma and was in and out of remission the rest of his life. A younger sister had undergone surgery to remove a tumor the size of a golf ball lodged above her eye. Melissa and her husband, after years of infertility, adopted a son who, at age five, was diagnosed with attention deficit disorder.

These events, alone or together, were capable of putting anyone under severe psychological, emotional, and physiological stress. Nevertheless, Melissa coped—she prided herself on that—but felt that at any moment "the lid might blow off." She was tortured by a constant, irrational worry of being incapacitated, "unable to conduct my life as I know it," and she had a longstanding preoccupation with disfiguration and death. "I've spent the last ten years preparing for the fact that my child will be living without a mother," she said.

As I listened to her story, I felt frustrated, wishing I could help. Why were the obstacles to Melissa's happiness so enormous? Melissa's greatest problems seemed to center on whether the symptoms were real or merely figments of her imagination and the fear that at any moment she could lose control of the painful, volcanic feelings boiling up inside her. Yet no internist, psychiatrist, or family member had been able to alleviate her suffering, a failure that is not unrelated to the mind-body dualism so entrenched in the system by which our society has chosen to care for its own.

Even today, with all the lip service paid to the integration of psyche and soma, our medical system continues to place the physical being at the focus of its diagnosis and treatment, while psychic pain is devalued, dismissed as imaginary or a character flaw within one's control. Why did it matter whether Melissa's symptoms belonged to a yet undiagnosed category of biologic disturbance or turned out to be an unusual manifestation of psychiatric turbulence? Was there really such a difference between the two? And hadn't the discovery of neurotransmitters provided a physiological basis for emotions, a kind of science of the psyche, if you will, which rendered this distinction quite meaningless? The health care system that could help Melissa, and should be obligated to do so, has divided itself into two camps, the mind specialists and the body specialists. So when issues aren't black and white, as they seldom are, people like Melissa, whose problems lie in that vast gray area between the physical and mental, fall between its cracks.

The Myth of the Psychosomatic Disorder

The term "psychosomatic" resembles hypochondria, with which it is often confused, in its ability to arouse controversy. By itself, it is neutral enough — psychosomatic literally means "pertaining to the mind and to the body." Only when you couple the word with others like "disorder," "illness," or "disease" does trouble start. Some health professionals claim that there is no such thing as a psychosomatic illness and would like to see the term thrown out of the medical vernacular altogether. Others in medicine view the term not as a distinctive *category* of disease but as an *approach* to disease and postulate that all illness, even death itself, is psychosomatic.

Culturally speaking, it's still preferable to have a psychosomatic disorder that is real, in the sense that it can be clinically certified by a doctor, than to be considered a hypochondriac, whose symptoms are merely imaginary. As a former editor of the *Journal of Existential Psychiatry* wryly noted, if there was such a thing as a cultural hierarchy of illnesses, "bacterial pneumonia would outrank peptic ulcers . . . and all illnesses known to man would outrank hypochondria."

Before body and soul were cleft from each other in the seventeenth century, a distinctly psychosomatic illness would have been unthinkable. If Melissa had consulted a healer in ancient Greece, or for that matter in modern China, she would never have had to face the distress and suspicion that her symptoms were all in her head. During the Renaissance a medieval midwife or herbalist would have treated her for an imbalance in temperament, prescribing hot liquids and exercise to "cook away" excess choleric fluids. Such remedies had been handed down over the centuries. Even the shamans of ancient times understood that illness has both physiological and psychological components. They might have employed a variety of tools to address Melissa's condition: consulting deities, examining dreams, offering massages, preparing herbal remedies and warm concoctions, and eliciting support from family members. Without modern medical weaponry, healers had to rely on naturopathic techniques, enlisting the patient's self-healing abilities to penetrate the mystery of illness and restore the unseen harmonies.

Today mainstream Western medicine, which for the most part has brought the Cartesian divide between thought and feeling, turns away from nonrational explanations for illness and the restorative power of the doctor-patient relationship to search for chemical and physiological abnormalities. Disease isn't real unless it can be physically proved. It is within this paradigm of illness that the roots of the "psychosomatic disorder" can be found. The assumption that mind and body are separate entities led to the cleavage of health care as medical versus mental health and to the implication that anything that could not be seen under a microscope was attributable to psychological factors alone.

The psychoanalytic movement seized on Freud's revolutionary theory, that unconscious emotions could be symbolically expressed in "body language," at a time of great transition in medicine. During the eighteenth and nineteenth centuries, discoveries in pathology had begun to bring about the division of maladies into diseases in which lesions could be found in an autopsy. The medical profession went to work classifying signs and symptoms into organizational constructs that could be diagnosed, treated, and cured. Then, from early in this century on, vaccines and antibiotics brought deadly bacterial illness virtually to a halt and life expectancy sharply increased, changing the face of medicine forever.

Yet despite the enormous impact scientific technology has had on the world, many believe that its myopic focus on curing disease has been damaging to medicine overall. With improvements in medical diagnostics during the late nineteenth century, physicians put more energy into measuring observable causes of illness and had little left for listening to patients. Vague, inexplicable symptoms, of scant interest to aggressive, high-tech medicine, were given short shrift, passed on to the practitioners of a new discipline, mental health. As author-physician Larry Dossey says in *Medicine and Meaning*, the medical profession lost something valuable when "X-rays, blood tests, and a myriad of other diagnostic tools . . . supplanted the eyes, ears, and hands of the physician."

Paradoxically, the rise of a new approach to illness known as psychosomatics—ultimately to be the crippling blow to hope for hypochondriacs—once held great promise for healing the splits in Western medicine. The psychosomatic movement grew out of a reformist initiative launched in the 1920s by a group of doctors to correct what they saw as a tendency among their colleagues to treat patients like machines and disease like a mechanical breakdown. Its vision was to build a bridge between the physiological and psychological approaches to disease and find ways to hold on to science while teaching practitioners the healing effects of paying attention to people. But the strategy didn't live up to its promise. The concept of the psychosomatic disorder took hold, and generalizations about "psychosomatic patients" began to sweep the profession. The legacy of 1930s mind-body research was the creation of a disparaging new category of ailments: the psychosomatic disorders, illnesses that were all in the head.

For much of this century there existed a group of diseases considered purely mental in origin, therefore inferior in stature, to illnesses that could be scientifically proven. These mind-generated diseases, sharing the wearisome traits of being chronic, enigmatic, and difficult to cure, included the so-called classic seven: high blood pressure, migraine headache, bronchial asthma, neurodermatitis, hyperthyroidism, ulcerative colitis, and peptic ulcer, each thought to reflect a distinctive personality type.

More than anything else, this medical myth, which assigned a group of "not-quite-legitimate" illnesses to mental health professionals, has helped fuel and perpetuate the stigma that surrounds hypochondria and continues to color our attitudes about what constitutes legitimate illness. For, despite the fact that a clear casual link between certain personality types and certain diseases has not stood up over time, the psychosomatic concept has been slow to die. Fear of being tagged with a psychogenic label continues to lead those who are sick and don't know why on frustrating and expensive wild-goose chases in search of organic diagnoses so as not to be held responsible—by loved ones, by employers, by insurance companies—for their pain.

THE ULCER STORY

Pity the poor ulcer sufferer. No physical ailment has ever been so closely tied to emotional turmoil. The diagnosis of this small, craterlike lesion in the stomach or duodenum has for decades been akin to wearing a badge that screams NEUROTIC! Franz Alexander, whose significant though ultimately flawed research at the Chicago Institute for Psychoanalysis had a major impact on the field of psychosomatic medicine, wrote in the 1950s that the central feature in the development of an ulcer is "the frustration of dependent desires originally oral in character." When the wish to be loved is frustrated, a regression takes place to an earlier wish to be fed. The shame and guilt associated with these dependent cravings, he said, leads ultimately to an ulcer.

In the next thirty years, the blame for ulcers would shift from the individual's psyche to his environment. A plethora of medical books published between the 1950s to 1980s describe ulcers as a psychic problem of tense, nervous people unable to adapt to the pressures of the modern-day world. One such, *The Mind Factor*, written by a psychiatrist in 1973, suggests that ulcers are generated by "constant pressure and an unwillingness to slow down and take time out for recreation, which erodes not only the stomach lining but peace of mind, too."

This time-honored psychosomatic theory of ulcers persists to this day. Everyone *knows* ulcers are brought on by emotional conflict, maintained and exacerbated by stress and poor diet. Or everybody did until recently, when researchers found a spiral-shaped bacteria, *Helicobacter pylori,* to be the culprit behind most ulcers. After all the aspersions cast upon "ulcer personalities," the disease, it seems, was more biological than psychological. Until the *H. pylori* breakthrough, standard therapy for ulcers was to block the secretion of gastric acid with medications. These acid-blocking drugs, notably Zantac and Tagamet, were effective in controlling ulcer symptoms which, however, recurred when people stopped taking them. New antimicrobial agents aimed at destroying the bacteria not only knocked out the symptoms but thwarted their recurrence. Sufferers had cause to celebrate: they could say good-bye to ulcers, *and* their stigma, for good.

Nonetheless, the debate is far from over. Though most people now receive antibiotics along with antacids to heal their ulcers, not all doctors believe that the mere presence of a bug is enough to explain the infection. A number of health experts applaud the discovery of *H. pylori* as an important cause of ulcers but argue that the germ is only one factor among many. The controversy lies in the fact that a high proportion of the population is infected with *H. pylori*. About 30 percent of thirty-year-olds and 80 percent of eighty-year-olds carry the bacteria, but only a small fraction of people worldwide develop an ulcer.

Medical experts and behavioral scientists with a more holistic vision of disease and health argue that biomedicine is too quick to dismiss emotional and psychological influences in illness. Says John W. Anderson, emeritus professor of anatomy at the University of Wisconsin Medical School, "I welcome the new finding that an infection is involved in peptic ulcer, but I decry those who crow about the defeat of New Age doctors when they have no data whatsoever to deny the involvement of stress in the etiology of the disease. . . . There is a massive amount of data to indicate the contribution of stress to the development of diseases, without calling it causative."

The ulcer debate and the vociferous disagreement it has provoked among medical theorists is just one of the many conflicts being waged by the medical establishment and those at the borders of medicine, between which the lines are becoming increasingly blurry. Traditional medicine finds itself embroiled on several fronts: between the alternative and conventional, the physical and emotional, the real and imaginary, the diseases that truly "happen to people" and those which people bring on themselves. The battles are as much philosophical and economic as they are medical, and the stakes are high. More than anything else, they are about whose version and vision of medicine can best lead to healing illness and alleviating human suffering.

The medical establishment, especially the old-line membership of the American Medical Association, would like you to believe that there is an "alternative" system of health care that exists only at the fringes of medicine. But according to a Harvard Medical School survey, one of every three Americans has taken this so-called unconventional path to health care, the majority of them willing to pay for it out of their own pockets. These people are searching for a new, comprehensive kind of care. They are tired of having their perceptions ignored, tired of being told their pain is imaginary.

Consider the plight of twenty-six-year-old Vicki Perryman, a speech pathologist in an Oklahoma school district. In early 1993, Ms. Perryman announced to parents, teachers, and friends that she had been diagnosed with ovarian cancer. Everyone felt terrible. So when Ms. Perryman began sloughing off—not completing paperwork, appearing disorganized, missing appointments—colleagues, attributing her behavior to cancer, tried to be sympathetic. The school board even renewed her contract. But when it was discovered that her problems stemmed from mental illness, a bipolar disorder that caused her to act erratically and believe she had cancer, she was summarily fired. This despite the fact that her condition was treatable with lithium and two psychiatrists testified that she was fit to work and posed no danger to students.

THE POWER OF CHRONIC FATIGUE

No wonder those suffering from chronic fatigue syndrome (CFS) are crusading so fervently to find the virus that will exonerate them from mental illness and the stigma of bringing the disease upon themselves! Even more than ulcers, CFS has become the poster ailment of the mind-body war, a symbol of the debate as to what constitutes "real" disease. At least ulcer sufferers can have their problem validated with an X ray; but with CFS, the complaints are so subjective and mimic so many other medical and psychiatric conditions that those afflicted with the disease become ripe targets for the psychogenic marksmen.

During the mid-1980s, when the first cases began cropping up in a small resort town near Lake Tahoe, CFS was disparagingly referred to as the Yuppie flu. Its telltale symptoms—exhaustion, muscle and joint pains, headaches, swollen lymph nodes, sleeplessness, poor concentration, and memory loss—seemed to strike fast-tracking, upwardly mobile young professionals, women twice as frequently as men. At first, it looked as if the Epstein-Barr virus, which causes mononucleosis, might be responsible, but when research couldn't bear this out, patients were accused of inventing the illness as an excuse to slow down. Casting further suspicion, studies began revealing a high correlation between the clinical picture of CFS and psychiatric syndromes — some 70 percent of patients suffer from depression and anxiety— sparking all kinds of chicken-and-egg controversies about which problems came first.

Of course, enigmatic ailments aren't alien to science, and CFS—for which there is no known cause, no simple diagnostic test, no known virus or infectious agent, and no known mode of transmission—isn't the first medical problem to defy explanation and cure. But few health riddles have become so political. For years a powerful lobby of sufferers—the precise number of CFS patients is unknown, but estimates of cases range from 10,000 to 5 million—exerted pressure on the federal government and the scientific community to track the epidemic. Their efforts led to a congressional directive that the Centers for Disease Control and Prevention (CDC) come up with a working definition of chronic fatigue for research and surveillance, which the federal agency did in 1987. (Since then, the case definition has been revised three times.)

The CDC now classifies chronic fatigue as a "syndrome" with a group of associated signs and symptoms that characterize its clinical picture. To qualify, patients must experience fatigue severe enough to reduce daily activity by 50 percent for at least six months and evince eight of eleven flulike symptoms. In addition, a panoply of other clinical conditions that produce similar symptoms, for instance, thyroid imbalance, neurologic disorders, connective tissue diseases, must be ruled out in a physical examination. While this case description, with its Chinese menu approach to diagnosis, doesn't exactly earn CFS an official disease label, it nonetheless validates the disorder: without federally approved diagnostic criteria, Medicare and Medicaid would not have to reimburse patients for treatment.

Today CFS is considered an important public health problem. Though the mysterious mechanism responsible has yet to reveal itself, a CDC research team with an annual budget of $3 million continues to investigate. In large part thanks to the grassroots patient movement, this once "imaginary" illness has spawned a multimillion-dollar industry. A growing number of practitioners specialize in the treatment of CFS. It has a nationwide support network, a national telephone hotline, and even a private research institution formed by top CFS investigators and clinicians to promote solid scientific inquiry.

The fight by CFS activists for legitimacy, and their refusal to allow the medical establishment to dismiss them, has given the mind-body debate a highly visible forum. For this still-puzzling condition, which challenges the traditional Western model of illness, namely, that one can't really be sick until observable biological processes take hold, will not go away. The majority of researchers and clinicians at prestigious scientific think tanks and medical schools remain convinced that the syndrome, in which the body appears to be battling itself, reflects the immune system's response to an invading infectious agent. But as infectious disease experts discard one viral theory after another, more holistic explanations of CFS are beginning to come to the fore. Some are admittedly flaky, like the claim that the illness is caused by a fungus or that it can be cured with injections of fecal material or intravenous vitamin C. But as the disease gains greater sanction, unsubstantiated "junk medical reports" and quacks prescribing ineffective, dubious treatments have become less problematic.

The latest thinking is that instead of a single cause of CFS, several conditions may converge in the syndrome to turn a benign, dormant virus into a malevolent one. Scientists suspect that people who become ill with CFS have an immunologic response to this latent virus at a time when they are particularly susceptible. The triggering events, as well as the specific virus that is reactivated, continue to be debated, but appealing candidates include exposure to environmental toxins, a response to another virus, and emotional stress, each of which may interact with the others to suppress immune function. But once the immune system is engaged, it can't be shut down, and the resulting activity consumes the body's energy, churning out antibodies and immunotoxins against an infection that cannot be licked.

The futility of the war CFS sufferers appear to be fighting within the immune system bears little resemblance to their battle with the powers that be of the medical establishment. For if anything holds promise for the transcendence of mind-body dualism, it is this baffling disorder, the answer to which seems to lie within the complex and as yet poorly understood connection between the mind and brain. The challenge of resolving and treating this physiopsychological riddle has been the catalyst for many clinicians and researchers to reject once and for all the narrow organic versus psychological paradigm of illness and replace it with a more holistic, multifactorial approach. "So much human suffering involves a psychological response to physical illness," says Dr. Anthony Komaroff, chief of general medicine at the Brigham and Women's Hospital and a leading CFS researcher, writing in the *Harvard Mental Health Letter*. "And we know that the mind can predispose a person to physical illness. So mind and body are inevitably linked, especially in this disease."

In the end, CFS may indeed be designated a psychiatric condition. Or a physical condition. Or it may turn out to be both. But regardless of its ultimate classification, the disorder is causing people to suffer. "Should we have to figure out which symptoms dominate the clinical picture before we pay attention?" asks Peter Manu, a psychiatrist who has long been involved in CFS research. In the absence of a cure, Dr. Manu says, the best thing health professionals and patients can do is to stop worrying about the cause or category and focus on alleviating distress. The truth is that even though most doctors view CFS as more complicated than simple depression, the most effective remedies appear to be a nutritional diet, exercise, and antidepressant medications, which help reduce CFS symptoms such as insomnia and muscle pain as well as the despair from chronic illness that can complicate recovery.

More than 70 percent of five hundred patients receiving treatment at a chronic fatigue clinic Dr. Manu directed at the University of Connecticut School of Medicine from 1986 to 1993 improved significantly on a moderate trial of antidepressants. "I've seen people begin antidepressant medication and within a week the lymph nodes in their necks have gone down," says Dr. Manu, the medical director of Long Island Jewish Medical Center's psychiatric hospital. "We're not supposed to think of the enlargement of lymph glands as a symptom of depression, yet when you see that kind of response you have to wonder how medicine ever bought the artificial barrier between mind and brain."

The triumph of mind-body approaches in chronic fatigue syndrome has placed a revealing spotlight on the tenets of conventional health care, and the attention surrounding the disorder has played an important role in holding health professionals accountable. In CFS, which lasts seven and a half years on average, a collaborative doctor-patient relationship is crucial. More than medical treatment, caregivers must provide emotional support and moral guidance to help patients cope with symptoms, adapt to chronic illness, and remain as active, physically, emotionally, and professionally, as they can.

Perhaps because CFS patients have achieved success in finally being heard, they have become more willing to listen to health professionals who don't view their problem as an either-or proposition. Kat Duff, in *The Alchemy of Illness*, a compilation of essays composed during her struggle with CFS, says it has been difficult for people who have been told in the midst of debilitating physical symptoms that their disease isn't real to consider the psychological aspects of their illnesses. But, she says, CFS patients must make the mind-brain connection in order to heal. During her own battle with chronic fatigue, she says, she came to realize that it was impossible for her to separate her illness from her recovery from childhood sexual abuse, because they were experienced simultaneously "in the dimensions of both the body and the psyche." Duff believes that while it's crucial for the medical community to pursue the organic basis for CFS and other diseases not yet grasped or treatable, it is equally important that "those living with these baffling illnesses give their whole stories, not just test results, but their thoughts, feelings, dreams, and histories."

BLAME STRESS, NOT YOURSELF

Hypochondriacs may not realize it, but their illness took a giant leap forward on the illness acceptability index when psychosomatic theories were replaced with the behaviorist notion of stress. Our modern-day mantra, stress, is an epidemic most everyone can deal with. Defined sixty years ago by the father of stress physiology, Dr. Hans Selye, as "a nonspecific response of the body to a demand," stress has a watered-down, deliciously ambiguous — not quite psyche, not quite soma — quality.

By now everyone's heard of the famous fight-or-flight response, the primitive survival mechanism that triggers an adrenaline surge which makes our muscles tense and hearts race when we face a stressful situation, be it money worries, marital discord, planning a wedding, or coping with pain. Stress, a great motivator, comes in particularly handy for short-term emergencies; without a little of it in our lives, our existence would be pretty bland. Nevertheless, too much stress can be paralyzing, even health threatening. "If you experience every day as an emergency," says author-neuroscientist Robert Sapolsky, "you'll eventually pay the price." Take the right concoction of genetic constitution, personality, and state of mind, introduce a demanding life event, and wham!

Stress is implicated in triggering or exacerbating just about every possible mental and physical insult: diarrhea, pimples, hair loss, sexual dysfunction, infertility, depression, high blood pressure, psoriasis, diabetes, heart disease, and even cancer. There is mounting evidence that chronic and repeated stress can impair immune function and lower resistance to disease. But scientists have yet to establish the specific pathways that lead from stressful events to emotional distress, to changes in immunity, to coming down with a so-called stress-related disorder. They are even more in the dark about the proportions of the stress-health-sickness equation, which, given the same stressors, vary markedly from person to person.

The good news about stress is that despite the endless ways in which it can disrupt lives, most of us cope fairly well with it physiologically and emotionally. "We do not all collapse into puddles of stress-related disease and psychiatric dysfunction," Sapolsky points out. Also, stress, like the old-fashioned notions of "hyp" and melancholy, is a socially acceptable state of being, practically bordering on fashionable. It's okay to tell people you're "stressed out" (undoubtedly they are, too), and you aren't required to divulge any more details unless, of course, you want to.

"Stress has a great clinical advantage because its moral implications are hazy," suggests Laurence Kirmayer, the McGill University psychiatrist. On one hand, we experience stress as "happening to us" because its physicochemical properties — the hormonal and neural systems that alert us to a crisis and deliver energy to help us cope — relieve sufferers of responsibility. On the other hand, stress is something we can identify, often predict, and to varying degrees gain control over, this hopeful message is the stuff of therapy sessions, self-help books, talk shows, and stress-reduction workshops.

The acceptance of stress as an organizing principle of health and behavior has ushered us into a new era, helping to change the way we think about, treat, and cope with illness and physical discomfort. Without necessarily being aware of it, we have, by adopting the stress metaphor, embraced a mind-body approach to getting well and staying healthy. And this approach is not so much about the impact of mental states on the immune system as about recognizing the subjective nature of distress and the importance of personal beliefs in shaping perceptions about how we feel.

A New Tolerance for Pain

Nowhere is this integrated vision more striking than in our growing understanding of the human pain response. Pain, especially chronic pain, has for centuries been an enigma to science and one of medicine's greatest challenges. The paradox is that at a time when biomedical research knows more than ever about the anatomy, physiology, and pharmacology of pain, more and more people are unable to find relief from prolonged, intractable pain.

Consider these statistics:

• One in five Americans report that they suffer from pain lasting six months or longer that has led them to seek a doctor's help.

• Nearly 12 million Americans are significantly impaired, and 2.6 million are permanently disabled by back pain alone.

• More than 550 million workdays are lost to pain each year.

Factors contributing to such statistics include an aging population, an explosion in repetitive strain injuries among users of word processors, and a cultural squeamishness about physical discomfort. The science of paleopathology, which investigates disease perceptible in skeletal remains, has revealed that our ancestors were impaired by many of the same chronic ailments that bother us today—arthritis, back trouble, bone deformations—without the benefits of modern pain relief.

Until relatively recently, medicine has focused on repairing injury and easing acute pain, virtually ignoring the burden of chronic pain, partly because its nature and treatment were so poorly understood. Cancer patients frequently have been undermedicated. Symptoms that didn't respond to medication or were deemed unsuitable for surgery have caused doctors to throw up their hands. Frustrated with a condition that had no clear organic explanation, doctors often told patients they were imagining their pain, causing chronic sufferers the further misery of doubting their sanity.

Then, in the 1960s, pain physiologists Patrick Wall and Ronald Melzack introduced their revolutionary gate-control theory, and old, dismissive notions of pain began to fade. The theory provided an explanation for the central conundrum that has puzzled scientists for thousands of years: how the brain interprets what the body has to say about pain. The theory, like pain itself, is maddeningly complex but can be simplified as follows. Pain impulses are flashed to the spinal cord, where they are modulated and sent through "gates," the neural mechanisms that open and close to let pain messages through to the brain or to block them. Once pain signals reach the brain, the sensory information is processed through the neural centers of mood, thoughts, attitude, memory, all of which can influence the perception of pain. Chronic pain sets up a vicious cycle, because when pain is prolonged, the brain itself begins to change, suppressing the production of the body's natural painkillers, such as serotonin and endorphins, just when they're most needed. The longer pain persists, the greater the molecular changes in the brain and spinal cord, which in turn make the cells more sensitive to pain.

Once it was widely accepted, the gate-control theory paved the way for further research and advances in pain treatment, and by the 1970s, a conceptual shift had occurred. No longer was pain considered merely a symptom, an alarm bell warning of pending illness or hidden disease; it had emerged as a dynamic process, a major component of disease, or even the disease itself. Health professionals began to regard pain not as an annoyance but a genuine affliction that called for a swift, aggressive multipronged attack. Pain clinics, which brought together neurologists, anesthesiologists, family counselors, psychologists, physical therapists, and other professionals to work as a team, became a symbol of this new paradigm in medical thought. Their emphasis was not necessarily on psychotherapy, or even medication, but on breaking the stress/depression/fear/ pain cycle by educating sufferers about how pain works and teaching them coping skills that would enable them to gain control over their symptoms and their lives.

The rethinking of pain, including the freer use of more specific, pain-relieving drugs, has contributed to a feeling of empowerment among chronic sufferers, bolstered by the proliferation of pain-management clinics, research institutions, and a strong patient-support movement. Self-help groups, bearing names like Share the Pain, Conquest Over Pain's Stranglehold (COPS), and Transformations unite, nationwide and overseas, people who endure all sorts of chronic pain conditions, from headaches and back pain to the agony of cancer.

Suzanne, a regional director of a Northeast pain support network, believes that if she hadn't found support to help her cope with chronic migraines seven years ago, she might have become suicidal. By then she had been through two worthless operations to correct a sinus blockage, experimented with powerful narcotics — quitting after she became addicted to Darvon — and suffered two bouts of major depression. It was becoming more and more difficult to care for her three school-age children and maintain a loving relationship with her husband.

At a friend's suggestion she contacted the American Chronic Pain Outreach Association. The Maryland-based nonprofit organization provided her with a "recovery workbook," which taught Suzanne skills like cognitive restructuring — using diaries to gain insight into dysfunctional thoughts that exacerbate pain—and problem solving—learning to identify situations that trigger pain—and steered her to a local support group. Within six months, she had found relief through exercise, biofeedback, and an antidepressant fellow sufferers recommended. The headaches still come, but less frequently. "I've learned to control how I respond to them, and when I don't drag them out feeling sorry for myself, they pass much more quickly," Suzanne says.

Still, she continues to be religious about attending group meetings, where a dozen or so people get together monthly to compare medications, keep abreast of research, and support one another via camaraderie and the solace of listening. "We aren't all best friends," she says, "but somehow we can cry, complain, shout, talk of our inadequacies and triumphs, and there's a keen level of empathy, as if we speak the same language. That's something that even the most supportive family can't always provide—there's too much emotional baggage."

Now that the news about stress and chronic pain—it's real, often debilitating, and can be controlled—has spread, the mind-body message is catching on. The idea that most human conditions involve complicated autonomic processes, in which both mental and physical mechanisms are at work, has become the new key to understanding just about any malady that defies simple cause-and-effect explanations and simple cures. Just how neurotransmitters and hormones combine with thoughts and emotions to wreak their havoc still eludes science. But investigators are making progress, and as mind-body revisionism gains strength, the notion of ailments originating in the mind is losing its grip.

Take the bizarre symptoms of so-called premenstrual syndrome—food cravings, insomnia, anger, migraines, depression, feeling out of control—that for generations have made women feel crazy. The prevailing view among researchers today is that PMS is, indeed, a bona fide organic disorder caused, as one expert put it, "by a defect in physiology, not in character."

Women with severe PMS, who represent approximately 5 to 10 percent of the U.S. menstruating population, appear to suffer from the same shortage of pain-dampening neurotransmitters — enkephalins, endorphins, and serotonin — that chronic pain sufferers do.

Then there's the widely accepted interpretation of irritable bowel syndrome (IBS), also known as spastic colon. This charming malady with its potpourri of unpleasant symptoms affects some 15 percent of the population and is the reason for half of all visits to gastroenterologists. Now experts tell us that although highly aggravating, IBS is basically harmless. (Surveys reveal that a large proportion of the population suffers its symptoms but does not consult doctors.) The basis for the dysfunction, researchers say, is the brain-gut connection, which, along with offenses like poor eating habits, too much alcohol, and too little sleep, can cause the gastrointestinal tract to go haywire. Current thinking about IBS runs along the same lines as pain perception and amplification theories, which are a bit like the Heisenberg principle of elementary physics: the very act of contemplating something changes its intrinsic nature. Those made miserable by an irritable bowel, the thinking goes, seem to have a lower threshold for picking up signals from the gut — the squeeze of peristaltic contractions, the rush of digestive juices. This ultra-awareness leads to psychic distress, which blunts neurotransmitters, which makes the brain more sensitive to visceral events — the vicious cycle once again.

Neurologist Oliver Sacks describes this phenomenon eloquently in his classic *Migraine: Understanding a Common Disorder*. The migraine — another malady undergoing mind-body revisionism — he writes, "is a physical event which may also be from the start, or later becomes, an emotional or symbolic event." Although Sacks is discussing a distinct and particularly debilitating form of headache, he could have been talking about chronic pain, asthma, eczema, stomach ailments, sexual dysfunction, or any of a myriad conditions, which like the migraine "cannot be conceived as an exclusively human reaction, but must be considered as a form of biological reaction specifically tailored to human needs and human nervous systems."

The gentle conceptual principles of stress, chronic pain, and other components of behavioral medicine are leading us back to some of the best of what the ancient Greeks taught us about the art of healing, like the wonders of nature; the strength of the placebo effect; the therapeutic value of diet, exercise, serenity, acts of kindness; the curative power of a collaborative doctor-patient relationship. We are beginning to come to a new understanding of human suffering: that distress reaches far beyond physical symptoms, that it has multiple meanings, causes, and implications, which vary from individual to individual; and that most people suffer from rather than profit from symptoms. This serene spirit of wisdom can be traced back to Hippocrates and is embodied in the Hippocratic oath. It states that physicians have an obligation to relieve suffering and that, above all, they must do no harm.

From a hypochondriac's perspective, a new day may be dawning. With the public demanding more personal, compassionate treatment, medicine, a consumer-driven industry, is beginning to listen. The entire health care profession is reevaluating its relationship to suffering, and in shifting from preoccupation with cause to an emphasis on care is expanding its calling, entering a new, less certain realm. This doesn't mean that we're turning back the clock to a time before antibiotics or aspirin, but rather moving ahead, combining modern technological know-how with attention to how people experience their illnesses — putting the sickness back with the patient.

The medical gray area that exists between the body and brain has created a vast diagnostic vacuum. Hospitals, clinics, physicians, and health writers are repackaging the notions of stress and chronic pain, creating a new holistic jargon. Phrases like "Take charge," "Seize control," "Mind over illness," "Heal thyself," "Change faulty thinking," represent a shift in semantics rather than a scientific breakthrough. But if people are altering their behaviors and finding relief from suffering, what's the harm?

Randy, a longtime back pain sufferer, credits a trendy mind-body diagnosis for sparing him from the surgeon's scalpel. This hard-working executive and father of three lay flat on his back for weeks, suffering from the third episode in two years. He had made the usual circuit of orthopedists, chiropractors, and neurosurgeons for relief of pain that radiated down his leg, making it difficult to walk. The specialists had alternately diagnosed him with sciatica, a herniated disk, a pinched nerve, and compressed vertebrae, for which one had recommended surgery. Then Randy read an article about John Sarno, a surgically trained physician who preached mind-body medicine, and specifically his own diagnosis, tension myositis syndrome (TMS).

The syndrome, which Dr. Sarno believes accounts for 99 percent of all back pain and explains a host of other chronic syndromes, is an excruciating but essentially benign physical disorder, not a mechanical condition but a problem of the soft tissue brought on by tension. The true source of pain in TMS is repressed unacceptable emotions, particularly anger, which have the physical effect of restricting blood flow to the brain and diminishing the supply of oxygen to the muscles, nerves, tendons, and ligaments in various parts of the body. The resulting sensations — pain, numbing, weakness — become a distraction against intolerable feelings.

Dr. Sarno, who is affiliated with the prestigious Rusk Institute of Rehabilitation Medicine, has written two best-selling books explaining the nature of TMS, which, he says, is a result of genetic, developmental, and environmental factors over which sufferers have little control. His theories are so popular that rather than seeing patients individually, he instructs them to attend two of his lectures at the Rusk Institute, which is what Randy did — and he swears it changed his life. Dr. Sarno's treatment strategy rests on two pillars: the acquisition of knowledge of and insight into the psychology and physiology of TMS, and the ability to act on that knowledge and thereby change the brain's behavior. The success rates he reports are impressive: in one study of 109 patients who had gone through the TMS program, all of whom had CAT-scan-diagnosed herniated disks, 88 percent were free of pain after a year, 10 percent had improved, and only 2 percent were unchanged.

Not so different from TMS is profound sensitivity syndrome (PS2), a theory presented by Dr. Neil Solomon and Marc Lipton, a clinical psychologist, in *Sick and Tired of Being Sick and Tired*. The book addresses itself to the thousands of people who suffer vague, inexplicable ailments—fluid retention, migraines, stomach and back trouble, fatigue, dizziness, yeast infections, PMS, sensitivity to chemicals, among other problems. These are people whose doctors have told them, variously, "There's nothing I can do to help you"; "No one disease could cause all this"; "It's got to be all in your head." Solomon and Lipton believe that there is something wrong, a biochemical phenomenon that is preventable and treatable.

In PS2 syndrome there is a cascade of intense physiochemical reactions. This "biochemical hyper-response" combines with destructive thought patterns to create a chronic state of stress, which further triggers biochemistry that erodes physical and mental health. The authors outline nine types of thought distortions. In one they call Expecting the Worst, a patient hears a news report of a dangerous disease that causes high fever, headache, irritability, and itching—and turns off the TV set before learning that the disease is confined to Europe. The next morning she awakens with a headache and concludes she has contracted the illness. "We sometimes label people who expect the worst as people with overactive imaginations," they write. "Often they spend so much time worrying about what terrible thing might happen that they neglect to enjoy the present. These people need to stop and smell the proverbial roses."

That's hypochondria! Despite the fact that the authors should realize that many expect-the-worst types already know that they should stop to smell those roses, it was heartwarming to read that hypochondria was an aspect of PS2, a real medical malady. Currently, hypochondria, for insurance purposes, is listed as disorder number 300.7 in psychiatric manuals. Ironically, it is not likely to be covered by most insurance plans, so to make hypochondria and other PS2 ailments diagnostically acceptable, doctors usually describe the problem on health forms as irritable bowel syndrome, migraine, or allergic sensitivity—whichever physical symptoms predominate. But this is confusing. Aren't IBS and migraine mind-body diagnoses? Yet most health plans reimburse for them. Surely insurance executives must be just as befuddled as we are about exactly which illnesses are all in our heads, which are partly in our heads, which start in the body but end up in our heads. Nevertheless, they're starting to cover us, and that's progress!

The rigid line between mental and physical is slowly dissolving, and someday the so-called Cartesian split will seem as ludicrous and arcane as the belief that the world is flat. In the meantime, medicine stumbles in search of a new paradigm. Somewhere between the mainstream medical establishment—lambasted for its arrogance, exorbitant fees, and mechanistic viewpoint—and the popular health movement—rebuked as New Age, flaky, and unscientific—between the psychoanalysts who heal the wounds of "toxic parenting" and biopsychiatrists who correct brain chemistry, lies a golden mean of medicine that will bridge the gulf between physical and emotional health, biology, and blame.

CHAPTER SEVEN

....

The Susceptibility Factor

I believe my consumption has grown worse. Also my asthma.
The wheezing comes and goes, and I get dizzy more and more
frequently. I have taken to violent choking and fainting. My
room is damp and I have perpetual chills and palpitations of
the heart. I noticed, too, that I am running out of napkins.
Will it ever stop?

—Woody Allen, *Without Feathers*

THE PREDISPOSITION to be anxious and compulsive about
health obviously isn't everyone's curse. Those of us who have to
struggle not to freak out about a pimple just to stay functional
may marvel at those stalwart, que será, será types who seem to
cope *so* sensibly. How do they *not* worry about their health
when people are sick and dying all around them? Why do they
see the cup as half full when we see it as half empty?

I often look at my friend Jill in astonishment. So stoic and
unalarmed that she might be considered a somatic denier, Jill
telephoned me one day with frightening news. A routine gyne-
cological exam had revealed a uterine fibroid tumor and a lump
in her breast. Moreover, while the doctor was examining her, he
noticed a suspicious-looking mole he told her she had better
have checked out. "Oh, my God, aren't you freaking out?" I
asked. I certainly was. Jill floored me with her response. "I refuse to kill myself worrying until the facts are in." The doctor's

report bore her out: the lump was a cyst; the mole nothing; the fibroid tumor still there but shrinking.

That some of us are more likely than others to perceive the worst is hardly news. Whatever the reasons—unconscious conflict, family dysfunction, ingrained bad habits, perturbed neurotransmitters—there are those who can take an EKG in the morning and be satisfied with a normal reading, and others who, by the afternoon, are wondering whether the reading was correct, whether the score was too close to borderline, and whether the test should be redone. But what accounts for these differences? Why do some people interpret the body's ambiguous signals and think vulnerable, and others think invincible?

THE SOCIAL PSYCHOLOGY OF SYMPTOMS

It shouldn't be surprising that hypochondriacs are susceptible to the power of suggestion. There is such a thing as the social transmission of illness, which can be even more contagious than the flu. Certain people get sick at the sight of blood, others when someone faints or vomits. Every year a small percentage of expectant fathers develop Couvade syndrome, from the French word *couver*, "to hatch," in which men anticipating the birth of a child experience symptoms of pregnancy—weight gain, food cravings, nausea, even labor pains.

Then there's the phenomenon of mass hysteria, which is increasingly showing up in the psychiatric literature as epidemic stress syndrome or collective illness perception. The syndrome occurs when a group of basically healthy people are suddenly stricken by a mysterious, vague ailment and fall ill like dominoes, though no clear biological basis is detected. Outbreaks have been observed in factories, refugee camps, hospitals, and schools, places where individuals work or perform in close physical proximity. A typical case appeared during a choral recital of junior and senior high schoolers in a California school auditorium. The band musicians had just tuned their instruments when an outbreak of headaches, dizziness, hyperventilation, stomach cramps, and nausea spread among the performers. More than a third of the six hundred students—girls outnumbered boys two to one—but none of the two thousand spectators, developed some combination of ailments; nineteen students were rushed by ambulance to hospitals. Nonetheless, a subsequent investigation found no evidence of any viral, infectious, or environmental problem.

Incidents of this sort are not common; a few occur every year. But one reason researchers study them is that they provide important clues to the type of people at risk for becoming somatizers. The outbreaks, in which disease phobia and amplification of bodily symptoms appear to play on each other, seem to be classic instances of hypervigilant individuals responding to subtle and ambiguous sensations.

What are the psychological and social factors, real or perceived, that contribute to making a person suggestible in this way? One of the greatest predictors of who becomes symptomatic during mass illness outbreaks is the immediate experience of observing a friend, or someone near to you, becoming sick. This is certainly true for AIDS phobia, rampant among members of homosexual communities who have seen too many healthy young men wither and die, as well as among doctors who treat AIDS patients. "These people are under severe stress in a heightened emotional climate, which makes them highly susceptible to the suggestion of illness," says Gary W. Small, a psychiatrist who has written extensively about mass illness. Other demographic and social variables correlated with susceptibility are an earlier experience with acute or chronic illness (a quarter of students in the California episode who fell ill had a chronic medical condition, most commonly asthma); early trauma; low income level; low level of education; and perhaps the most important factor, being female.

The Feeling Sex

No question, women are more attuned to matters of health. They have a greater awareness of changes in their bodies, are more apt to gripe about aches and pains, talk graphically about symptoms, doctor-shop, and take to their beds. We've all heard nasty remarks about how women can't be president because of their high-strung temperaments and lack of rationality, unmistakably tied to their hormones. And while women have come a long way since the days when their Victorian sisters had to communicate their rage and helplessness against domestic confinement and male domination in the language of fits and paralysis, still they don't feel well.

• Three times as many women as men suffer from migraines.

• Women are two to three times more likely than men to experience depression, a statistic that holds true across all continents and cultures.

• Women are twice as likely as men to have panic attacks.

• Women make up 80 percent of chronic fatigue patients and 99 percent of fibromyalgia sufferers.

• Being female puts one at ten times greater risk than men for developing anorexia nervosa.

• Three quarters of patients who seek medical attention for irritable bowel syndrome are women.

What's going on? When it comes to bodily symptoms, women win hands down. Is it those troublesome hormones? Subtle differences in brain chemistry? Greater life stresses? Or are we women truly the "weaker" sex, the fragile gender that just happens to live an average of nine years longer than men?

In spite of the gender's seeming frailty, being female in the contemporary world doesn't exactly mark women as an endangered species. The fact is that women *aren't* any sicker than men. Indeed, men at any age are more likely to be in poorer physical health than women but are less likely than women to report, or admit, it. It doesn't take much digging to realize that one reason these ailing men may feel so hardy is that their physical and emotional needs are being met by women, society's nurturers, who are a third as likely as men to have a spouse as a caregiver. But there's also some truth to the adage "Men act, women feel." Just as men and women vary in their conversational styles, there are vast differences between the sexes in the way they notice, interpret, and react to ambiguous sensations in their bodies. Deborah Tannen, a professor of linguistics at Georgetown University, describes the gender-based distinctions in men's and women's conversation, which she labels "genderlect." "Women speak and hear a language of connection and intimacy," Tannen writes, "while men speak and hear a language of status and independence." This dynamic, both the spice *and* poison of male-female relationships, applies to communicating about pain and sickness.

Tannen illustrates this asymmetry with an example of a woman who notices that her husband is favoring the use of one arm and asks why. He responds that his arm hurts. When she inquires how long his arm has been troubling him, he tells her, "Oh, a few weeks." To his surprise, his wife reacts with hurt and anger. She feels pushed away and distanced by his silence. Later the husband explains that he had only wanted to protect her. "Why should I worry her, telling her about my pain, since it might be nothing and go away anyway?" Apparently women just aren't on this wavelength. They feel comfortable talking about their bodies, verbalizing the pain of menstrual cramps as well as of personal crises and misfortunes. They may even find such talk prescriptive. When it comes to sharing distress, women tend to respond to troubles by offering matching troubles: "I know how you feel," they say. "I've felt the same way." Men, on the other hand, prefer to respond to suffering by offering solutions and mapping out a course of action. They are annoyed when a woman analyzes her negative feelings instead of taking steps to master them.

The mapping of brain differences between the sexes is beginning to show scientifically that women may be more sensitive than men. A study at the University of Pennsylvania School of Medicine compared male and female ability to identify emotions in others by showing both sexes photographs of actors' facial expressions. While women had little trouble recognizing distress in the faces of either men or women, men were much more adept at noticing men's unhappiness. "A woman's face had to be really sad for men to see it," said Dr. Ruben C. Gur, who led the study and directs the brain behavior laboratory at the medical school. "The subtle expressions went right by them."

The fact that women are more intuitive when it comes to others' pain may help to explain why they feel more of it themselves. (Interestingly, women don't seem to *fear* sensations any more than men do. Questionnaires probing for hypochondria — disease phobia in particular — have found cases to be equally split between the sexes.) Men and women, it seems, travel along different perceptual pathways to arrive at their own internal states. For the most part, men rely on such visceral sensations as a racing heart or sweaty palms to define how they are feeling, while women respond to situational cues — the time of day, room temperature, how others say they feel — according to psychologist James W. Pennebaker, who has been studying gender differences in emotion for the last fifteen years. Consider something as universal as hunger: men usually determine they're hungry by a gnawing in the pit of their stomachs, while women are more likely to eat when the clock tells them it is time.

It may not be that women exaggerate or overreport emotions and symptoms, but rather that men repress them, making them guilty of the common charge that they deny their true feelings. The reproductive capabilities of women, which span half a lifetime, put them on familiar terms with bodily changes and keep them cycling within the health care system. They examine their breasts, schedule Pap smears and pelvic exams, give birth, and are more likely than their spouses to take children to a pediatrician regularly. Men, on the other hand, are often squeamish about physicians and medical procedures. Talk to a woman trying to get a reluctant husband to undergo a vasectomy. "I've been through three pregnancies, three labors, two caesareans, and he refuses to make an appointment!" is a common sort of lament, even among women whose husbands are anxious about the prospect of unwanted pregnancy.

When men do get sick, they often ignore their symptoms until they become severe. Two famous examples are the late baseball commissioner Bartlett Giamatti, who may have waited too long after the onset of chest pains to seek help, and Jim Henson, whose own doctor said his life could have been saved had he sought treatment for pneumonia just twenty-four hours earlier.

Men also tend to make passive patients, and their health may suffer as a result. Researchers at the Primary Care Outcomes Research Institute at New England Medical Center analyzed 296 doctor visits and discovered that in the typical fifteen-minute session men asked one or no questions; women asked six. In addition, men displayed less emotion than women and were less forthcoming about the reason for their visit. "Our studies indicate that when patients are more communicative with their doctors, they have better health," says Sherrie H. Kaplan, a senior scientist who is codirector of the institute.

The fact that women sense how they feel and are able to express pain and frustration not only contributes to physical health but may protect them from the kinds of troubles that seem to haunt men. While it is true that women suffer more depressive and anxiety disorders than men—but there is some evidence that the gender gap in depression is narrowing—when it comes to overall psychiatric illness, the sexes aren't far apart. Men outnumber women in suicide deaths by a ratio of four to one, and they are five times more prone to drug or alcohol abuse and to display antisocial behavior. Women bear the brunt of this violence—an estimated 4 million women are severely assaulted by their male partners each year—which may partly explain their tendency to somatize.

The consequences of women's victimization frequently show up in the health care system, in psychiatric illnesses, and more often in physical complaints, particularly chronic pelvic pain and gastrointestinal ailments. Physical and sexual abuse are the chief reasons women seek treatment in emergency rooms, and numerous studies have found that women with a history of sexual assault are incapacitated by illness longer and more often than those who have experienced no such trauma.

Dr. Douglas Drossman, professor of medicine and psychiatry in the division of digestive diseases at the University of North Carolina School of Medicine, who has conducted research on the emotional aspects of gastrointestinal (GI) ailments, calls female victimization the hidden factor within GI referral practice. In a study of 206 women with GI disorders attending the university's clinic, Dr. Drossman and colleagues found nearly half had experienced some form of traumatic violence.

Despite statistics showing that up to a third of women will become victims of domestic violence at some point in their lives, physicians rarely inquire about patients' abuse history. A study at two Boston hospitals found that while more than two thirds of 164 patients favored routine inquiries about physical abuse, only 7 percent had been questioned by a doctor during an initial or subsequent visit. Nearly all patients in the study who had experienced sexual or physical trauma, 16 percent of the sample, said they thought doctors could help with medical and psychological problems stemming from abuse. The irony is that the doctors also believed they could assist these patients, but for various reasons—reluctance to ask personal questions, fear of alienating patients, time constraints—chose not to get involved.

Is it any wonder that feminists are raising the issue of whether women's health needs can be met by a profession that is still overwhelmingly dominated by males? Just as it may be easier, in the short run, for victimized patients, to remain in denial about what their symptoms signify than to make difficult life changes, doctors may find it less complicated to distance themselves, by viewing these women as somatizers, than to respond to their masked appeals. But in the long run, doctors, uniquely able to assist these patients, may be the key to helping them get well. Recognizing this, the American Medical Association (AMA) in 1992 issued guidelines advising that physicians routinely ask female patients if they have been abused. The guidelines also recommend that health professionals be trained to identify signs of violence, discuss it with patients, make appropriate referrals, and generally become more comfortable in dealing with abuse.

STEREOTYPICAL IMAGES AND DOUBLE STANDARDS

The troubled relationship between women and their doctors is fast becoming a volatile political issue as a debate looms over whether women should be entitled to a medical specialty of their own. Women, likelier than men to seek care for minor symptoms as a preventive measure, are often humiliated by condescending male doctors who dismiss their complaints and label them hypochondriacs, crocks, and hysterics. Male doctors also tend to view female patients as demanding, bitchy, and noncompliant, terms rarely applied to men. Even when physicians observe similar symptoms and behavior in men and women, the implications aren't the same. Studying gender differences among patients with multiple somatic symptoms, researchers at the University of Arkansas for Medical Sciences found that doctors are more apt to perceive women as somatizers and the same symptoms — fatigue, digestive distress, chest pain — are seen in men as something else — organic illness, seeking compensation, or trying to get out of work.

The bias against women in medicine is increasingly being

exposed by medical journalists and outspoken insiders like Dr. John Smith, whose indictment of the health care system in *Women and Doctors: A Physician's Explosive Account of Medical Treatment, and Mistreatment, in America Today, and What You Can Do About It,* has been widely applauded by feminists. Smith, a gynecologist, writes of the debasing attitudes, sexism, and outright abuse that women have endured at the hands of male doctors. He tells of a colleague who invited him to do an examination on a patient because "she has a body you won't believe." Of doctors who waltz into an operating room and matter-of-factly lift up a sheet to peek at a patient's breasts. Smith goes so far as to say that men have no business being gynecologists, the primary physicians for two thirds of women in this country. The role, he says, properly belongs to women, "the only sex truly able to understand, empathize with, and appropriately relate to women in the already difficult doctor-patient relationship."

Not taking women's health complaints seriously and making false assumptions based on sexual stereotypes is degrading—and dangerous. Recent evidence confirms that because women are neglected in medical research, they often receive inadequate or inappropriate treatment and fail to get definitive diagnostic tests for many life-threatening illnesses. A growing awareness of these inequities led the National Institutes of Health in 1990 to establish the Office of Research on Women's Health, which oversees investigative studies into how diseases and the drugs that treat them may manifest themselves differently in women. Even the clubby AMA, a male bastion some claim may have reinforced gender bias by supporting doctors' complete autonomy and unparalleled authority, is beginning to recognize the poor treatment of women within medicine. In a 1990 statement, the AMA urged physicians to "examine their practices and attitudes for influence of social and cultural biases which could be inadvertently affecting the delivery of medical care."

Proponents of women's health care are particularly incensed about studies which show that heart disease is treated less aggressively in women than in men. Physicians continue to see cardiovascular illness as a man's disease, although as the number one killer among American women, it is six times as deadly as breast cancer. Estrogen may protect women somewhat from developing coronary disease, but their hormone levels drop after menopause, and by their sixties, women are more likely than men to die from a heart attack. Nevertheless, women who come to an emergency room with chest complaints wait longer than men to see a doctor and are twice as likely to be told that their symptoms stem from anxiety or emotional upset. When problems are indicated, women are half as likely as men to receive clot-dissolving drugs or to be offered bypass surgery.

Such biases can lead to nightmarish experiences like that of Elizabeth Rigdon, whose story was recounted in *The New York Times*. When Rigdon, a surgical nurse from Connecticut, was forty-seven, she began to experience a crushing pain in her chest for which she consulted a cardiologist. For a year the doctor insisted that her heart was fine; except for a few peculiar "blips" when she exercised, her electrocardiogram was normal, as was her angiogram, the X ray of her blood vessels. "Everyone should have coronary arteries as good as yours," Rigdon recalls her doctor saying. "He told me to go home and calm down, that it was all in my imagination, my nerves." Fortunately, Rigdon sought the opinion of another cardiologist, who diagnosed her with syndrome X, a cardiovascular abnormality more prevalent among women than men. Unlike classic male heart disease, which manifests itself in the large blood vessels, syndrome X shows up in small blood vessels that fail to dilate in response to physical and emotional stress.

Frightening stories like these are frequently given play in popular magazines, ostensibly to empower women and give them incentive to take charge of their health. But the message women increasingly hear is distrust doctors, be skeptical — then, when a crisis arises, they don't know where to turn. The prospect of being told, by a harsh, authoritarian male physician who makes it clear she is wasting his time, that her symptoms are imaginary can cause even the most confident woman to doubt her instincts about her body, although most women really can tell when something isn't right.

Even when it is impossible to separate the physical and emotional factors, taking one's turmoil to a physician isn't necessarily inappropriate. The doctor's office, whether that of a GP or fancy specialist, should be a safe place where one can bring any problem and not have to worry about being ridiculed. So what if the wellspring of one's pain turns out to be emotional? A conscientious doctor, after a brief exam and an extensive chat, should have a reading on what's wrong and an idea of what course of action to take. But that rarely happens in medicine these days, when problems are less than transparent.

One woman related the story of a confused period in her life when she became quite hypochondriacal. "It was a choice between tranquilizers, beating my kids, or eating around the clock, and I chose to freak out about my health and run to physicians, most of whom treated me as if I was some kind of a nut." After months of doctor-shopping to cure numerous ailments she thought she had—"At one point I even believed I had dutch elm disease," she joked—a nurturing female physician finally helped set her in the right direction. "She was a wonderful, warm woman with kids, to whom I could relate. She reassured me that my body was fine, though I could lose a few pounds, and helped me face that I needed to go back to the working world, and into therapy. Something I knew, but was terrified of."

The data on the impact of balancing split roles—wife, mother, worker—are not clear. Some studies have found that women who stretch themselves in many directions are happier than traditional homemakers. Others have found that working mothers suffer more stress-related ailments, like stomachaches and premenstrual tension, than either childless career women or stay-at-home moms. Nevertheless, a common problem for all women, at home or in the workforce, is that they often become so involved in caring for others that they ignore their own needs. Illness, for some women, then, provides an acceptable though unconscious means of relief. "Saying 'I'm sick' may alleviate some of the guilt women feel for not being all-giving at home and superachieving in the workplace," says Sylvia Pollack, a psychologist at Beth Israel Medical Center in Newark, New Jersey. "It allows them to nurture themselves." But because the medical system, for the most part, gives short shrift to psychological and social issues, "the symptoms, rather than being a signal, become self-perpetuating." The cost, Dr. Pollack says, is that "these women never confront the fact that the demands they've placed on themselves are outrageous."

Women juggling multiple roles and contradictory goals tend to experience stress and conflict to a greater degree than men do. Indeed, physiological studies show that while the flight-and-fight response is similar in men and women, the situations that provoke anxiety vary according to gender. In men, the level of stress hormones generally rises more sharply in response to competitive and intellectual challenges, while women's pressures increase more dramatically during stressful personal situations. In an ongoing study of Volvo employees, known as the five o'clock study, Swedish researchers found that men began to wind down at home after work as soon as they walked in the door. In contrast, women, who were also managers, continued to be agitated after work and during the evening, mostly in response to family responsibilities.

Women are gaining more control of medical care, interestingly, at a time doctors have become more regulated and less autonomous; more than half of all entering medical students are female, but health care remains essentially an old boy's game. As bad as that is for women, it cannot be that much better for men, who may find themselves in cahoots with male doctors to keep up manly appearances. Men don't cry, kvetch, wallow, or reveal too many secrets. They play out their pain on the sports field, corporate ladder, or in combat, and if that isn't enough, they drink, smoke, confront, become workaholics, and commit suicide.

The same cultural values that peg women as emotional "flooders" — a term employed by neurologist Richard Restak to describe "people [women, of course] for whom problems and complexes gush out of every pore, drowning the listener" — don't allow men to experience, much less show, emotions or vulnerability. Traditional culture makes it difficult for them to present their inadequacies, and when they feel crazy, they have few places to go. It is hard for men to be outwardly hypochondriacal; it isn't particularly macho. Yet if studies are correct, men worry about illness as much as women; they're only better at hiding their fears. One reason is that women, absorbing the mores of their culture, often disdain men who show their fears too openly. Listen to how one woman responds to a hypochondriacal husband: "His obsessions drive me crazy," she says. "The way he keeps one of those symptom books by his night table and is always checking it. When he gets a cold there is no talking to him. He's certain he's going to die. It gets real tiring after a while."

Seeking a kind of emotional gender equality, enlightened men are beginning to rebel against a patriarchal social system that demands they stand tall, grit their teeth, and take it like men. The burgeoning men's movement rejects the notion that men can't cry out for help, experience psychic pain, and speak of feelings simply because they are men. Traditionally, women have been the ones who have helped men get in touch with deep feelings, and so it is with women doctors. Studies show that men are more willing to open up to female physicians, who tend to spend more time with patients than male doctors, interrupt less often, and be less authoritarian.

ETHNIC AND CULTURAL CONSIDERATIONS

The delicate art of transforming emotional turmoil into physical complaints is a universal phenomenon, occurring in many if not all cultures. When a culture stifles the ability of people to communicate feelings to one another directly, illness can serve as a way for them to let others know of their unhappiness. The rules for expressing emotions and sickness vary, depending on where you live and who you are.

In Hispanic cultures, for instance, men and women alike are subject to *ataques de nervios*, a malady characterized by headache, trembling, abdominal pain, palpitations, muscle weakness, agitation, and loss of control, symptoms infinitely more acceptable within a culture that tends to prize machismo and look down on mental illness. In certain regions of New Guinea, people who are sick withdraw from the community, cover their bodies with ashes and dirt, refuse food, and remain isolated. If you reside in England and someone asks how you're doing, you're likely to report "just fine" because of the cultural expectation that one ought to remain stoic and contained about physical and emotional health problems. The famed stiff upper lip actually results in more parsimonious medicine. The British spend half as much as Americans on health care, have fewer screening examinations and surgical procedures, and take less medication. They even consume fewer vitamins. "The British patient is less likely to be labeled as sick by his doctors," writes Lynn Payer in *Medicine and Culture*, a comparative study of medical treatment in four countries. "You can't be diagnosed having hypertension if nobody ever takes your blood pressure."

In contrast to the British, other cultures view illness as an intimate and appropriate part of everyday life and conversation. On Manhattan's Upper West Side, where therapy and candor are the rule rather than the exception, one can comfortably discuss psychoanalysis, Prozac, abortion, or chemotherapy with equanimity. In India and other societies, where people may not be quite as open, sickness is still a community event in which friends and relatives join forces as a management team, administering lay therapy, offering special foods and indigenous medicines. The Navajos of the American West, who view the body as being in moral harmony with the physical landscape, have dozens of communal open-air ceremonies in which tribal folk gather in a circle, the symbol of wholeness and perfection, to drive out ill health.

The cross-cultural study of how people of different ethnic and religious backgrounds communicate pain and anguish provides a mirror reflecting rich and diverse values, traditions, expectations, and attitudes, of which the participants are largely unaware. Just as societies vary in expressions of physical suffering, they differ in their hypochondriacal concerns. In eastern Africa, for instance, "brain fag" is a common syndrome involving heavy, hot sensations—described as peppery feelings or crawling worms in the head—associated with the effort of studying. Typically, it strikes students who are the first in their families to become literate and, in the process, experience separation from their loved ones and communities.

Koro, or *suk-yeong*, a frightening preoccupation that one's genitals are shriveling and will disappear into the abdomen, is another culturally related syndrome occurring chiefly in Southeast Asia. One of the unusual things about koro is that it often appears in clusters within villages. Abrupt terror descends upon its victims who, in mass panic, may use clamps, string, rubber bands, and clothespins, anything, to prevent the shrinkage. The syndrome most frequently involves the penis, but when it occurs in women, it is characterized by frigidity and the perception that the nipples, breast, and labia are vanishing.

Western-trained physicians and social scientists may view koro as a deviant, albeit colorful, psychiatric disorder. But it is really little more than a temporary alteration in body perception—acute castration anxiety with hypochondriacal overtones.

In most cases, victims of collective koro return to a normal state of health soon after being convinced that the illness is over or never existed. The physical perception of shrinkage, often triggered by physiological changes caused by cold, physical exertion, aging, or illness, makes sense within a frame of reference that draws on folklore and mores of a society in which sexual weakness is extremely feared. Koro-like symptoms, in some Asian societies, are linked to spirits or ghosts, supernatural powers, and the folkloric belief that penis retraction results in death. In regions within Indonesia and Malaysia, for instance, there is a superstition that the soul of a woman who dies in childbirth becomes a malicious spirit who may present herself in the guise of a vampire and tear off her husband's penis or testicles.

Koro, brain fag, and *dhat*—a common preoccupation of men in Hindu cultures who fear losing semen—are some of the more exotic transcultural syndromes that, in an age of multiculturalism, are beginning to be known to our health care system. Not surprisingly, a medical bureaucracy that has slighted women in treatment and care also falls short in dealing with symptoms related to ethnicity and race. For as difficult as it is for anyone to disentangle ethnicity from other influences, a white male clinician trained in biomedicine is particularly handicapped by unintended biases that can lead to misinterpretation and misdiagnosis. This is particularly problematic in urban areas, home to large numbers of immigrants who, lacking health insurance, frequently show up in inner-city clinics and emergency rooms with symptoms and health beliefs that doctors cannot understand.

In the name of political correctness, however, a new ethnic and multicultural perspective is gradually following feminism into the medical school curriculum. A growing sensitivity to what transcultural psychiatrists call idioms of distress has made its way into courses offered at inner-city medical centers and urban hospitals. One such program is Cultural Diversity in Medicine, started at Mount Sinai Hospital in New York a few years ago. The courses, taught by professors of varying ethnic backgrounds, focus on the differences among Asians, African-Americans, Latins, and Orthodox Jews, the primary patient population at Mount Sinai.

For example, students learn that Asian patients may not tell their doctors that they are taking herbal remedies which could interact with other medications because they don't consider herbs as drugs. And that Orthodox Jews tend to consult a rabbi before submitting to surgery and will not schedule an operation on the Sabbath. In California, where a number of Iranian refugees have settled since the Islamic revolution and the Iran-Iraq war, health professionals are becoming aware of *naharat*. This medical syndrome, expressed by Iranians through silence, sulkiness, avoidance of food, and bodily discomfort—most commonly chest pain, digestive problems, and pains in the limbs—appears to serve as a camouflage for depression that may be a result of upheaval and cultural and social loss.

Psychiatry, long criticized for ignoring minorities in its epidemiological studies, is making up for past transgressions, leading the way toward bringing a multicultural dimension to health care. Special efforts were made in the most recent edition of the *Diagnostic and Statistical Manual* to incorporate an awareness of the nuances in the way ethnic groups experience sickness, distress, and physical symptoms. For the first time, the manual includes an appendix of culturally influenced syndromes to help clinicians step beyond Western beliefs and attitudes in approaching and evaluating illnesses.

For example, neurasthenia, the once-popular syndrome of nervous exhaustion essentially gone from North America, is still a common and important diagnosis within China. The psyche-soma aspect of neurasthenia—its primary symptoms weakness, headache, fatigue, and extreme hopelessness—is not compatible with traditional Chinese medicine, which approaches problems in terms of flow of *ch'i*, "vital energy," and imbalances of yin and yang elements in the body. The diagnosis enables the Chinese to weave narratives of personal trauma, loss, and emotional suffering into their medical encounters in a society that continues to stigmatize mental illness severely.

However, the powerful influence of culture in shaping and interpreting symptoms is not limited just to foreigners and the immigrant experience. The same preconceptions exist in judging and assessing people whose ancestry goes back generations in our diverse nation. The misdiagnosis of "hidden" popular folk illnesses was demonstrated in a study conducted at a primary care health clinic attended by blacks and poor whites in rural Appalachia. Anthropologists interviewed patients, eliciting the source of their distress following visits to physicians who had come from the Northeast to work in the clinic. The five most common complaints were high blood, weak and dizzy, nerves, sugar, and muscles swelling up, ailments peculiar to the Appalachian dialect that connote a complex array of physical and emotional troubles. When these folk maladies were compared with biomedical diagnoses, the two interpretations had little in common. Physicians, unable to decode complaints, simply took them at face value. The result: unnecessary testing, patient and physician dissatisfaction, and little improvement in the patients' physical or mental health.

NERVOUS AND KVETCHY: ARE JEWS FATED TO BE HYPOCHONDRIACS?

When it comes to hypochondria, there is a fine line between translating idioms of distress and unfairly stereotyping certain ethnic groups. But as I spoke to people across the country about hypochondria, questions about prevalence of nervous ailments and complaints voiced among Jews came up again and again. More than one person struggling with undiagnosable maladies and illness fears said, "Maybe it's because I'm Jewish" or "It must be my Jewish upbringing." Some researchers have taken note of the phenomenon: a smattering of studies in the 1960s and 1970s on nationality and illness behavior found that Jews, along with Italians and Greeks, had the lowest tolerance for pain, the most physical complaints, the highest ratings for hypochondria, compared with other ethnic and racial groups.

Jewish hypochondria, noted for the last hundred years and more recently made famous by Jewish comics, deserves some exploration. If anything, the propensity of some American Jews to kvetch openly and make fun of their neuroses, regarding health and just about everything else, has played a part in keeping hypochondria less hidden. The formal labeling of hypochondria as a Jewish foible may smack of anti-Semitism and have something to do with perpetuating its stigma.

In popular culture, Woody Allen's antics have been updated in the character of George Costanza, Jerry's sidekick on the popular television series *Seinfeld*. George, played by actor Jason Alexander, has many Allenish features: he's insecure, neurotic, bald, cheap, a sort of nebbishy mensch—a perpetually unsuccessful but lovable man—who still lives in Queens with his Jewish mom and Italian dad. For example, in a 1993 episode George was obsessed with a white discoloration above his lip. "What's this white discoloration?" he asks a variety of people. "It's a white discoloration," each answers. George consults a physician who says he's never seen such a discoloration and orders a biopsy. Of course, George must anxiously await results. Later, George recounts his conversation with the doctor to his friends. "So I ask him point blank, 'Do I have cancer?' And he didn't give me a 'Cancer, get outta here!' I'll be dead," George whimpers. "I'll have no dignity." (The biopsy is negative.)

Edward Shorter, the Canadian historian, argues that the collective Jewish experience of upheaval, dislocation, and anti-Semitism is inseparable from Jewish hypochondria. In *From the Mind into the Body*, Shorter traces the belief that Jews are prone to hypochondria back to the mid-18th century, when nervous diseases were first described. By the turn of the century, American physicians were labeling Jews noisy, troublesome patients and doctor-shoppers. The term "Hebraic debility" was employed in northeastern hospitals to designate the condition of the Jewish patients who frequented their clinics complaining of "burning" or "sticking" pain in the stomach or chest.

Acknowledging the shortcomings of using anecdotal evidence, Shorter ponders the question of whether the perception of Eastern European hypochondria was more anti-Semitic slander than behavioral reality. But any reservations Shorter has about the preponderance of hypochondria among wealthy Jews who could afford private care were apparently quelled by his observation that Jewish and non-Jewish physicians have noted the Jewish predisposition to worry about nervousness and illness. In 1907, Hyman Morrison, a Harvard medical student who spoke Yiddish, conducted an in-home study of patients, mostly recently arrived Russian immigrants, who had received the diagnostic label Hebraic debility at Massachusetts General Hospital.

Morrison noted that the chief complaint among the majority of the patients was constipation. But more important, he observed an extreme collective anxiety about illness—cancer, TB, and heart disease in particular. He concluded: "The Jews, always a highly imaginative people, have been for centuries cradled in fear, so that it has become one of their keenest emotions, provoked by trifles." The internalization of pain was also surmised by a French-Jewish psychiatrist who treated Holocaust survivors in 1947 and 1948: "The general inclination of the Jew towards hypochondria ... must be allowed for," wrote Henri Stern after interviewing Jews who had survived the Belsen concentration camp in Germany. "It is another manifestation of the insecurity which tortures the Jewish spirit, and I found it expressed most often in the anxious preoccupation shown in the case of illness."

Although today's Jews are only one generation removed from the Holocaust, it is possible that awareness among them of the historical roots of suffering might combine with a generally freer expression of physical and mental anguish. Jewish descendants of immigrants undoubtedly have heard parents and grandparents speak freely of their *tsoriss*, "troubles," and *michegoss*, a catch-all for "intense aggravation." "I'm feeling well, *kineahora*," is another Yiddish expression, the Jewish equivalent of "knock on wood" that Eastern European immigrants used. Don't tempt the heavens by feeling too good; rather, pair any declaration of pleasure with a magic phrase to ward off the evil eye. And what better mental inoculation against disaster than a dose of self-inflicted hypochondriacal misery that can protect one from a harsher punishment?

Such reflections of guilt and retribution through sickness and disability have been noted among famous Jewish hypochondriacs. Al Jolson, who emigrated from Russia as a boy and worked his way up from vaudeville to become a star of film and the stage, was both the "world's greatest entertainer" and the "world's greatest hypochondriac," according to his biographer Michael Freeland. Jolson was haunted by a fear of tuberculosis, an illness he had had as a boy, and a phobia about losing his voice that "had him on familiar terms with doctors all over the country," Freeland writes. At the first sign of a cough, he consulted a dozen doctors; then, if he still felt ill or thought it likely he'd develop TB, he'd phone the William Morris agency and ask to be booked into the Saranac Lake sanatorium, where he'd give a show.

Another Eastern European Jew whose hypochondria was legendary is Jerzy Kosinski, the tortured intellectual and Polish born novelist, who killed himself in 1991. Says Kosinski's self-proclaimed friend, theater mogul Rocco Landesman, as reported in a *New Yorker* magazine article, "Jerzy had the ultimate hypochondria suicide. He had a heart problem, and he thought he was going to end up paralyzed and in a vegetable condition, and kept worrying that that was going to happen, and so finally—and this is the ultimate hypochondriac move—in order to keep himself from getting sick he killed himself."

But is there any evidence stronger than anecdotal? One of the most interesting cross-cultural studies of illness behavior was conducted in the 1950s, comparing attitudes toward pain among World War II veterans. Over a three-year period, Mark Zborowski, a staff anthropologist at a San Francisco hospital, evaluated pain responses among four ethnic groups: Jews, Italians, Irish, and "old" Americans—not senior citizens but white Anglo-Saxon Protestants. Zborowski's research, published in a 1969 book, *People in Pain,* found old Americans to be phlegmatic and stoic about pain. They hid or denied discomfort and rarely complained. Similar to the immigrant Irish, old Americans tended to attribute pain to something safe, like a cramp or a sore muscle, and left further speculation about its meaning to physicians. But the Irish patients, particularly, displayed a distinct cultural pride in refusing to surrender to pain. Typical laconic responses from Irish veterans: "Well, what can you do? Have to take it"; "Just have to take it, that's all"; "I don't mind taking it." By contrast, Jews and Italians had a lower tolerance for pain and tended to respond to it emotionally, crying, complaining, or becoming more demanding. But while Italians were concerned with relieving their immediate pain, Jews tended to focus on the implications of their symptoms and what they meant for future health and welfare—their own and their family's.

In *The Culture of Pain*, a study of pain over two millennia, David Morris points out that early Jewish Scripture and teaching regarded pain as a possible punishment for sin, a divine test of faith, or a means for redemption. (Consider the Hebrew Bible's story of Job who, when covered with boils, wonders aloud and eloquently why God has punished him.) But a more dominant tradition in Judaism views pain and disease as challenges for which God has provided the means and right to treat. Pain is not to be borne but *must* be treated to restore wholeness of body and soul.

Morris relates how Zborowski countered criticism in his day that his research was offensive and promoted or concealed a racist agenda. In defense of his work, Zborowski offered a rationale similar to what Shorter argues today. Pain is contextual, a construct as well as a sensation that takes on the meanings which each social group assigns to it. "The physiology of pain," Zborowski wrote, "acquires cultural and social attributes, and its analysis calls for investigation not only in laboratories and clinics but also in the complex maze of society."

Jews may not suffer more disease or receive treatment differently from non-Jews. What sets Jews apart could be a longstanding pattern of describing disease in detail as well as a more positive attitude toward seeking help. Some of their willingness to seek expert advice is the veneration Jews have expressed over centuries for medical authority. In Western Europe, medicine became the vocation of choice for sons of Jewish immigrants. In America, where Jewish men and women alike were subject to the Hebraic debility label, Jewish women, in particular, earned a reputation for their penchant to consult with prominent physicians. Shorter claims that for Jewish women in America, doctor and hospital visits acquired a certain cachet owing to their being a status symbol in the New World. The availability of private care for those with earnings allowed the Jewish woman to feel pampered and to focus attention on herself. Taking action was a strong departure from the Old World attitude that "a woman keeps dying all the week, but recovers on the Sabbath," a saying in Russian Jewish households. This new notion of the Jewish woman, fastidious about her body and appearance in a time of tremendous fear of TB and diphtheria, was dovetailed with the caricature of the Jewish American princess in popular literature. A later generation of writers depicted somatization in the person of the symptomatic Jewish mother—overprotective, selfsacrificing, and suffocating her children with guilt.

But such simplifications are dangerous. Linguist Deborah Tannen addresses the tendency of people from different cultural backgrounds to have varied ways of speaking and conversational styles. She describes Jews, particularly Jewish New Yorkers, as "high involvement speakers," which causes them to be perceived as interrupting conversations with speakers who expect longer pauses and less frenetic give-and-take, like New Englanders or mid-Westerners. Anti-Semitism classically attributes loudness and aggressiveness to Jewish people, she says, making the leap from a manner of interacting with others who have a different style to negative stereotyping of character.

When referred to affectionately, high-involvement speaking becomes a symbol of ethnic tradition and philosophy, like the British tendency to queue patiently in long lines and talk about the weather. Applying Tannen's way of thinking, the tendency toward hypochondria should not be judged in moral terms. It is merely a cultural trait or behavioral temperament that is, like anything else, a matter of preference, taste, or opinion—and to a certain extent, degree. True, in large doses preoccupation with health can be paralyzing and problematic for hypochondriacs and their loved ones. In smaller doses, hypochondria can give people a boost in taking care of their health and serve as a "safe" outlet at a time in life when distraction is necessary.

Health concerns can also provide a mode of social communication. I remember as a kid listening to the ladies who huddled in lounge chairs outside my grandmother's Brooklyn apartment building. They'd talk: about their kids, their health, the meal they'd eaten the previous night. The banter, that of a close-knit family, was not depressing. In their golden years, aches, pains, and trips to physicians—the realities of the aging process— were on these women's minds, and conversing about health had become a natural part of their social landscape. It was not really hypochondria but a way to rally a sense of community.

GROWING OLD GRACEFULLY

No one should minimize the pain and anguish that can accompany old age. The chronically ill elderly face problems that the young and healthy can only imagine: physical and mental disability, loss of income and status, social isolation, the prospect of hospitals, nursing homes, eventually becoming a burden to one's family, and ultimately death. The stresses of aging are enormous and utterly terrifying. It would be no surprise if after sixty-five people tended to become hypochondriacal, preoccupied with bodily functions, and to believe themselves in poor health.

Studies, however, don't bear this out: hypochondria doesn't appear to advance with the years. To be sure, the elderly suffer more disease and chronic physical ailments than the rest of the population, but when it comes to assessing one's health and well-being, age, it seems, takes a back seat to personality. "The public's impression of rampant despair, depression, and hypochondria among the elderly is a myth," says Paul T. Costa, Jr., chief of the laboratory of personality and cognition at the National Institute on Aging's gerontology research center. "The person who makes excessive and exaggerated complaints in old age is probably the same person who has made them all his or her life."

Psychologist Martin Seligman, whose research is in the area of optimism, has found that whether a person sees the glass as half full or half empty changes little as he or she grows older. Optimists tend to view misfortune as temporary and surmountable, nothing more than bad luck, while pessimists are apt to feel hopeless and helpless when faced with adversity and perceive setbacks as personal defeats. In one study, Dr. Seligman compared the teenage diaries of senior citizens to self-accounts of their current lives. He found that men and women who were fearful, depressed, and self-doubting were, in their teens, fearful, depressed, and self-doubting. For example, women who as teenagers wrote that boys weren't interested in them because they were unlovable, wrote fifty years later that they were unlovable when their grandchildren didn't visit. Another study of middle-class residents of San Francisco in 1928, who were located and surveyed again forty years later, found that those who felt sickest in old age were those who at age thirty fretted and complained most about their health.

The tendency to experience distress and evaluate experience accordingly is related to what Seligman calls a pessimistic explanatory style and others have called neuroticism, a trait that appears to have no connection with age. Fear, rumination, self-consciousness, anxiety, anger, and low self-esteem are all aspects of neuroticism, which is strongly associated with overmonitoring biophysiological reactions, excessive complaining, and hypochondria, as well as depression. "Ruminators who are pessimists are in trouble. Their belief system is pessimistic, and they repeatedly tell themselves how bad things are," Dr. Seligman writes in *Learned Optimism*. "Even when things go well for the pessimist, he is haunted by feelings of catastrophe."

How pessimistic beliefs and hypochondria feed on each other can be seen in the following case. Phil, a retired sixty-six-year-old industrial engineer had looked forward to his retirement for years. He'd been unhappy and resentful that he had never received the recognition or money he thought he deserved. He was also out of shape and not sleeping well. But he believed that all this would change once he stopped working and could relax with his wife. They would read, see movies, visit grandchildren, and spend the winters down South, he told himself.

Instead, Phil is spending his retirement running to doctors — something he's been doing on and off for twenty years. His heart just doesn't feel right; he has night sweats and sometimes a stiff neck. Despite the fact that physical exams have revealed nothing dire, he feels certain he's going to die. The couple had to cancel a trip to Florida because Phil was afraid of having a heart attack on the airplane. "The doctors say my health is fine, but I can't enjoy it," Phil says. A childhood friend who has been trying to get Phil and Millie to Florida for some time is aggravated, but not as angry as Phil is at himself. "My friend is two years older than I am and had a heart attack in his fifties. He's doing great — playing golf, swimming, dancing the polka with his wife — while I'm living like a cardiac patient."

It isn't that there are no elderly hypochondriacs, but given the group's large burden of illnesses and debility, it is remarkable that over the years their attitudes toward life have held so steady. In fact, research suggests that the elderly may appraise their health more optimistically than younger people. The Baltimore Longitudinal Study of Aging, which has been tracing hundreds of men (since 1958) and women (since 1978) whose ages range from seventeen to ninety-seven, found that as people aged they experienced an increase in cardiovascular, genitourinary, and sensory problems. But surprisingly, the study found that general, diffuse bodily complaints did not escalate after sixty-five. "It may even be that medical complaints decline relative to actual impairment with age," Dr. Costa says. "What may be indicative of hypochondriasis in a thirty-year-old may be accurate self-assessment for an eighty-year-old."

Many studies corroborate the elderly's realistic assessment of their health and relatively stable mental health. In the National Institute of Mental Health's epidemiological catchment area (ECA) survey, higher rates of virtually all psychiatric disorders were found among younger age groups, primarily in individuals under thirty-five. The only mental disorder with higher rates in persons sixty-five and older was severe cognitive impairment. The surveys also revealed that somatization—unfounded, vague somatic complaints—does not appear to increase in old age.

The ECA studies didn't specifically test for hypochondria but suggest that the peak years for hypochondria are typically not old age but the third to fifth decades. In a study comparing hypochondriacal patients sixty-five and older to younger hypochondriacal patients, Dr. Arthur Barsky found that the older patients had lower scores than younger patients on both disease-conviction and disease-fear portions of tests for hypochondria despite the fact that they were sicker.

That the complaints of the elderly appear to be remarkably low-key and valid may be attributed to several factors. One is what sociologists call the reference group phenomenon or what gerontologist Stephen Crystal has dubbed the Henny Youngman factor. The effect is depicted in the comedian's classic joke: asked "How's your wife?" the comedian replies, "Compared to what?" Dr. Crystal, a professor at the Institute for Health Care and Aging Research at Rutgers University, explains: "The elderly have a different frame of reference than the young for assessing how they feel, namely their friends, who may be worse off than they are."

It is natural for health expectations to decline with age. Older people expect fatigue after exercise or indigestion after a large meal. Another factor that may mitigate hypochondria in the aged is a conscious attempt to work against the stereotype of the doddering senior who collects symptoms like postage stamps and drives doctors and children crazy with insufferable complaints.

Geriatric physicians and others who are involved with older patients point out that we are in the midst of a revolution in the way society views and responds to the elderly and the manner in which they perceive their capabilities. "The image of the senior citizen waiting to die is being replaced by a vision of the grandmother or grandfather who takes an aerobic class or plays golf, attends Elderhostels, is vigorous, spirited, and glad to be alive," Dr. Crystal says. One additional aspect of health realism among the elderly may be that those past eighty-five, who make up the fastest-growing segment of the population, tend to be genetically hardy, strong individuals who literally do grow old gracefully.

....

CHAPTER EIGHT

Family Ties—
in Sickness and in Health

> The reason so many family dilemmas defeat us is that we fail
> to recognize that every family member's behavior is influenc-
> ing and influenced by the behavior of the rest.
>
> —Salvador Minuchin, *Family Healing*

"I NEED a Band-Aid," whimpered my friend's two-and-a-half-
year-old, Alex, tugging at his mother's sweater. We were spending a beach vacation with another family, and it was the cocktail
hour. The little boy's mother jumped up to fetch a Band-Aid
despite protests from her husband, who explained that such demands had become habitual. Some weekends, he said, Alex
asked for no fewer than a dozen Band-Aids, usually when he
was not getting attention. Sure enough, through the ensuing
week, when Mom and Dad were preoccupied with his older
brother or relaxing with friends, Alex complained that his stomach, head, and finger hurt. For these ills he demanded *Sesame
Street*, hot-neon Band-Aids, or a teaspoon of syrupy red Tylenol,
over which a family dispute inevitably broke out.

Alex's complaints were disruptive, but no more so than any
child's whiny behavior, and the first aid worked as a palliative,
at least for a few hours. Clearly, the little boy wasn't faking. He

really felt rejected and needy, experiencing his emotions on some level as physical pain. Medical care had become associated with comfort. Whether Alex will grow up to be a hypochondriac or a chronic pain patient is impossible to predict, but a foundation for dealing with his emotional discomfort was already being laid. Administering to his anguish was provoking great dissension between Mom and Dad, yet neither of them seemed capable of taking action to change their way of interacting with their child, or with each other. In truth, Alex seemed to enjoy all the fuss, and sickness as a means of communication was becoming well established in the household.

Soon afterward, I observed an episode involving my own son, which confirmed that children discover the power of illness at a young age. I like to believe that I have shielded our children from my obsessional concerns, hypochondriacal and otherwise, and consciously try not to express inordinate worry when they get sick. If my daughter points out a black and blue mark or complains of a canker sore, after a moment of fright I calmly respond, "Don't worry. It will be gone in a few days" — and so far so good. I'm not happy about the eczema which sporadically attacks my son's feet, but I've allowed his doctor to reassure me that it's a benign condition which he will probably outgrow. When the kids get yearly checkups, I dread the nervous wait for laboratory results as much as I hate waiting for my own. Nonetheless, I don't think my worries are pathological. I cannot be the only parent who on returning home gives herself a mental inoculation — "I know she's had ten stitches" — before walking in the door.

But once I did lose it with my son. Three-year-old Michael was home with a fever, lying lethargically on our bed, watching a superhero videotape. All of a sudden this uncomplaining kid yelled out, "Mommy! My eyes hurt!"

"What do you mean?" I responded, peering into his big blue eyes, now squinting in pain.

He began to cry. "My eyes hurt."

Sure enough, a few weeks earlier I had read about a doctor who performed risky brain surgery in children whose tumors were otherwise inoperable. There had been an anecdote about a little boy with pain so excruciating that he used to bang his head against the wall — because *his eyes hurt*! I continued to examine Michael, looking for signs of God knows what. As I wondered, Should I take him to the emergency room? Should I call 911? Am I overreacting? Michael rolled over and fell asleep.

When he awoke, I asked how his eyes were. "Good," he replied. "Are you sure?" "Yes." "Are you *sure*?" "Yes." What else can you ask a three-year-old? I watched him closely for a day or two. He seemed fine and I forgot the incident.

Apparently Michael didn't. Nearly a year later, we were in a new phase. He was climbing into our bed at night, refusing to stay in his room, which he "hated." One morning at two, my husband put his foot down and decided to make him stay in his room. Michael wailed for half an hour, shouting all kinds of nasty remarks, like "I hate my bed. I hate my toys and my books. I hate this house." I lay in bed listening to his tirades, almost amused. Each time the episode seemed to be over, he would have a new brainstorm: "My pajamas aren't comfortable." "I'm having a bad dream!" And then came the ultimate weapon: *My eyes hurt!* He remembered.

THE PHANTOM PAINS OF CHILDHOOD

Children are not born hypochondriacal, which is not to say that they do not have the propensity to become so. Anyone who has had contact with newborns realizes that they come into the world with distinctive temperaments, which they manifest through their personalities and behaviors. Infants also vary in physiological vulnerability and genetic predisposition toward illness. Jerome Kagan, the distinguished Harvard University psychologist, has demonstrated that 15 percent of children are born with a tendency to be anxious or fearful; they inherit a neuro-chemistry that makes them overly sensitive to touch and sound and excitable when exposed to the new and unfamiliar.

The pain a child encounters on the journey to adulthood is an exquisitely rich blend of both the physical and the emotional, and making sense of it can be a complicated process for children and parents alike. Assessing the hurt young children feel is particularly difficult because their vocabulary and experience are limited. How does one know when a small child is really sick if there are no telltale signs like fever and rash? Teething and ear infections are sometimes difficult to distinguish from simple crankiness. Toddlers experience separation anxiety and feel it as physical pain. Try getting an accurate description of pain from a four-year-old. "What hurts?" "I don't know." "Is it your ear?" "No." The pediatrician's diagnosis: a double ear infection. As parents search for clues to help them decode their children's messages of distress, they become familiar with individual temperaments and needs.

By age six or seven, children are capable of talking over their difficulties reasonably, but they cannot differentiate between bodily and emotional pain as well as an adult should be able to. It is hard for them to separate their stomachache from not wanting to go to school because a boy in class makes fun of them. Because they are still learning to verbalize feelings, their unsettling emotions tend to be acted out in such behavior as tantrums, hitting or biting other children, withdrawal—and being sick. Parents need to help children of this age learn to identify distressing feelings and to cope with frightening or unpleasant situations. If parents fail to teach their children the emotional language to express unhappiness, they may have difficulty sorting out the tummyache from what's really bothering them. And unless a child can make that connection, he or she may not get better.

Phantom pains that seem to spring from nowhere in childhood and adolescence are not uncommon. As they grow, many children complain of vague pain and discomfort—in the stomach, head, chest, any part of the body—without being sick. Loving parents are naturally concerned. What with the threat of Lyme disease, lead contamination, childhood cancer, any complaint can be terribly worrisome. But luckily, the majority of these complaints signal transient stress, not serious disease.

It is not necessary to run to a doctor every time a child complains. The majority of ailments to which children fall prey heal themselves, and serious illnesses are relatively rare, the exception rather than rule. Pediatrician Robert S. Mendelsohn, in *How to Raise a Healthy Child . . . In Spite of Your Doctor*, argues emphatically that medical attention should be a *last* resort for most children's illnesses. Mendelsohn maintains that 95 percent of pediatric office visits are unnecessary and possibly harmful because they expose a child to tests, X rays, drugs, and theories that in most instances are "no substitute for the common sense that you, as an informed parent, can provide."

Nevertheless, a child of any age with persistent complaints should have a thorough physical examination to rule out any condition of medical significance. If findings are negative or out of proportion to the complaints, the next step is to consider emotional causes. Your pediatrician should be able to guide you as to whether symptoms require further evaluation. Childhood is anything but stress free, and periods of transition can trigger "growing pains," which should resolve on their own. One caveat: if children remain stuck in symptoms for longer than a few months, if symptoms worsen or begin to intrude into other areas of a child's life, the same underlying emotional problems one might suspect in hypochondriacal adults—depression, panic disorder, obsessiveness—should be considered.

Twenty years ago, doctors thought that children could not become depressed—an official diagnosis for childhood depression did not exist until 1980—but childhood depression has become the object of much research. Various studies estimate that between 2 and 10 percent of eight- to thirteen-year-olds experience major depression in the course of a given year, and the numbers rise in adolescence, especially for girls. Childhood depression is not merely transitory unhappiness or disappointment, but a deep sadness lasting several weeks or more. As in adults, depression in children can manifest itself not just in sadness, but in loss of appetite, sleep problems, belligerence, apathy, or withdrawal. It can also show up in vague physical complaints, typically stomachaches, headaches, and bowel problems. Children with chronic medical conditions, such as asthma, often suffer from depression caused by having an illness that intensifies family stress and makes them different from their peers.

Though panic disorder, the full-fledged, four-symptom adult variety (see Chapter 3), isn't all that common in childhood, youngsters can have exaggerated stress reactions and exhibit panic symptoms such as clammy hands, pounding heart, chest pain, twitching or trembling, and a feeling of impending doom. By ninth grade, one in ten children has had at least one panic attack.

Obsessive-compulsive disorder (OCD) most typically emerges in midadolescence but can begin at a younger age. Half of all adult sufferers of OCD can trace the start of repetitive thoughts or rituals to childhood. A serious psychiatric disorder like OCD, however, should not be confused with the "magical thinking" — nightly bedtime rituals, coveted blankies, or superstitions like not walking on sidewalk cracks — common in childhood. However, if a child continues to exhibit ritualistic tendencies after age six, he or she may be trying to quell some powerful fears or phobias magically. By definition, phobias are long-lasting and intense. Unlike normal fears, says psychologist Norma Doft, "they cannot be soothed away by a parent checking under the bed for monsters, or promising to be back by four."

Nonetheless, the cycle of fear, reassurance, and medical attention characteristic of hypochondria in adults isn't apt to be seen in the phantom illnesses of children. After all, the young are not usually in charge of such decisions as whether to seek a doctor's care. Children tend to be more consumed by the wish to get rid of pain than with its significance. Researchers say that youngsters don't officially begin to worry like adults until the age of seven or eight, when they have the cognitive capability to construct what-if scenarios and mentally represent the future. A realistic concept of death, for instance, emerges at about age ten, though surveys reveal that half of fourth-graders do not clearly understand death's irreversible nature. Ages twelve through eighteen are prime times for worry. Adolescence is a period of heightened introspection, which leads to a greater awareness of emotions and physical sensations. Sexuality is burgeoning, and there is much curiosity and insecurity about the body. Yet fear of failure, lack of acceptance among one's peers, or of not being invited to the prom is more real for most teenagers than the possibility of falling ill. Adolescent girls struggling with dependency/independence issues are more likely to fend off anxiety about attaining adulthood through the self-starvation of anorexia nervosa or the binging and purging of bulimia than to gravitate toward hypochondria as a symptom of distress. Boys tend to play out their pain in aggressive conduct or other behavioral problems.

At different stages, most healthy children have one or more bouts with anxiety, fear, vague pain, or discomfort, and perhaps even hypochondria. Most pass through these episodes quickly and unscathed if parents soothe and reassure and, even more important, help them label their feelings. Persistent symptoms may not signify a serious physical or psychiatric disorder but may be a cue that parents need to listen more and show greater patience, understanding, and support.

Some parents are better than others at sensing the emotional meaning of their children's pain. Symptoms can be a way of defending against frightening emotional experiences, or they can help a child to feel more important in the family. A child in pain may symbolically be sending out a nonverbal communiqué: "Take care of me. I hurt. I need your attention." Some children embrace pain because it allows them to escape situations and responsibilities they dislike or find threatening. Their being sick reduces parental expectations of achievement and can relieve stress or pressure. Powerful, unconscious anger may also underlie symptoms in children who use pain to punish a parent for rejecting or pushing them or for being rigidly authoritarian. If a child prone to panic attacks ends up time after time in a hospital emergency room because he can't breathe, it may be because he finds that the emotional concern he gets for his physical problem is a substitute for the attention he is missing otherwise. By then, a parent who plays into health concerns may contribute to hypochondria. Being pushed into extensive testing—blood tests, urinalysis, MRIs—by anxious and unobservant parents and doctors can reinforce a child's perception that he is sick.

In her essay "Enough to Make You Sick," pediatrician Perri Klass describes a case of a woman who brings her seven-year-old to an emergency room one night. The child has been complaining of abdominal pain, so wrenching that it makes him groan and cry out. The mother worries that it might be appendicitis. But she is also suspicious because she knows that her son faces a spelling test the next day, and her husband has warned the boy that if he brings home any more bad test grades his computer will be taken away. The boy is examined, a few blood tests are done, the problem does not seem to be appendicitis. Nor does it resemble any other treatable medical condition. Klass asks, "Is the boy pretending to have stomach pain so he can get out of going to school, or does the prospect of taking the test, facing his father, and losing his computer terrify him so thoroughly that his stomach is hurting?" In extreme cases, she says, both types of behavioral patterns can be evidence of psychological disorders. "But both patterns, to one degree or another, fit almost all of us." So, Klass asks, "when do you stop working him up? There's always another test you can do, another even more unlikely diagnosis to rule out."

These are questions parents must ask themselves when a child suffers from symptoms that cannot be ascribed to any disease.

For some families, encouraging the sick role may be easier than delving into their own emotional lives. Focusing on a sick child can turn down the volume of family tensions, detour a crisis, or mask another problem. A mother doesn't have to face her depression. A father temporarily stops drinking. A couple avoids marital conflict.

David Sherry, a specialist in psychogenic musculoskeletal pain in children, says that in some families of children who have persistent symptoms, the home atmosphere is unmistakably chaotic and stressful. There has been a divorce, a death, a traumatic relocation. The lack of stability is palpable. But more frequently, he says, family stress is covert. "Ask Mom and Dad and they'll say everything's fine. The child plays the violin, is enrolled in ballet. I saw a kid recently with inexplicable leg pain who had received trophies for swimming, cross country, and track." These children seem to have something in common: they are overly compliant kids who are treated as brighter, stronger, and more mature than they actually are. They are likely to be put in inappropriate roles in the family, like a ten-year-old girl who is her mother's best friend. "They bend over backwards to meet other people's needs, but their needs don't get met," says Dr. Sherry. "They can't break away from an overly protective family and become their own person."

MÜNCHAUSEN BY PROXY: CREATING ILLNESS IN A CHILD

Inadvertently reinforcing somatic behavior in children is easy enough, but the process is reversible. If parents recognize the problem or someone sensitively brings it to their attention, they frequently make great efforts to change. Quite different, however, is the parent who purposely induces sickness in a child. Chapter 2 introduced the phenomenon of Münchausen syndrome, an extreme form of psychogenic illness in which a healthy person invents a physical disease where none exists and misleads doctors into believing he has it. Just as there is a world of difference between the Münchausen patient and the hypochondriac, so there is between Münchausen by proxy parents and parents who unconsciously encourage the sick role.

Münchausen by proxy parents, the vast majority of them mothers, go to extraordinary lengths to convince health care professionals that their children are sick. In a mild form of the disorder, a parent might exaggerate the symptoms, say, of a child's allergic condition. In more extreme forms, parents pursue the abusive behavior compulsively. They heat thermometers, feed or inject children with laxatives, sedatives, or diuretics, contaminate urine specimens, or cause them to stop breathing temporarily.

The bizarre behavior that is the hallmark of Münchausen by proxy, which is considered a form of child abuse, has received much attention of late. The public appears fascinated by the grotesque idea that a parent could make a child sick, an act that violates every instinct and ethical standard imaginable. Sensational cases have been featured in newspaper and magazine articles, portrayed in television dramas, and even in a best-selling mystery novel. And though the self-induced illnesses of Münchausen are rare—about four hundred hospital patients are diagnosed with the syndrome each year—Münchausen by proxy is apparently more common, perhaps because pediatricians are getting better at recognizing signs of abuse. A 1991 survey of 1,200 pediatric neurologists and gastroenterologists uncovered 273 confirmed cases and 192 suspected cases among patients of the 316 physicians who responded.

The motives of Münchausen parents are not easily understood. The perplexing behavior seems to be without tangible benefit. The parents are usually not trying to win a custody battle or to extort money. "The Münchausen by proxy mother has an insatiable need to play the role of the heroic caregiver," says Herbert A. Schreier, chief of psychiatry at Children's Hospital in Oakland, California, and coauthor of *Hurting for Love*, a book about the disorder. But beyond that, there seems to be an aggressive component to the parents' interaction with health providers that involves "dependency, control, and revenge for past slights and humiliations." These mothers are extremely skilled at posturing good mothering, but the child is less important to them as a person than as a pawn to manipulate in their intensely ambivalent relationship with doctors.

Most psychiatrists agree that, in Münchausen by proxy, normal boundaries were never formed between parent and child; the two identities become fused for a variety of reasons. Münchausen parents, similar to Münchausen patients, seem to have an "exquisite sense of what is going on in a person's mind," says Berney Goodman, a psychiatrist who has written about the disorder. There is almost an element of telepathy in their cat-and-mouse game with the hospital. The parents seem to know intuitively when the hospital staff is on to them, and often they flee. "The life stories of Münchausen patients seem to be embellished with episodes of tragic loss and attempts to elicit sympathy and extra care," Dr. Goodman says. A common scenario is that one or both parents was a sickly child who required attention or care and encountered engulfment, abandonment, or abuse. It is not uncommon for Münchausen parents to have undergone hospitalizations as children, which they recall as positive experiences. They typically comment, "The doctors were good to me" or "The nurse brought me ice cream."

The sadomasochistic tendencies of Münchausen patients make garden variety hypochondria and somatization look fairly tame. Nevertheless, it may take several months, even years, before doctors are able to distinguish between misguided parental concern and a potentially lethal disturbance. If there is any similarity between Münchausen and somatizing families, it is in symbiotic overinvolvement, an inappropriate attachment between parent and child. In families whose children have somatic illnesses or recurrent unexplained pain, parents' emotional needs are often met by the same symptoms or disability. There are, however, some key differences between the two. Parents who make frequent visits and phone calls to physicians and overreact to minor symptoms in their children do *not* want them to be ill and express relief, even if only temporarily, when reassured that the youngsters are well. They do not push for invasive tests and procedures and are pleased when laboratory results are negative. "The overanxious parent responds well to a social services or a psychiatric referral, taking advantage of the opportunity to express her fears, explore her concerns, and admit to her high anxiety level," Dr. Schreier says. In contrast, Münchausen parents have difficulty acknowledging any personal problems and, unlike overanxious parents, often lie about their backgrounds, medical histories, and life experiences. While the overanxious parent may irritate physicians, she is rarely experienced as controlling, manipulative, or peculiar.

THE WEB OF CONNECTION

Children come into this world innocent and are quickly enlisted in the family arena. Things happen, and the family that was once our greatest hope for intimacy and connection becomes our greatest source of disappointment. Dysfunctional behavior patterns, like hideous heirlooms, are handed down from one generation to another. Thus we absorb character traits and defining labels: he's moody, she's demanding, a hypochondriac, just like Grandpa! Parents focus on decoding a child's conduct but ignore their contribution to it. Spouses loathe behavioral tendencies in each other but refuse to look at the purpose they serve in the marriage. The bigger picture is lost.

The joke about sending a hypochondriac to a desert island to make his symptoms disappear is meant to be facetious. But there is some truth to the notion that hypochondriacs are trying to say something, something that family members may be unaware of, unsympathetic to, or refuse to hear. Sickness exists in a social setting: the caring and cared for, the helpful and helpless. Partners, spouses, and others involved with a hypochondriacal loved one have several avenues of response available. They can coddle and comfort, become distant and withdraw, express overt anger, or pull out, among other options. How a family reacts to complaints can influence the nature of an illness and how sick or disabled a person becomes.

Each family constructs its own culture to make sense of its life and to make the system work. Sometimes in the struggle to maintain balance, or what family therapists call homeostasis, one individual gets elected "the patient." Though that person may not be, and often isn't, the most troubled person in the household, he or she has the problem—or *is* the problem. As the late Carl Whitaker, one of the pioneers of the family therapy movement, put it: The symptomatic individual becomes the "family scapegoat, whipping boy, Christ—someone who agreed to suffer openly the stress of the entire family so that the family could remain stable."

Paradoxically, while hypochondria has the potential to tear a family apart, it can also maintain stability, protecting the members from more serious disturbance. A wife's anxious caretaking may encourage dependence in a remote husband she is terrified might leave her. For a child with chronic migraines, the ability to detour bickering parents who might otherwise divorce or harm each other can serve as a reinforcement for the illness.

The family systems movement, devised by psychiatrist Murray Bowen in the 1950s and 1960s, departed radically from previous theories of human emotional functioning. Pioneering family therapists, including Bowen, Whitaker, Virginia Satir, Jay Haley, and Salvador Minuchin, carved out new ground from which to view people and explore problems. Rather than diagnosing people as sick or well, the new family therapists dispensed with deciphering the cause of the problem and concentrated on responses within the emotional environment. They asked questions like, How is the family organized? How do symptoms fit into patterns of family interaction and communication? Who holds the power in the family? What is happening between people? Thus, systems therapy shifted the focus from individual dynamics to group processes that had become predictable generational blueprints for family unhappiness.

Family systems was a tailor-made vantage point for the exploration of illness dynamics within families. Most of the early research in this area was done by Salvador Minuchin, the Argentinean-born pediatrician turned family therapist who began his work in somatization during the 1970s while treating asthmatic children who were virtually crippled by their illness. The psychosomatic notion endorsed in the 1930s by the Franz Alexander school, that asthma represented a repressed cry of the rejected mother within, was no longer in vogue; the disease was declared "too physical" to be caused by psychological factors alone. Emotional distress, along with genetic predisposition, exposure to allergens, and other triggers, such as smoke, cold, physical exertion, were thought to play a role in provoking and maintaining the inflammation and constriction that would leave the sufferer wheezing, coughing, and gasping for air. But the asthmatic child was viewed as a passive recipient of family stress; thus, the therapy of choice for many years was to separate the child from the family, to perform what was known as a "parentectomy." What often occurred was that children would sustain long periods of remission undergoing individual therapy in a hospital, only to have the symptoms return when they went home.

Minuchin had the novel idea that rather than simply treat sick children, why not empower their parents to become a stabilizing force in the emotional regulation of the illness? Working from a systems perspective, he launched a family research project at Children's Hospital in Philadelphia, treating the families of children with asthma, diabetes, and anorexia nervosa, whose illnesses appeared to serve many purposes in the ecology of their families. In a safe, therapeutic setting, parents learned to initiate and negotiate conflicts without involving their children. As they gained new coping and communication skills, they began to resolve long-standing problems and repair the emotional damage they themselves suffered in childhood. Dramatic improvements or remissions of children's symptoms were achieved in nearly all forty-five cases of the pilot study, which was successfully repeated.

As Minuchin and his colleagues continued their work with parents and children who presented their problems in a variety of somatic disguises, they realized that certain transactional patterns among family members seemed characteristic. The family of a "psychosomatic" brittle, or difficult to control, diabetic functioned very much like the family of a psychosomatic anorectic or psychosomatic asthmatic, which differed markedly from the functioning of the families of so-called normal children who came into therapy for other problems.

Throughout Minuchin's work, a common set of background findings emerged in families with psychosomatically ill members. No one pattern of family involvement alone, he found, was enough to cause an illness, but when mechanisms that allowed families to avoid or anesthetize emotional pain were clustered together, they encouraged somatization. According to Minuchin, the four transactional characteristics that provide context for the use of illness as a mode of communication are:

Enmeshment. In the highly enmeshed family, members are overinvolved, intruding on one another's thoughts, feelings, and communications. The boundaries that define autonomy are so weak that an individual's life space is impinged upon. Triangles form in which family members gang up against one another, promoting rivalry and hostility. One parent enlists a child's support in the struggle with the other parent. Children may join with one parent in criticizing other family members or take inappropriate parental roles.

Overprotectiveness. In the overprotective family system, everyone is hypersensitive to signs of distress, continuously on guard for the approach of dangerous levels of tension or conflict. Nurturing and protective responses are constantly elicited and supplied. A sneeze sets off a flurry of handkerchief offers; complaints of fatigue and discomfort punctuate communication. Parental overconcern retards a child's development of autonomy, competence, and interests outside the family, and the child, in turn, feels great responsibility for protecting the family.

Rigidity. Authoritarian families exist in a "chronic state of submerged stress." They deny any need for change and are heavily committed to maintaining the status quo. Issues that threaten change, such as negotiations over individual autonomy, are not allowed to surface to the point where they can be explored. Even in therapy, the families typically present themselves as untroubled, except for the one child's medical problem. Such families are highly vulnerable to stress. Almost any outside event may overload their coping mechanisms, precipitating illness.

Lack of conflict resolution. Here the family threshold for friction is very low. Problems are left unresolved to threaten again and again. Typically, one spouse is an avoider who manages to detour conflict that would lead to problem recognition and perhaps negotiation. A husband may simply storm out of the house when his wife tries to bring up a problem. Some families bicker continuously, but frequent interruptions and subject changes obfuscate issues before they come to the fore.

Subsequent research has confirmed Minuchin's theories. Indeed, it is a rare case of severe familial somatization in which home life isn't turbulent. Studies have demonstrated that mothers who have experienced abuse bring their children to the pediatrician more often than nonabused mothers. Other research has found that children whose parents somatize are subject to more emergency room use, disability, and suicidal behavior than medically ill children in normal families. In a three-year study of one hundred children, ages three to twenty, admitted to Children's Hospital Medical Center in Seattle with unexplained musculoskeletal pain which had persisted for more than a year, the researchers found that 90 percent reported conflicted family situations—alcoholism, marital discord, abuse, parental anxiety or depression—or had experienced traumatic events. Two-thirds had a role model with chronic pain, usually another family member.

It is difficult for somatizing families to take a step back. The resolution of symptoms can expose problems that children may be afraid to let surface. But when parents realize that a child's pain is a result of the burden he carries, they become open to examining the stress in their lives. The parents begin to work on their own issues, altering school expectations, engaging in individual or marital counseling. In the end, the entire family benefits.

HYPOCHONDRIA AS A THREAT TO MARRIAGE

The scapegoat in illness dynamics doesn't necessarily have to be a child. One of the spouses in a marriage may unconsciously agree to be the "problem." In some marriages, hypochondria can be the glue that holds the relationship together; one partner worries and complains and the other responds with sympathy and attention. In others, health preoccupations can cause deep rifts and resentments.

No couple *purposely* walks into a problematic relationship or plans to create a dysfunctional family. Nevertheless, emotional chemistry—the shock of recognition that "it's as if I've known you all my life"—is rarely blind accident. Something draws people together. Strengths complement weaknesses: he's gregarious, she's shy; he's ambitious, she's laid back; he's a complainer, she's so stoic. Whether a childhood was stable or turbulent, falling in love stirs up early feelings of safety, comfort, and dependency. At its worst, marriage travels a path of parental mistakes, unleashing a torrent of unmet childhood needs. At its best, it be-

How Not to Encourage the Sick Role

What we learn in childhood has a powerful influence on how we care for ourselves as adults. Studies have shown that as adults, people tend to develop the symptoms of their childhood to which their parents paid attention or the symptoms they witnessed in their parents. With so much at stake, how does one know what example to set? How do parents respond to illness complaints without encouraging hypochondria later in life? What follows is some advice that may help you tread the line between heeding a child's pains and making too much of them.

• **Resist the temptation to take action.** Any persistent complaints should be evaluated by a doctor. But after a meticulous physical examination, including neurological and musculoskeletal tests that reveal there is no disease present, stop seeking reassurance. If you don't think a child is sick, don't offer medications, even sugar pills or candy, as a child will believe she feels better because of something external rather than something she herself initiated.

• **Don't overreact when a child complains.** Be appropriately concerned. Ask a few questions. Feel a forehead. If intuition tells you there is nothing to worry about, encourage the child to go about his normal tasks. A child's autonomy can be curtailed by parental overconcern.

• **Deal with illness matter-of-factly.** It certainly makes sense to provide rest, comfort, and sympathy to an ill child. But if you regularly reward that child with new toys, favorite foods, and treats, you may deliver the message — to the child and siblings — that the way to command attention at your house is to become sick.

• **Don't use minor complaints to avoid work or other unpleasant tasks in your own life.** Parents can unknowingly teach children behavior that may lead to hypochondria. William Whitehead, a psychologist at the University of North Carolina, and his colleagues developed scales to determine how the illness habit is learned in childhood. They found that children whose parents missed work, canceled social obligations, or focused on symptoms of trivial illnesses, such as a brief bout with diarrhea and the common cold, were more apt to be hypochondriacal about the same symptoms later in life.

• **Dig Deeper.** Look for nonverbal clues to a child's pain, such as tone of voice, facial expression, body language. Are emotions being expressed by complaints of pain and regression from activities? Why doesn't the child want to go to school? What issues are going on in the family?

• **Ask yourself questions.** Is dependency acceptable for your children in other aspects of life, not just illness? Do you show your child more affection when he is sick than at other times? If your child is hurting emotionally, are you afraid you won't be able to make it better? Are you anxious that your child will grow away from you?

The French novelist Marcel Proust suffered from hypochondriacal symptoms and from asthma. The son of a doctor, he was aware of illness dynamics within his family and in his writing accused his mother of contributing to his illness. "The truth is . . . that the moment I'm well . . . you demolish everything until I am ill again . . ." Proust wrote. "It's very sad not to be able to have affection and health both at once."

• **Get the facts.** When it comes to health concerns about children — sudden infant death syndrome, Lyme disease, cancer, choking — the statistics are on your side. Critical illnesses tend to be freak occurrences that often cannot be averted, but accidents can be. Take safety precautions: keep ipecac in the house, insist on helmets for bicycling, post emergency phone numbers — then relax. Children can benefit from the facts, too. One psychologist told of an eight-year-old boy who feared that if he played in his basement a cricket would bite him. The psychologist assigned a report on crickets and the boy learned everything about them. "They don't bite, so I can't be bitten!" he proudly told his parents.

• **Use common sense.** Trust your instincts. If you think there is something wrong with your child, call the doctor. If stomachaches seem to crop up on school exam days, then disappear miraculously when the television is turned on, something else is probably going on. As pediatrician Robert Mendelsohn says, "Mothers, grandmothers, and mother nature are the best doctors."

comes a source of mutual support and satisfaction, a secure emotional base from which the partners can change and grow.

In the early years of becoming a couple, hypochondria that was previously a problem for one partner may go underground. Fears and symptoms may remain unexpressed, go unnoticed, be solicitously attended to, or taken at face value. The marital adventure is an exciting and absorbing one, and couples at the outset tend to put their best foot forward. Dependency longings and emotional turmoil that served in the past as a trigger for hypochondria may be temporarily gratified. It can take some time for the seeds of hypochondria to become embedded in the soil of a new relationship and for a dynamic to take shape.

In the early years of their marriage, Susan recalls, her husband, Peter, joked about his fear of disease, which he called his six-month brain tumors. At least twice a year, health anxiety would strike, usually at a time of great stress. In fact, part of what had attracted Susan to Peter was his vulnerability and Woody Allenish ways, so different from the stoic men in her family. When Peter got over a period of worry, he would admit how silly he had been. "We both recognized his apprehension as ridiculous," Susan recalls. "We'd laugh it off."

It took a while for it to dawn on Susan that Peter's behavior was a "thing." Peter would try to hide his anxiety, but fear would build. "I could tell when it was happening," Susan says. "He would become noncommunicative, short-tempered, and spend a lot of time in the bathroom." She could sense that he needed something, but she didn't know what. Susan came up with a rule: if the tense mood lasted more than two days, she would ask what was bothering him. At first, he'd say nothing. Then, with a little prodding, the fear came pouring out. She would try to reassure him — "Well, the test looked good" or "The doctor doesn't seem too worried" — but such statements only set them up for an argument. Susan began to realize that no matter how many times she reassured him — "Gee, I have the same brown mole on my arm" — it made no difference. Once hypochondria established itself, Peter would erect a wall between them, pulling Susan into his worries, then pushing her away. There was no reaching him. All she could do was wait it out. When the phase was over, there would be a good period, for which she began to live.

My husband, too, was indifferent to hypochondria during our whirlwind courtship. Before we met I had recovered from my earlier fixation with lupus; the entire episode seemed far away, as if I hadn't been the person involved. I was healthy and in love. David paid no heed to the telltale signs of trouble ahead, like my phobia about flying. He didn't seem to mind when I asked what he thought a spot or pimple was, just as I managed to ignore the fact that he squirreled away every ticket stub and stuffed dirty laundry in his closet. We also weathered an early medical crisis: a breast lump that turned out to be benign. The morning I freaked out about a delay in getting the final biopsy report, he was calming and supportive. But after all, it *was* a lump in the breast.

One incident early in our marriage stands out. We both remember it well. It was a Friday, and we were about to leave for a romantic weekend at the New Jersey shore. That night I returned home to find a message on my answering machine from a doctor asking me to call about blood work done during a probe for what I thought might be an ulcer. I reached the doctor, a gastroenterologist, who told me there was nothing to worry about, but one of the tests revealed that my white cell count was a little low. "Let's retake it to be sure," she said.

That was all I had to hear. I knew: I had leukemia, a disease that killed my grandmother's brother at twenty-one and my grandfather at eighty. I had read that the disease was marked by an abnormal white cell count, but whether it meant high or low I wasn't sure. All weekend long I obsessed about leukemia — how I would react when I got the diagnosis, the tragedy of dying before having a baby.

My husband was thinking something else. "*I* knew that there had to be some kind of mistake," he recalls. "Here was an active, healthy girl, whom *nobody* had said had leukemia! But you had me doubting myself. You would gaze sadly in the mirror, asking me things like, Do I look like someone with leukemia? Is that a black and blue mark? The weekend was essentially ruined by your obsessive thoughts, and in those days I naively thought that no one would destroy a weekend unless something really serious was going on."

That Monday, David accompanied me to the doctor, but a retest proved unnecessary. My doctor had discovered that Zantac, a medication she had prescribed for my supposed ulcer — which never did show up on X ray — had temporarily depressed my white count. She took me off the drug and suggested I take another test in two months, which she assured me would be normal. I cried tears of relief. A death sentence had been lifted.

David said, "It was after that episode that I knew something was not right, that you were a hypochondriac, even if I didn't know precisely what the word meant. No question, the doctor was an idiot not to realize the effect of a medication she prescribed. She was also insensitive for leaving that message, on a Friday, no less. But your immediate fear that this was evidence of leukemia was excessive, and after that I began to doubt a lot of what you had to say about your symptoms."

Such are the early signs of hypochondria. There may not be one defining moment of awakening in a marriage, when a spouse finally says, "Ah-ha, it's hypochondria." The awareness may rise to the surface gradually or smolder silently underground, but hypochondria is an elusive problem. While some sufferers fit the stereotype of the ailing, bedridden invalid, the majority do not. A spouse who has never lived with hypochondria may be mystified by it and be afraid to question symptoms in his mate that seem so, well, serious. Another problem for the spouse of a hypochondriac is that the symptoms tend to wax and wane, shifting with life circumstances, with physical and emotional changes, and with tensions within the marriage. If the hypochondria is related to depression, its severity may vary from season to season — a depressed mood can be brought on by lack of sunlight. For some women, emotional and physical symptoms fluctuate with the hormonal cycle, causing hypochondria to become more prominent at certain times of the month.

Pregnancy also seems to have an impact on hypochondria. Though it is not true for everyone, several women, myself included, have noticed that their fears of illness abate somewhat during pregnancy. Laura, a thirty-year-old interior designer and mother of a three-year-old, recalls being terrified during the seven months it took her to conceive that she had a physical abnormality or disease. She consulted an infertility specialist after trying for three months, only to be told to come back in six. There was a period when she thought she had an ovarian tumor. Yet from the moment Laura learned that she was expecting, she "never worried another minute during the pregnancy that my body, or my baby's, wasn't healthy."

When Val, thirty-four, an aspiring actress whose problems with agoraphobia and illness fears stem from her early twenties, went into early labor at twenty-two weeks, her obstetrician ordered bed rest for the duration of her pregnancy. She felt wonderful. "I was calm, stable, and surprisingly chipper," recalls Val, who gave birth to a healthy girl a day before her due date. "Everyone complimented me for my attitude. Part of it, I know, was that my husband, who worked a lot, tended to be impatient with my complaints. So here was something legitimate. My health suddenly became very important."

Susan Baur addresses this phenomenon in *Hypochondria: Woeful Imaginings*. Aside from the excitement and joy that accompany having a baby, pregnant women are universally praised and admired for their important role. "Pregnancy's most powerful weapon against hypochondria seems to be its ability temporarily to resolve a woman's confusion about dependency," Baur writes. The ambivalence that pulls a wife in two directions — toward autonomy and worldly achievement, on one hand, and a wish to be dependent and protected on the other—is temporarily put on hold.

It is also a time when certain behaviors, unacceptable in everyday life, are condoned, even encouraged. "A pregnant woman is expected to be demanding, restless, and indecisive," Baur continues. She can send her husband for pickles and ice cream in the middle of the night and eat cheesecake and pizza without worrying that her jeans will be too tight. She also has the unique opportunity to indulge herself with medical attention without fear that her concerns will be dismissed. In fact, the carefully monitored regimen advocated for healthy pregnant women—routine checkups, diet, exercise, vitamins, schedules for further treatment—has much in common with the traditional medical wisdom for managing hypochondria. Physicians have been advised to give hypochondriacal patients regular appointments regardless of their symptoms so they needn't worry that their getting better will terminate the doctor-patient relationship.

Throughout the ups and downs of hypochondria, many couples never recognize the emotional pas de deux for what it is. As hypochondria becomes more entrenched in a marriage, husband and wife may experience an escalating sense of disenchantment and tension. There is often a distancing and a disaffection that take place, and the couple may find themselves in a troubled relationship but be unable to sort out the predicament. Though one spouse generally does not cause the symptoms, he or she becomes intertwined in them by virtue of merely responding to them. The more rigid and predictable the psychodrama, the more trapped the participants feel, until the emotional environment becomes inseparable from the problem.

For some, the hypochondriacal pattern may work temporarily, providing the homeostasis family therapists speak of. The couple becomes locked into patterns of interaction regulated by hypochondriacal symptoms. Fear and reassurance. Fear and resentment. Fear and withdrawal. Fear and anger. Anger and anger. But such a foundation is tenuously constructed, and when a crisis or disappointment arises, the enmeshed couple falls apart.

For Val, the respite of pregnancy did not last long. When her daughter was six months old, she noticed herself becoming preoccupied with little things about her body. She had taken off the pregnancy weight rapidly without trying. She was tired and her joints ached. When she looked in the mirror, she saw someone she hardly recognized. "I didn't look healthy. My face looked haggard and old." She had just turned thirty. It can't be that I'm unhappy, she thought to herself. She adored her little girl, had enrolled in an acting class, and her tryout for a role in a community theater production looked promising.

That's when Val developed the irrational fear that she had AIDS. The thought began with a lingering sore throat, and by the time the condition cleared up weeks later, Val had worked herself into a panic. She could not stop thinking about the two men with whom she had made love during a summer trip to Europe ten years earlier. Could they have been AIDS carriers? Could she have passed the virus on to her baby? Now a slight cold, an unusual spot on her skin, or simple exhaustion sent her running to doctors. The two physicians she consulted gently pointed out that her lifestyle did not put her at risk for AIDS: she had been monogamous for five years, and the chance of AIDS turning up after a decade was small. One suggested she take a blood test, a prospect she found too frightening. At one point Val fantasized that her symptoms might be related to Lyme disease, for which she didn't mind being tested. She was disappointed when the test came back negative and pushed for a second one because she had read somewhere that the disease screening delivered many false negatives.

Her husband, Jeff, tried to be supportive, but was losing patience. He could not forget a similar episode during their engagement when she was convinced that her stomach pains were cancer. Her obsessions increasingly became a wedge between them. The record kept playing again and again. Val would be doing well, enjoying her daughter, getting back to her acting. Then some trivial symptom would set her off again. Worried and frantic, she would look toward Jeff, who would automatically suggest she see another doctor. But there was no warmth there. Jeff felt used, hurt, and confused. He no longer had any control in the relationship and began putting in more time at the office. No longer wishing to get sucked in by the good times just to have them turn sour, he withdrew from Val, who began to fear she was losing him.

This is a pattern any couple who has had marital problems may recognize. All of a sudden you're wondering, Who is this person? How did we ever decide to get married? Hypochondria can be depressing. For one, it's a turnoff, a real romance killer. It's as if a person is saying, "How can you love me? I'm damaged goods." Being the "healthy" partner is also draining. Who wants to be reminded of one's physical vulnerability, the aging process, and the inevitability of death all the time? Hypochondria also seems selfish. No problem *you* might have could possibly be worse than bad health. On the other hand, a person who finds hypochondria so offensive and threatening to the point of shutting out her partner is sabotaging any chance at communication. Partners of hypochondriacs thus find themselves torn between the belief that their mate's fears are dishonest and can be controlled and what they know in their hearts: that the person with whom they fell in love is truly frightened and miserable. Not knowing whether to confront the problem or leave it alone, the spouse sometimes finds withdrawal the easiest path, and so becomes an accomplice in maintaining a pathetic status quo. Pain and isolation are continuous as the marriage spirals downward.

My husband and I were almost at this breaking point during the fifth year of our marriage, following the birth of our second child. He was tired of being supportive. I was racked by guilt, but so angst-ridden that I couldn't focus on anything except my symptoms. I was also angry that he wasn't there for me.

He was angry, too. "The first couple of years I didn't question things much," David says. "But then I began to notice the litany of complaints and think of the boy who cried wolf. I admit, if pressed, I probably would have said you were making things up. I remember thinking that if only I had kept a list of the different ailments you had freaked out about over the years—ankles, stomach, irritable bowel, carpal tunnel, hair loss, multiple sclerosis, lupus—you would have to realize it didn't add up. I thought you would see with dispassion what was never possible in conversation. I think you refused to remember certain things, a trait I observed when you recounted your medical history to your friends or the few times I accompanied you to doctors. The hair loss was the last straw. We used to have these ridiculous exchanges. I would try to tell you your hair didn't look significantly different to me and you would thrust the brush in my face. Every morning you would scream, 'It's coming out' and point to your pillow. I remember being livid with you. Then when we went to visit your parents, they were trying to be supportive, and I thought it was all a bunch of shit."

Marital discord is never pretty, and there is no end to the disastrous methods couples can employ to make each other miserable. Couples caught in the entangling web of hypochondria, as well as other problems that become entrenched in marriage, cope with the situation in accordance with who they are and where they have been.

Here are a few variations:

The Humpty-Dumpty syndrome. Charles Ford, the University of Alabama psychiatrist, describes this syndrome in which a "good egg" suddenly becomes hypochondriacal despite having no history of the problem. The person is often a hardworking and conscientious sort who married young and has been a source of support, financial and otherwise, for children, parents, siblings, or other dependents. Frequently in childhood, often because of the death or illness of a parent, he was thrust into a position of early responsibility. Then an illness or accident forces the good egg to discover his dependency needs for the first time. His fragile defenses crumble, he perceives himself as disabled, and no matter how hard family members and physicians try, he cannot be put together again. Unfortunately, Ford says, the price is high: the patients are usually chronically depressed, marital and sexual problems are common, and finances are almost always more of a problem than they had been.

As a boy, Alfredo, a forty-year-old mechanic, moved with his family from Puerto Rico to New York. He didn't finish high school, married at twenty, and quickly had three children, who are teenagers. Three years ago a doctor suggested back surgery for a herniated disk. After all, there was more pain. Not only in his back, but in his chest, where he felt "a needle or sharp sting." His internist suggested he see a cardiologist, who diagnosed mitral valve prolapse, a potentially serious but, some say, overdiagnosed disorder of the valve controlling blood flow between heart chambers. Alfredo sought the opinion of another heart specialist, who insisted he didn't have the condition. A third doctor agreed, but Alfredo followed the advice of the first and began taking medication to slow his heart rate. He became increasingly anxious, afraid to go anywhere alone. Twice he ended up in an emergency room convinced he was having a heart attack. "When I get a pinch in my heart, my body gets scared. My doctors say it is nothing to worry about, but I'm not leading a normal life."

A year ago he quit his job at the garage. His wife, who works in a handbag factory, is the family's sole support while Alfredo stays close to home, trying desperately to finagle disability payments. Financial problems and his fear of leaving the house are causing friction between them. "We never used to have arguments, but now we do. Because of my problem, my family does not respect me."

The sympathizer. This spouse has a vested interest in the continuation of symptoms. He or she fluffs the pillows, fetches tea, and waits on the "patient" hand and foot, unconsciously encouraging invalidism. By being overly helpful, the sympathizer constructs what Minuchin calls a cage of love, which becomes a jail for the entire family.

Terry, an only child, remembers her parents' lives revolving around her father's illness. "My dad's arthritis was like a fourth member of our family," she says. "My mother tended to his every whim." She brought him food in bed, drove the car. Washed his clothes, paid the bills. After her father retired, Terry says, his disability got worse. "If he had a temperature of ninety-nine, he would go to bed." He rarely did anything on his own. One day the family received a big shock! Terry's mother was diagnosed with a brain tumor. No one could believe it. That wasn't the way it was supposed to be. Terry, recently married, moved back into the house to take care of both her parents. She became a conduit between two people who could no longer carry out their prescribed roles. "My father was lost and needed more support than my mother did. She was still being strong for him."

For years Terry was angry with her father, who died of a heart attack shortly after her mother's death. Eventually, through therapy and the experience of having her own children, she gained insight into their marriage. It wasn't her father's fault alone. Her mother had encouraged his passivity. His dependence had pumped her up, made her feel strong and competent, and given her significant leverage in the marriage. But the symbiotic entanglement had sapped Terry's relationship with both parents, and she grew up isolated, afraid to let her needs and feelings show. Terry will always wonder why her mother needed so much power, or what in her father caused him to be childlike. But she no longer blames them. "It would have been wonderful if they could have shown more love. But they weren't able to, and in the end it dwarfed their lives more than mine."

The intolerant. For many couples struggling with hypochondria, resentment and anger are balanced by spurts of love or passion. The glimpse of the person they married keeps them plugging away at the relationship. But in some marriages, the

defenses partners erect against each other are made of stone. It
is not just that the couple is distant and guarded or has stopped
confiding in each other. One spouse, the "healthy" one, is full of
pent-up anger and contempt, mocking the other. The demoral-
ized hypochondriacal spouse, racked by guilt and inadequacy,
cannot fight back and practically disappears into symptoms.
This dynamic is typical of emotional abuse, and unless the couple is jolted out of this pattern, the behavior is likely to escalate
into physical violence before divorce.

Sara, forty-two, grew up nervous and high-strung. Her mother
died from diabetes when Sara was sixteen. Shortly after high
school, desperate to get away from being a domestic servant to
her father and brother, she became engaged to Tom, a salesman.
A week before their wedding, she began to experience chest pains
and palpitations. A cardiologist tested her and said her heart
was fine. Sara is convinced that her body was trying to warn her
of marital danger.

Soon the couple had two children and moved from the city
where her father lived to a faraway suburb. Sara was lonely in
early motherhood. With Tom on the road much of the time, the
responsibility of raising the children fell to her. When her son
and daughter were small, she would take them to the library in
the afternoons, and while they played in the kiddie room, she
would read up on disease. One day she was devouring an article
about the actress Sandy Duncan, whose doctors had initially
missed diagnosing a tumor behind her eye. "Suddenly a fear
came over me like I never knew was possible." She felt a twinge
in her own eye and could not get the actress's story out of her
mind. She began to have headaches. She made an appointment
with a neurologist, and although he saw no problem on her
physical exam, she begged for a CAT scan. Insurance didn't
cover all the cost, and Tom was furious.

In succession, she believed her gallbladder, an ulcer, her ovaries
troubled her. Her internist prescribed Valium and told her
to seek psychiatric help. She kept going for tests. "I've had so

much radiation I probably glow in the dark," Sara says. "The weird thing is I'm terrified of getting cancer from X rays. But I am addicted to getting the hundred percent reassurances that it's nothing." Once she felt something under her ear that seemed thicker on one side. The doctor shot dye into her. As the examination proceeded she kept asking herself, "Why am I doing this?" When the test result was normal, she wanted to look further, but the doctor refused. He was satisfied that she was well.

The worst part, she says, is what her obsessions have done to her family. "The last thing I wanted to do is screw up my kids. But I think I've made them nervous. My little girl has nose bleeds, and I keep thinking it is something serious and taking her to the doctor. Tom yells at me and says that I'm on the road to making her as loony as I am." Sara makes excuses for her husband. He works so hard and when he is sick he handles it well. That is why she thinks he doesn't have patience with her. "Not long ago he was diagnosed with diabetes, but you don't hear him complaining. When he doesn't feel well, he shuts the door, turns out the light, and wants to be left alone."

Three years ago, her father was stricken with Alzheimer's disease and she brought him to live with them. That caused many arguments between her and Tom, and when she decided to place her father in a nursing home, she thought things would improve. They didn't. Now that she wasn't caring for her father, she found herself worrying about her health again.

On Christmas Day Sara had an anxiety attack. She was certain she was in the midst of a stroke. "My husband didn't think it was real. When I go to doctors he doesn't even ask me what they say anymore. When I complain, he says, 'I don't have time for nonsense.'" Sara wants to get better, not for Tom but for the kids. She is taking a new antidepressant. "I know that a lot of this stuff about my health is psychological. Tom says I bring it on myself. It's probably true, but I can't help it. He doesn't believe me when I say I want it to be gone as much as he does."

*

Illness challenges any marriage. Couples fail to realize when they walk down the aisle that at some point in their life's journey, illness will strike, perhaps prematurely. Arthritis, cancer, heart disease, depression, any ailment that enters a relationship adds complication and stress.

Studies show that even in the most successful marriages, when one partner's health takes a turn for the worse, marital satisfaction often declines as well. Few spouses are prepared for the emotional demands of sickness, the adjustments, the turmoil, the fear, the exhaustion of picking up the pieces. The well spouse, particularly, is likely to report a decline in the quality of the relationship following illness, and there is an increased tendency toward divorce.

Hypochondria has to take an even bigger toll. When a spouse believes his partner is exaggerating the extent or severity of an illness, or questions its existence altogether, resentment is sure to follow. The well spouse doesn't know what is expected of him. Too often, lines of communication are crossed. But even though the terrain of hypochondria can be quite perilous, by recognizing the minefields, couples can discover islands of safety. If people are to grow old together, they must learn each other's language of illness and find new ways to communicate.

Josh and Renée: "I see sun. She sees clouds."

This couple's encounter with hypochondria almost destroyed their marriage. It was a journey begun in ignorance, guilt, and anger, but through love and an ardent desire to make the marriage work, they have come far in recognizing, understanding, and grappling with the problem. Their story could be a script for any couple battling hypochondria.

Renée: All my life I've been a nervous, worried person, but my problems exploded ten years ago after a close friend suddenly died of a blood clot. She was thirty-six, four years older than I. After Maura's death, I began experiencing vague but constant aches and pains. I am the daughter of a hypochondriac, so at first I joked with my husband that I was becoming my dad. But the problems persisted until I got to the point where I couldn't concentrate on anything else. I was irritable and depressed, and I missed Maura terribly. One day I had a big fight with my boss, which led to my first panic attack. I woke up in the middle of the night with this pain in my chest. I couldn't breathe.

Josh: That was the night before I had to defend my dissertation. I was upset that I couldn't go to the doctor with you. I thought about you all day. God knows how I got through the defense, but I did. I remember coming home afterward to find you remarkably calm. The doctor at the university clinic had said it was probably a muscle spasm and suggested you might benefit from seeing a mental health professional. You told me you had talked with the doctor about Maura's death and it had felt good. That was the first time, I think, we ever really looked at your physical problems in psychological terms.

Renée: A couple of years later, Josh got a job as a professor in Virginia. We bought a cabin outside the university town, and in the spring of 1990 I opened a dessert shop that had been a fantasy for ten years. Shortly after I went into business, my symptoms started up again. I had mystery pains throughout my body and numbness and tingling in my hands and feet. I was sure I had MS. I began reading up on the disease, talking to people about it, visualizing life in a wheelchair. I even mapped out the first floor of our house for ramps. About this time we took a vacation to Washington, D.C. I didn't have the strength to tour the city. I found myself sitting in the lobbies of museums while my husband did the sightseeing by himself.

Josh: This was truly a period of hell. I loved my job, you had the shop you had always dreamed of. But it made no difference. In fact, I remember thinking that the happiness associated with your new venture was related somehow to the symptoms, but I didn't know why. No doctor would say you had MS, and I kept telling you it was stress, that tightening up your muscles was causing you pain. You'd snap at me and ask how it could hurt so much if it's stress. You cried a lot, too.

Renée: After the Washington fiasco you practically ordered me to see a therapist. I think you said if I didn't, we were through. I kept arguing I wasn't crazy, that it really hurt. But I also could see how painful this was for you. I knew you loved me and were only telling me this for my own good.

Josh: You can't imagine how frustrating it is to live with someone who has this problem. Someone you deeply love. You get up in the morning and say, "It's a sunny day. Let's go out and do something." Then Renée comes down from bed and says: "It's not sunny. It's going to rain." "Wait a minute," you say, "it's not raining." She says, "But it's going to. I see a cloud." All of a sudden you realize she's using a totally different logic. It's as if you are not living in the same universe. And the worst part is you wake up to it day after day after day.

Renée: There came a point when I knew that if I didn't get better I would lose Josh. That I would have to let him go. This was a time of our lives that should have been glorious. He had a wonderful job doing research he loved, which allowed him to travel all over the world. He wanted me with him. I could have gone. We had made the decision early in our marriage not to have children, and I had the flexibility of my own business. But I was stuck in . . . I didn't know what. Then Josh got a chance to spend a summer in France. He begged me to go with him but ended up alone. I stayed home, worked in the shop, and moved from one malady to another.

Josh: What kept me going is that, through it all, once in a while I'd see that the Renée I married was still there. She'd laugh a certain laugh. We'd eat Chinese food in bed. She would forget her troubles — for five minutes, an hour. But then it was gone, and I got angry, worn down. What would really kill me is when I'd telephone her in the shop and ask how she was feeling and I'd hear *that voice*. I knew that the next moment, when we hung up, she'd be all sweetness and light with the customers. She seemed to save the worst for me, but I guess that's natural. Sometimes I'd look at her and say, "Okay, there's something wrong here. We're going to lick it." But I was frightened that we would never find out what it was and it would go on forever. No question, Renée's going into therapy saved us.

Renée: I had decided after the summer apart that we couldn't go on this way. I had to get well. If I couldn't I wanted to die so I could stop being such a burden. I began seeing a psychologist. At first we talked about the symptoms and Maura's death. Then we moved to the topic of my growing up in an alcoholic household. When my father wasn't drinking, he was decent enough. But when he was drunk, there would be yelling and screaming and everything was horrible. I spent my childhood never knowing whether things would be good or bad, and I never felt comfortable when things were good because I knew that sooner or later they'd be bad. The better things got, the more afraid I got. Then, in his fifties, my father developed gout, an inflammatory disease made worse by drinking. Things got even worse. Now he complained about pain all the time, but he still drank anyhow.

Josh: The thought of hypochondria occurred to me early on, but it really takes a while to realize the implications of it and what it really means. After her weekly sessions, we would talk. A few times we went to the therapist together. I knew about Renée's childhood, but I guess I never really understood the connection between what happened then and Renée's feeling the way she did as an adult. As I began to appreciate the emotional pain that was behind her symptoms, I became more tolerant. My background was more stable, but I could identify a little because my dad had a hot temper and would fly into rages. I've had to struggle with keeping my temper under control as an adult.

Renée: It wasn't as if the symptoms went away as soon as I started therapy. They'd come and go. I even tried Prozac for a while, but I felt that having to take a mind-altering drug meant I was weak, so I went off it. I'd be lying if I said I was totally better. I have occasional headaches and joint pains. I read about a middle-aged person with Alzheimer's or hear someone has cancer, and I start worrying. I see a few doctors, get a round of tests, but the difference is that now I have more control. I am able to say sooner, *Enough of this.* I realize earlier in the game that after a certain point, the search for a medical explanation causes more problems than it solves.

Josh: Life is definitely better. I'm realistic enough not to expect the problem to suddenly go away, never to darken our doorstep again. The problem was a long time in the making. I am willing to accept that we're in it for the long haul. We've suffered brain tumors, cancers, MS, strokes, and heart attacks together, and now hypochondria. But, somehow, this time it's an easier foe to battle. For the first time the problem feels real.

When Someone You Love Is Suffering

WHAT NOT TO SAY

• "Stop acting like a hypochondriac; there's nothing wrong with you!" No matter how strong the impulse, don't say this. It will hurt. Until the stigma of hypochondria disappears, it's like calling someone a liar or fraud. Besides, the person probably won't believe you. He or she is convinced something is wrong, and *something* is.

• "Snap out of it." This implies that the pain and suffering is within the person's control. When it comes to depression or anxiety disorders—the underlying cause in the majority of cases—one can't simply decide to get better and have the problem disappear.

• "You'd better get psychological help." The hypochondriac needs to cling to the belief that a physical disease lies at the root of her problem, specifically to avoid a psychiatric diagnosis. Depression or any other mental disorder is just one more ailment to worry about.

• "Don't worry; it's probably stress." Now we're getting somewhere, but only temporarily. A hypochondriac craves reassurance. Such words may comfort him for an hour, or maybe a day, then they are rejected. So whether you say them once or fifty times, the problem won't be solved.

WHAT YOU MAY SAY

• Tone is important. Be warm, empathic, and nonjudgmental. You don't want to convey anything that lowers self-esteem; it only makes the symptoms worse. But avoid coddling or playing into the fears.

• Try gently to link the symptoms to stress or conflict, especially if you can identify a recent event or strain that might have contributed to your loved one's state of mind. If you see that this approach isn't working, however, stop. Hypochondria is a long time in the making and doesn't go away easily.

• Relate an episode in your own life when emotional upheaval caused physical problems. During my bout with hypochondria, a friend told me how in the midst of a stressful period her eyelid wouldn't stop twitching. I also remember being comforted by an article I read about a woman whose hair thinned after her divorce.

• Encourage the person to verbalize health fears and problems, then respond with increased interest when talk turns to personal, as opposed to physical, issues. But be aware of your limits and patience. Don't try to play therapist or you'll find your emotions and energy being sapped. Your friend or relative needs to build confidence and self-reliance, not an unhealthy dependence on you.

CHAPTER NINE

Between Doctor and Patient

To write prescriptions is easy, but to come to an understanding with people is hard.

—Franz Kafka, "A Country Doctor"

THE FAMILY who can sympathize with the fears of hypochondria and look beyond complaints without anger and judgment may serve an important function, providing a loved one with strength to cope and courage to seek treatment. But as sensitive and accepting as family members may be to the plight of their hypochondriacal relative, they can go only so far in reassuring and guiding the sufferer through the daunting world of symptoms. That role properly belongs to the physician.

It only makes sense: the doctor who possesses knowledge of disease and medical science, who touches the body, observes the spirit, and can decipher the meanings of signs and sensations is best equipped to unlock the mysteries of hypochondria and work with the patient to separate the real from the symbolic, the alarming from the benign. Yet, although the doctor–patient relationship can be a source of support, knowledge, comfort, and healing, this rarely happens. In fact, quite the opposite occurs.

Hypochondriacs live in a world of cataclysmic uncertainty, that limbo of uncertain wellness. If they feel well, they cannot enjoy good health for fear that it will end. It is easy to see how, at times, illness might be preferable to the agony of incessant doubt. Hypochondriacs, as they waver in regard to the status of their health, need and depend on doctors, but they also fear their power. It is doctors who can grant the sick role, of which hypochondriacs are terrified, or take it away, about which they are tremendously ambivalent. No wonder that, when it comes to hypochondriacs and their doctors, there is little room for anything but disappointment.

For physicians, whose self-esteem is deeply rooted in their ability to cure disease and dispel symptoms, hypochondriacal patients can be a worst nightmare. They are difficult and demanding; they solicit reassurance only to reject it; and they switch doctors frequently. Anxious, even desperate, they demand relief from refractory symptoms or a definitive diagnosis, causing those who can't help them to feel baffled and impotent. Doctors can't wait to get rid of them, don't return their phone calls, refer them to other professionals, and under pressure to do *something*, may end up subjecting them to repeated diagnostic tests and invasive procedures.

The hypochondriacal patient, like a demanding, whiny child whom parents want to shut up, is skillful at getting doctors to do what she wants, or think she wants, and in the end, she is more miserable for the "cure." Patients with severe unexplained symptoms undergo two to three times as many operations as the average patient, which pushes up the likelihood that they will fall victim to iatrogenic illness, a disease caused by medical treatment. These are the all-too-frequent cases in which physicians, out of ignorance, greed, or the human wish to relieve anxiety, remove organs that should be left intact, mutilate healthy tissue, inject, implant, anesthetize unnecessarily, and inevitably injure, sometimes even kill, a certain percentage of their patients.

Mack Lipkin, Jr., an internist who directs primary care at New York University Medical Center, became interested in treating somatic disorders during the 1970s while working in a community hospital in rural North Carolina. "You could often tell the somatizing patients by looking at their bellies," said Dr. Lipkin, president of the American Academy on Physician and Patient, a professional society dedicated to enhancing the doctor–patient relationship. "These were people who had virtual warfare played out on their bodies. They had multiple scars from invasive, exploratory surgery; uteruses, gallbladders, parts of the intestines removed; operations for pinched nerves. Doctors were treating their symptoms without having objective evidence of disease," Dr. Lipkin says. And worst of all, the patients were still in pain.

How could something like this happen within a profession whose cornerstone principle is "First, do no harm"? Certainly, the physician who ends up cutting biologically healthy tissue does not wish to do harm. Most probably he started out acting in good faith. But in spite of efforts on both sides to communicate and get to the bottom of the suffering, something went terribly wrong. Thus, the difficult, troubled patient who is most in need of the physician's help becomes the one for whom medicine is least effective, sometimes even fatal.

A RELATIONSHIP AT THE CORE OF MEDICINE

The doctor–patient relationship has been described as the heart or art of medicine, and for all patients, sick or well, establishing a continuous and dependable alliance of mutual trust is the key to getting better care. When you are sick and frightened, much more than your body is exposed. The seriously ill or seriously worried patient entrusts life and limb to the doctor's hands; in turn, the doctor proffers expertise and compassion. Whether or not the doctor likes you or you like the doctor, he or she has a professional obligation: to make an accurate diagnosis and prescribe a course of treatment that alleviates your pain and suffering. There is no getting away from this. No matter how many times a patient switches doctors, no matter if the patient is an alcoholic, drug abuser, sexual molester, or hypochondriac, the relationship exists.

In the best of all worlds, what transpires between doctor and patient becomes crucial to the healing process. As the renowned psychiatrist Michael Balint wrote in *The Doctor, His Patient, and the Illness*, "By far, the most frequently used drug in general practice is the doctor himself." The manner in which a doctor gives of himself—his tone, his touch, the atmosphere in which a "drug" is dispensed and taken—seems to have as much, if not more, therapeutic value as the treatment itself.

The positive impact of this relationship is well documented. Balint, who devoted his career to helping physicians understand the psychological implications of their interactions with patients, was not the first to note the power of the so-called placebo effect, in which the patient improves even without treatment because he believes the physician is helping him. Since the days of Hippocrates, enlightened practitioners have recognized that their behavior alone, even the simplest laying on of hands, could wield curative power. Long before the arrival of vaccines, antibiotics, and other modern miracle drugs, patients were visiting their doctors and managing to get well.

Even in our present age of biotechnology, the human dimension of healing remains one of medicine's most potent weapons. Proven treatments are enhanced when patients have an optimistic doctor in whom they trust. New findings, in fact, show the effect of the doctor–patient relationship to be far stronger than originally thought. The placebo response has been demonstrated in 30 to 60 percent of patients who receive medicine or other therapeutic treatments.

Despite the proven effectiveness of placebo treatment, medical investigators tend to denigrate it because it confounds their ability to isolate the specific benefits of particular drugs and therapies. Because placebo responses originate in the mind, if patients report relief from them, doctors interpret the recovery as evidence that the pain had no physiological basis, says Andrew Weil. "Instead of paying enthusiastic attention to the placebo response as a major clue to the interworkings of mind and body, and as a potential key to activating true healing, most doctors and researchers regard it as a nuisance, as something to be screened out or eliminated." Dr. Weil, a Harvard-trained physician who writes extensively about holistic medicine, is only one of a vocal minority of doctors who believe that the medical community has yet to appreciate that the placebo phenomenon is the most effective, life-enhancing medicine doctors can offer their patients.

The role a physician plays in eliciting the placebo response is indeed mysterious. The improvement or disappearance of symptoms, which occurs after one takes a pill or adheres to a regimen that has no demonstrable medical value, has long been attributed to the magical expectations of medicine. But why does the effect continue to be observed in a population of patients who consistently question the motivation, level of caring, and expertise of the physician?

In *The Silent World of Doctor and Patient*, Jay Katz, a physician who left clinical medicine to teach medical ethics at Yale Law School, suggests that the power of the placebo may be unconsciously mediated. Through personal suffering, from illnesses and the death of loved ones, patients on a conscious level are aware of the shortcomings of medicine and the fallibility of physicians. "They may hope for miracles but they are also resigned to the reality of their rarity." Yet despite this awareness, embedded in the unconscious is the image of physicians as miracle workers, not unlike the fantasied all-caring parents of infancy. "Medicine, after all, was born in magic and religion," Katz writes, "and the doctor-priest-magician-parent unity that persists in the patients' unconscious cannot be broken."

When the relationship works, when there is what Katz calls a positive transference, what follows is a therapeutic alliance, a bond that is essential to healing. It is not physicians' promises to do the impossible that patients find so comforting. What patients have sought in doctors since antiquity, Katz says, is "the promise of nonabandonment, of a caring and honest presence that can underlie faith, hope, and reassurance in the face of limitations of medical knowledge."

But what happens when the alliance doesn't work? If doctors

themselves can act as placebos and produce dramatic cures, it follows that, like any potent medication, what they do or say can have adverse reactions. In fact, the influence a doctor has on a patient's illness has as much toxic capability as cortisone, chemotherapy, or any other drug used in medical practice. Yet as Balint noted in the very first edition of *The Doctor, His Patient, and the Illness*, published in 1957, the lack of information about the possible hazards of this "most frequently used drug" is "appalling and frightening," a problem which, some forty years later, is only beginning to be addressed. He writes, "No guidance whatever is contained in any textbook as to the dosage in which the doctor should prescribe himself, in what form, how frequently, what his curative and his maintenance doses should be . . . or the various allergic conditions met in individual patients which ought to be watched carefully."

That the interaction of a doctor with his patient affects treatment for better or worse is beyond doubt. That this relationship is of particular importance to those suffering from hypochondria makes sense because the anxious, frightened patient, with his sensitivity to bodily changes and bits and pieces of medical knowledge, is the one most likely to get lost in the high-tech jungle of clinical care. The hypochondriacal patient needs a conscientious and compassionate physician, ideally someone who can validate pain and suffering, tolerate uncertainty, and protect him from harm, but at the same time recognize when to turn on the heat in a biomedical investigation. Too often, however, any hope for a collaborative alliance turns into a power struggle over whether symptoms are organic or not. The doctor–patient relationship, which could help demystify symptoms and alleviate fears, instead becomes untenable: the doctor is perplexed and frustrated, unable to interpret what's wrong; the patient, rejected and misunderstood, is generally worse off than before.

The questions and dilemmas posed by Balint about the doctor-patient relationship continue to perplex. "Why, so often," Balint asked, 'does the prescription not work as intended? What causes the patient and his doctor unnecessary suffering, irritation, and fruitless efforts? Why do these two people who need each other speak two different languages?"

To understand what went wrong between hypochondriacs and their doctors and begin to repair the damage, it is important to try to see the problems from both sides.

FROM THE PATIENT'S POINT OF VIEW

Physicians, long the darlings of the health care system, have fallen from grace, and not just in the eyes of hypochondriacs. For years medical consumers hadn't wanted to upset their doctors who, they were afraid, would refuse to take care of them. Then came the 1960s and the toppling of many icons of authority. The era of unchallenged faith in the medical profession, deference to medical authority, and the belief that the doctor knows best, which had flourished in the post–World War II period, was replaced by the era of patients' rights.

Thanks to the ability of computers to analyze vast quantities of data, the public gained awareness of the inexactitude of tests and of wide variations in procedures and costs. Think tanks began churning out "outcome studies," sorting what treatments do and don't work. Doctors who had long managed to evade economic forces became accountable. At the same time, patients found themselves facing restrictive medical coverage, higher deductibles, and greater out-of-pocket expenses.

Disillusioned with high-tech, high-cost medicine and empowered with knowledge, medical consumers finally let it be known: they were tired of paternalistic, power-mongering doctors. Doctor-bashing became not only acceptable, but fashionable. As the trust between physician and patient continued to erode, the doctor-patient dyad was put under the microscope of academic scrutiny. Researchers set out to examine the dynamics of this relationship, developing an entirely new discipline to assess the causes of patient dissatisfaction. Study after study revealed that medical consumers were unhappy, not with their doctors' proficiency but with their people skills. Doctors didn't listen very well, were insensitive to patients' needs, weren't respectful, and communicated poorly.

In a well-known study of patient malaise, investigators examined more than a thousand grievance letters to a large Michigan health maintenance organization. The most common complaints concerned the physicians' lack of compassion and the brusque speech of the medical staff. Patients complained that physicians never looked at them during an entire office visit, made them feel humiliated, and used medical jargon that left them confused.

Other studies of medical encounters uncovered these problems:

• Physicians on average interrupt patients eighteen seconds into their opening statements.

• Patients get the chance to tell their doctors fewer than half of their complaints.

• Fifty percent of the time doctor and patient do not agree on the main problem.

• The typical general practitioner spends only seven minutes with the average patient, down from eleven minutes twenty years ago.

• A significant proportion of patients misunderstand medical advice or forget what doctors tell them within moments after leaving the office.

Despite the medical community's fear of litigation and huge malpractice premiums, the harshest criticisms lobbed at physicians do not involve incompetence. Mistakes, misdiagnoses, and foul-ups occur; the public, perhaps cognizant that for every life lost, hundreds of thousands are saved and prolonged, seems willing to cut doctors some slack on this front. But if medical consumers are not taking action to shield themselves from bad doctors, what protection do they have from the subtle slights, insinuations, and insensitivity that do not make headlines?

Like the doctor who blithely told my friend on a Friday that her breast biopsy contained "a few abnormal cells." Not until she telephoned the office on Tuesday morning did a nurse inform her, "Oh, yes, that turned out to be fine." Or the story of a social worker who, struggling with cancer phobia, discovers a lump on the back of her neck. Her internist tells her it is a small calcification, nothing to worry about. "A little extra knowledge bone," he jokes, but she can't stop touching it. She decides to consult an ear, nose, and throat specialist for extra reassurance. "I tried to alert the doctor to how anxious I was. I wanted him to know I kept focusing on the thing and that I was making myself crazy." This doctor rolled his eyes, conveying the clear message that he was not her man. He was not going to walk her through this. "He minimized everything I felt," she says.

Physicians themselves, even some of the most old-fashioned and conformist, have become critical of their profession. Nearly half of American doctors say they regret their career choice and would opt against medical school if they had to do it again. Edward Rosenbaum, former chief of rheumatology at Oregon Health Sciences University, does a great deal of soul-searching in *A Taste of My Own Medicine*, which was made into the 1991 film *The Doctor*. In it, William Hurt plays a surgeon immune to his patients' hunger for emotional support until he himself gets throat cancer. The film is based on Dr. Rosenbaum's experiences after he was diagnosed, at age seventy, with cancer of the larynx. On becoming a patient, Dr. Rosenbaum experiences the impersonal and distancing care of his profession and is personally and professionally transformed.

In one of the book's many poignant vignettes, Dr. Rosenbaum undergoes a CAT scan before beginning radiation. As he lies on the narrow steel table, without even a sheet beneath him, two young technicians begin to discuss his anatomy. "It won't work, too thick-necked," one comments as she attempts to place a large plastic block under his neck. "Damn," the other says. "Now his big shoulders stick up in the way." Driving home after the procedure, Rosenbaum recalls the scene, which brings back painful memories. A little boy trying on a suit, he hears the salesman say to his mother, "Won't fit. Too thick-necked," at which his mother storms out of the store. He is also reminded of Hazel, a former patient. When she was thirteen, Hazel accompanied her mother to a doctor's office and overheard him say, "She's got big boobs for a little kid." The insult remained with her the rest of her life. Another example, Dr. Rosenbaum sadly reflects, "of a member of my profession talking about patients as if they weren't there."

That there are less-than-caring doctors out there isn't new. The question for us is, Why do hypochondriacs all too frequently seek out doctors who are wrong for them? Like people who wouldn't want to join any club that would have them as members, they gravitate to physicians who ignore their individuality, make no effort to relate warmly, and focus on their own agenda. One possibility is that hypochondriacs mistake authoritarian for omniscient. If they find a doctor who listens empathetically but doesn't offer them a firm diagnosis or refer them for yet another test, they begin to doubt the doctor's competence. As the social worker with the cancer fixation explains, "I start off on a good foot with the doctor, but if I'm reassured I'm in good health, I quickly manage to find something wrong. I decide the doctor is too young to have had enough experience. Or too old to be up on the latest research. I don't know what it is I want . . . and somehow we never click."

When it comes to my own experiences with the medical profession, one encounter that seems to exemplify the sorry state of hypochondriacs and their doctors stands out. The incident took place during the period that became the wellspring for this book. I had been upset about my painful wrist, and a gentle orthopedist—whose reassurances, of course, I rejected—suggested I consult a hand surgeon, "the best in his field." Let's call him Dr. Gold. I went to see Dr. Gold, lugging X rays, bone scan and medical records. Silently he examined my wrists and evaluated

their motility with a tape measure. "The left one is twenty percent less flexible than the right," he told me.

Validation of *a* problem, but *what* problem? I thought. "What
does that mean?" I asked.

"Don't know," he replied. "It's not mechanical or structural.
There's nothing I can do for you."

Nervously, I mustered up courage to ask what had been prey-
ing on my mind. "Is this possibly the sign of an early rheumato-
logical problem, a disease like lupus?"

The doctor, unmistakably uncomfortable, shrugged, looked
me in the eye, and said flatly, "Could be."

I stood up and suddenly felt faint. The room went dark. I fell
to the floor in a cold sweat. I must have been out for a few seconds. When I opened my eyes, a nurse was wiping my brow
with a cloth. Where was Dr. Gold? Mortified, I told the nurse I
could drive home. She asked me for ninety-five dollars. The
hand and wrist specialist had done his job.

The episode with Dr. Gold left me feeling not only confused
about my medical status, but negated, flawed, and crazy. The
hypochondriac who must be punished, not worthy of checking
up on. Yet once I put my fragile ego aside it occurred to me that
even mean old Dr. Gold might be a victim, a symptom of the ills
of a health care system that is set up to fail.

We patients, hypochondriacs in particular, expect so much
from the medical profession. For starters, we want our doctors
to diagnose us accurately, prescribe appropriately, and make us
better, if not well. On top of that, they are supposed to instill
trust and confidence, rekindle hope, and relieve fear and doubt.
Now they are being asked to spot emotional problems and prof-
fer psychiatry as well. Not every doctor can have all the skills.
The all-around physician who can make you laugh as she tends
to a sore throat or sprained knee in the examining room may
not be the crackerjack surgeon you want in the operating room
when a child needs an appendectomy or a parent faces heart
surgery.

Somewhere down the line, society made some errors in assigning godlike characteristics to doctors and promoting the idea that they are infallible miracle workers. By becoming the dispensers of the overblown promises of high-tech science, physicians, as Katz points out, "all too unquestionably accepted the burden of being healers to all the ills of mankind." Small wonder that the doctor–gods of technology, whose power has been cloaked in secrecy and mystique, would come tumbling from their pedestal. Sadly, the casualty of the demythologizing has been the doctor-patient relationship. Patients see themselves as duped victims, the doctors as evil perpetrators, when the truth is that doctors are the all-too-human prey of a culture that expected more than medicine could deliver.

Patients, no less than doctors, have been seduced by the biomedical model and send signals that they expect to be treated accordingly. In this age of high-tech care, physicians have a hard time convincing some patients that the best thing to do is watch and wait. One half of those who consult a physician anticipate a test; three-quarters want medicine, according to a study by Kurt Kroenke, an internist affiliated with the Uniformed Services University in Bethesda, Maryland. Sometimes "it is simpler to give the patients what they want," Dr. Kroenke says. "The reflex of many doctors, still, is to schedule a lab test or reach for the prescription pad."

In addition to feeling some compassion for the godlike roles we ascribe to physicians, it can be helpful for hypochondriacs to realize how the "difficult patient" affects a doctor's ability to do good.

FROM THE DOCTOR'S POINT OF VIEW

It is not entirely a doctor's fault when a relationship goes sour, as it does in as many as one of every six medical encounters. Difficult patients, often viewed as demanding, dependent, manipulative, self-destructive, seductive, hysterical, and hypochondriacal, are not merely those with whom the physician may have an occasional personality clash. They are, in the words of one doctor, those "whom most physicians dread."

Such patients, who have been described in medical literature as "hateful," are capable of mobilizing intense and disturbing feelings of rage, despair, impotence, and downright malice in their doctors. Even more confusing is that the wish to avoid, get rid of, or transfer the patient may alternate with feelings of love, sexual arousal, wishes to rescue the patient or give him exceptionally good care.

A doctor's perception that a patient is difficult inevitably leads to burnout that affects the care the patient receives. Physicians who cannot identify the source of their anger often act out their feelings with their patients by overprescribing medication, asking for a larger than usual number of consults, proposing aggressive diagnostic procedures, or simply being rude.

In a 1993 study of one thousand patients who visited four academic medical centers, investigators found that those whom doctors rated as "difficult" — roughly 15 percent of the sample — were twice as likely as less troublesome patients to suffer from a psychiatric disorder. They were more prone to depression, substance abuse, eating disorders, hypochondria, and other somatic behaviors. Not surprisingly, difficult patients were as miserable as their physicians were frustrated; they made twice as many office and emergency room visits as other patients, yet reported greater dissatisfaction with medical care.

Most clinicians would agree that of all the possible chemistries between provider and patient, few are as combustible as that of the hypochondriac and her doctor. Hypochondriacs make their doctors feel persecuted. Their relentless attachment to symptoms, perceived self-centeredness, mistrust, irrationality, and clingy demandingness create an urgent atmosphere that threatens both patience and authority. The dynamic is worthy of study because, in the words of Don Lipsitt, chief of psychiatry at Mount Auburn Hospital in Cambridge, Massachusetts, "in an intense way, it highlights everything that can possibly go wrong with the doctor–patient relationship."

The majority of patients, when told that a problem is benign or not serious, react with relief. So does the hypochondriac, but only temporarily. The reassurance may last hours, days, even weeks, but inevitably the doubt resurfaces and, in the end, the hypochondriac discounts any shred of security a physician's words or a diagnostic test can offer. Worse, patients may have such a strong attachment to symptoms that at first signs of improvement, new symptoms appear. "The hypochondriac's doubt has an exact complement in that of the practitioner, who knows at heart that, in spite of trying to convince the hypochondriac to the contrary, he can never be completely certain himself that the patient doesn't have the disease," writes Arthur Kleinman in *The Illness Narratives*. "Clinical work is a matter of probabilities, as is biology, unlike physics. . . . The hypochondriacal patient elicits the physician's doubt and makes him decidedly uncomfortable; perhaps this is one of the reasons why physicians often find such patients irksome."

Yet not every clinician is equally nonplussed by difficult hypochondriacal patients. Certain doctors seem to possess innate characteristics that make them prey for hypochondriacs and predispose them to enter long-term, counterproductive relationships marked by excessive testing, unnecessary hospitalizations, and iatrogenic disasters. The physician who requires omnipotence and uses the admiration of patients to gratify that need may find that the hypochondriacal patient taps into his own conflicts concerning dependency, insecurity, and anger.

Charles Ford, discussing the psychology of physicianhood in *Illness as a Way of Life*, suggests that, like hypochondriacal patients, physicians exhibit a high frequency of obsessive-compulsive characteristics. Physicians tend to be exacting and perfectionistic. They are taught to be meticulous in examining patients, leaving no stone unturned. Indeed, the ability to inhibit personal gratification and control one's emotions and vulnerability is regarded as a necessary virtue of physicians, perhaps one reason they have more than their share of hidden troubles. They suffer from higher rates of depression, suicide, addiction, and marital discord than the general population and are five times as likely to abuse sedatives or tranquilizers. Defending against many of the same anxieties experienced by their patients, they tend to erect counterphobic defenses, particularly against dependency needs and fear of disease. This can make them uncomfortable with and unsympathetic to the needs of clingy, demanding hypochondriacal patients and unable to establish a trusting bond.

Of course, what goes awry for hypochondriacs and their doctors has *something* to do with who the doctors are. But the barriers to a productive relationship have more to do with the manner in which physicians are trained and molded by their clinical experience, which has little to do with the mystical qualities of the doctor–patient bond.

Most doctors start out with a sense of intellectual excitement and a genuine desire to help others. They then suffer the trauma of residency training—sleep deprivation, isolation, menial chores, low wages, demanding hours, and bureaucratic politics, which quickly effaces idealism.

Terry Mizrahi, who spent three years observing the house staff of the department of internal medicine at a large southern university medical center, says it is primarily this tough induction into the practice of hospital-based and clinical medicine that causes doctors to lose their compassion. In his classic book, *Getting Rid of Patients: Contradictions in the Socialization of Physicians*, Mizrahi describes the socialization process within a rigid, hierarchical system that devalues patients. The system abets the acquisition of what Mizrahi calls a getting rid of patients (GROP) mentality. The GROP mentality thrives in the atmosphere of the overcrowded, understaffed public hospital, where the sheer numbers of patients and shortage of beds force the residents to dispose of patients as quickly as possible. It is a system in which those admitted to the emergency room are called hits, train wrecks, scumbags, dirtbags, crocks, GOMERs (get out of my emergency room), and SHPOS (subhuman pieces of shit). In this system, the most efficient resident is applauded for "dispo-ing" (discharging) and "turfing" (transferring). Peer allegiance becomes all-important, while patients, reduced to the enemy, become targets on which to vent hostility and frustration, especially if they are difficult to control. The ideal patient is a compliant person with an interesting disease the doctor can cure. Or as one resident put it, someone who is "sick as shit and gets better."

The detachment process that feeds the GROP mind-set is intensified by medical jargon that further creates distance and separation from patients. The hospital setting is one in which a diagnosis is a DRG and disease an ICD-10 code. Physicians speak in an idiom that is not only frightening to patients but condescending and insensitive: the LOL (little old lady) in room 230. In describing the public hospital as a dumping ground for unwanted patients, Mizrahi recounts a gripe session among hospital interns irritated about the number of nursing home admittances. One complains about getting "stuck" with "five dehydrated UTIs" (nursing home patients with urinary tract infections). "There's not much you can do. If there's ever going to be a *disaster* you'll have it with them." His colleague sympathizes. "There's no satisfaction . . . no reward. Their IVs run out, and it takes a half hour to stick them again. Then just as you're ready to discharge them, they develop bedsores."

Perri Klass, in *A Not Entirely Benign Procedure*, an account of her clinical training at Harvard Medical School, discusses the penchant among students and faculty for the fascinoma— "oma," the suffix for tumor—a one-of-a-kind, difficult-to-diagnose disease. This is a subculture in which the excellent diagnostician is held in the highest esteem, and the "best and the brightest" are pushed toward specialization and research. The general attitude, she says, is that "rare diseases are somehow real prizes in the grab bag of clinical medicine." Dr. Klass worries whether the emphasis on great cases will cause medical students to stop caring so much for patients with mundane illnesses, or at least give less credit to doctors who concentrate on them. And if doctors who treat bread-and-butter ailments are getting low marks, how can the patients who suffer them be getting the attention they deserve? And what of those pariahs whose "medical" problems turn out to be emotional?

Until a few years ago, hypochondriacs and somatizers were not part of the medical school curriculum. *Maybe* doctors read one or two paragraphs about them in a textbook. The big shock comes in the real world when these patients make up one third to one half of their practices. "A week doesn't go by that someone doesn't come in begging me to perform a hysterectomy I don't think is necessary or I get a hysterical call about a chronic yeast infection the patient is certain is something else," says a New Jersey gynecologist. In medical school, he says, they don't prepare you. "I did a rotation in psychiatry, but we learned about schizophrenic and psychotic patients, not neurotic ones. Who was to know I'd be dealing with them practically on a daily basis? I don't know how to help them, and to avoid an unproductive relationship for both of us, I either refer them or get them to abandon me."

The prevailing attitude seems to be that it is one thing to *recognize* anxiety or illness phobia, quite another to *confront* the patient with the finding. Many physicians interviewed for this book admitted that they virtually never make a "mental" diagnosis. On one hand, they said, they fear offending the patient if they suggest that there is a psychiatric problem. On the other, they dread the prospect of opening a Pandora's box by broaching emotional topics themselves. Why, these doctors wonder, are such patients wasting their valuable time? Hypochondriacs, depressives, neurotics, have always belonged in therapy, the "soft" side of medicine.

A psychiatric diagnosis is not something about which patient and doctor can talk comfortably. A number of insurance companies print forms with diagnostic boxes in which a doctor can designate a suspected psychiatric illness like depression or panic disorder. A few even list hypochondria as an option. "I might think it, but I've never checked it," said one internist. "I would first have to ask patients questions like, Do you believe you suffer from an undiagnosed disease? Are you preoccupied by a fear of death? And if they said yes, I'm not sure it is an area I would feel qualified to deal with." But it is not simply patient reaction that causes a doctor to steer clear of a psychiatric diagnosis, it is the insurance companies. "I'm afraid to put down anything other than a physical problem, even when I recognize depression, hypochondria, or what have you," another internist commented. "It is unlikely that mental problems will get covered at the same rate as medical ones, and I don't want to risk it for me or the patient."

HEALTH REFORM'S CONFUSING IMPACT

As the nation's health care delivery system is torturously transformed, physicians are not the only ones who have to make adjustments. Patients do, too. Research reveals that some 25 percent of them consume 50 percent of all services, much of which may be inappropriate. These so-called high utilizers suffer psychiatric problems that more than half the time doctors fail to identify. So while the country moves toward a more "universal" system of health care, hypochondriacs and somatizers, patients deemed to be "misusing" the system, face the prospect of constraints.

The promise that biotechnology would relieve uncertainty and lessen doubt has had a backlash effect on doctors and patients alike. Lured by state-of-the-art science and lofty incomes, physicians abandoned primary care for specialties like neurosurgery and cardiology. Then, after years of out-of-control medical costs, both government and industry have combined to slash expenditures and reform the system. The problem, policy analysts conclude, is too much emphasis on medical heroics and not enough on preventive care and old-fashioned doctoring.

There is a huge surplus of specialists—about 70 percent of all physicians—and not enough doctors practicing frontline medicine. These specialists have acquired high-tech skills for procedures many will never use. Furthermore, they find themselves herded, along with their patients, into a maze of preferred provider networks and health maintenance organizations.

Medical consumers are understandably confused. Bombarded with bewildering terms like "managed competition" and "risk selection," patients feel frightened as they watch their options narrow and confront ever more baffling decisions about care. While many may pine for a romanticized vision of the GP who made house calls and managed family problems, as Robin Toner points out in *The New York Times*, the phrase "the best in the field" still has a powerful allure. Not only do today's patients have to "worry about losing a primary care doctor with whom they have developed a long-standing relationship—they may worry about never getting to see the specialist they want."

Also muddying the picture is the contentious issue of alternative medicine. What is and what isn't? The main characteristic appears to be that the "alternative" methodology hasn't been subjected to rigorous scientific review, but that, too, is changing as the National Institutes of Health attempts to bring unconventional treatments into the mainstream. Since 1992, its Office of Alternative Medicine, established under a congressional directive, has been evaluating the merits of dozens of alternative therapeutic practices, from music therapy for victims of brain injury to yoga for obsessive-compulsive disorder.

The probable merging of traditional and alternative systems of care is exciting and long overdue, but revolutions are always perplexing for those in their midst. Indeed, the same Harvard survey which discovered that one in three Americans rely to some extent on nontraditional methods to treat their illnesses also found that the same patients were afraid to tell their regular doctors about their unprescribed activities. This love-hate ambivalence toward medical authority is not unlike the conflicting emotions a rebellious adolescent might feel toward parental control.

One visible candidate for sacrificial lamb to medical turmoil is Gilda Radner, whose tragic and perhaps avoidable death from ovarian cancer at forty-two should convince any hypochondriac, whether doctor-shopper or avoider, of the merit of the doctor-patient bond. The comedienne, who endured nearly a year of fatigue, abdominal pain, and medical tests before her cancer was detected, might still be alive if she had had that special doctor with whom she could have forged an intimate relationship. Like many of us, Radner did not have a physician who knew her family medical history. If she'd had one, he might have realized the significance of an aunt, a cousin, and possibly her grandmother having suffered from the disease—information that might have saved her life. Instead, Radner traveled the medical carousel of gastroenterologists, gynecologists, internists, and holistic healers, who, she felt, paid the most attention, collecting diagnoses that ranged from the Epstein-Barr virus to depression to constipation. She experimented with all kinds of medicines, food supplements, and concoctions, although at one point, when her alternative doctor suggested a colonic, a huge enema, to clean out her bowel, thinking it was too "weird," she returned to the mainstream. The next internist gave her a shot of gamma globulin to help alleviate symptoms of Epstein-Barr, then felt her stomach and wrote a prescription for laxatives.

"Suddenly I began to wonder how to please so many people," Radner wrote in her autobiography, *It's Always Something,* completed before her death in 1991. "Do I take the magnesium citrate? What about the coffee enema? . . . Do I tell the doctors about each other? East meets West in Gilda's body: Western medicine down my throat, Eastern medicine up my butt."

The changing face of medicine presents unique opportunities. But until competing interest groups can compromise on a clearer national vision, fragmentation will continue to spawn inconsistent medical messages and contradictory impulses that could prove detrimental to health. At the moment, there seem to be two trends developing and their impact on the worried well remains uncertain. One reflects the biopsychosocial approach with its emphasis on the whys and whats of ailments, prevention, and support of behavioral changes that will lead to improvements in health. The other trend is more sinister. Sickness, after all, is a business, and as American health care moves aggressively into managed care mergers and networks, time constraints and money pressures on health care professionals will undoubtedly increase. Many fear that the job of managed care physicians will become that of a policeman, to weed out somatizers and limit access to second opinions, specialists, and procedures. There has been a lot of talk about the economic benefits of teaching doctors to recognize the hidden emotional problems of their patients, but the additional training of professionals to treat these conditions may not be cost-effective. The result may be to deny hypochondriacs medical access. Somatization and hypochondria are tremendously time-consuming and vexing problems for physicians, but how detrimental are these elusive maladies, really, in the grand scheme of things?

CREATING COST-CONSCIOUS DOCTORS WITH A HUMAN TOUCH

No question, digging beneath symptoms and addressing the cause of a hypochondriac's unhappiness demand lots of time, energy, and patience from doctors. The counterargument, of course, is that "quality" time with troubled patients early on reduces costs down the line. Dr. Mack Lipkin, who specializes in treating the "difficult" patients other doctors refer, spends a minimum of four one-hour sessions with such new clients. A physical exam is done in each case, but more important, there is listening, talking, easing fears, encouraging, and in the end coming up with a plan that puts a halt to doctor-shopping and repetitive procedures and tests that generate costs and cause harm. "Most of these patients are fundamentally healthy," Dr. Lipkin says.

"What they need is psychological growth or adjustment, a new method of relating that doesn't involve illness and fear." If it is done correctly, he says, "a collaborative doctor-patient relationship should allow for a corrective emotional experience that will have a spillover effect into other parts of their lives."

As Dr. Michael Balint realized years ago, the ability of doctors to perceive and address patients' needs is not always a gift, nor are these skills necessarily acquired through experience and intuition. But the art of the doctor-patient interaction can be effectively taught. Debra Roter, a professor at Johns Hopkins School of Hygiene and Public Health who has made a career of studying the doctor-patient relationship, says that when doctors are trained to better recognize and handle patients' emotional stress, the consequences are far-reaching. A controlled study of 648 patients cared for by 68 family practitioners and internists found that as patients became more willing to disclose sensitive, personal information, psychiatric symptoms and overall disability decreased. Physicians who gained skills in treating emotional problems felt a greater sense of personal satisfaction than did those in the control group. What surprised researchers was that the patients' improvement could not be attributed to a specific mental health treatment. Rather, it was the act of engagement itself that appeared to be therapeutic. Simple, humane gestures — active listening, acknowledging sadness and isolation, reinterpreting signs and symptoms, becoming an advocate for the patient — appeared to be the active elements in the recovery process. And though some physicians initially worried that getting more emotionally involved would open a "Pandora's box leading to unmanageable and interminable visits," the fears proved to be unfounded. Patients under the care of trained doctors were able to reduce emotional stress for as long as six months following consultation, with virtually no increase in the frequency or duration of their visits.

Dr. Kurt Kroenke, like other advocates of psychiatric training for general practitioners, believes that the tremendous improvements in psychiatric diagnosis and pharmacology should make it possible for family doctors to treat patients' psychosocial problems, in tandem with their medical complaints, 80 to 90 percent of the time. "We are not asking these doctors to treat schizophrenia and suicidal depression," he insists. Patients who wouldn't dream of seeing a therapist are much less resistant to having emotional problems addressed or taking medication prescribed by a nonpsychiatrist. After all, he says, these patients have presumably developed a relationship with the doctor, and they are already there. In addition, when doctors become confident about working with emotional issues, they order far fewer medical tests and procedures, which streamlines costs and avoids iatrogenic complications. Compare the price of a $600 CAT scan or a $1,000 MRI with a $75 counseling session.

Merely supporting a doctor's intuition that a given patient is experiencing distress seems to go a long way. In an oft-cited study, psychiatric researchers at the University of Arkansas Medical School asked family physicians to refer to them patients with long-standing, unexplained physical complaints. After evaluating the referrals, the researchers sent consultation letters to fifty-six physicians, confirming the diagnosis of somatization disorder in seventy patients. The letter, which included recommendations for treatment, was associated with a 50 percent reduction in annual median charges for medical costs per patient, which remained stable for two years. More important, a year later nearly all the patients reported that they felt better physically and emotionally.

Granted, nonpsychiatrists have to be wary of applying "cookbook" medicine in the treatment of mental distress. But the push to include mental health within general medicine has already produced some promising developments. Consider the SF-36 questionnaire being tested in medical settings, which measures physical well-being and quality of life. It gives doctors clues about how a patient is doing emotionally, how a disease might be affecting her relationships, job performance, and state of mind.

PRIME MD (Primary Care Evaluation of Mental Disorders) is another new procedure, developed by Dr. Kroenke and Dr. Robert L. Spitzer, a professor of psychiatry at Columbia University, to assist physicians in recognizing mood, anxiety, eating, alcohol, and somatoform disorders, problems most commonly seen in primary care settings. Medical schools are changing, too. Hoping to produce more empathic graduates with better interpersonal skills, they are redesigning curricula, mandating courses on the doctor–patient relationship, or requiring students to teach preventive medicine in public schools.

Perhaps the most pronounced changes have come in the field of family practice, which prides itself on producing compassionate family- and community-oriented physicians, well rounded in just about every health issue individuals and families face from birth to death. Family practice grew during the 1960s as an alternative to internal medicine, which many believed had become more organ than person centered. Trained in pediatrics, obstetrics, and gynecology, family practitioners differ from general practitioners in that they have three years of speciality training after medical school while GPs have one.

"We try to impart in residents that you don't have a piece of skin, a heart, or a stomach walking into the office. You are treating a human being, and what is happening to this person physically affects, and is affected by, what's going on psychologically," says Dr. Joseph Connelly, who has directed the family practice residency program at St. Josephs Medical Center in Stamford, Connecticut, for the last fourteen years.

The manner in which medicine is taught to residents at St. Josephs, one of three sites where Dr. Brian Fallon's ongoing hypochondria study is based, is a good example of just how well the merger of psychiatry, behavioral sciences, and primary care can work. While the majority of family practice residencies utilize mental health professionals, primarily psychologists or social workers, St. Josephs is one of a small number of residency programs nationwide to have a psychiatrist on staff. Dr. Robert Feinstein, a psychiatrist whose formal title is director of behavioral science, divides his time between St. Josephs and private practice. Part of his job at the hospital is to teach residents the basics of psychiatry—diagnosis, treatment, and short-term counseling—and to support them in their relationships with patients.

"When a doctor feels 'I can't do it, I don't know how to do it, I can't make this person feel better,' " that's where psychotherapeutic intervention comes in, Dr. Feinstein says. The philosophy, based on Balint's teachings, is for practitioners to be aware of their ambivalent feelings and to know when prejudice is getting in the way of treatment. "It's okay to say to a colleague 'I hate this patient,' but that sentiment doesn't belong in the room with the patient." For the most part, psychotherapeutic interventions, in which the mental health practitioner meets with the physician and patient, are limited to five sessions, after which the physician continues with the case or decides to refer the patient.

Dr. Lipkin, who spends a great deal of his time helping residents work with hypochondriacal and somatizing patients, says that the physicians have a common fear: What if a patient really is, or gets, sick? "It is certainly true that a tendency to somatize by no means confers immunity to physical disease. Somatizers die too," Dr. Lipkin says, and one must always be alert to new symptoms and changes in behavior patterns. But, he adds, in case after case, when somebody has what turns out to be a serious organic illness, the presentation is different even if the problem is in the same organ system. He tells the story of Marianne, a woman in her thirties, who for years complained of colonic pain and had a recurring phobia about blood in her stools. She ran the gamut of New York doctors and emergency rooms, subjecting herself to test after test. "The year before she became my patient," Dr. Lipkin recounts, "she had put herself through eight barium enemas." One night Dr. Lipkin received a call from Marianne, saying that she was in agony with stomach pains. But this time there was a different affect. "Her voice was clear, strong, and direct. I heard the message: something serious was really happening." Dr. Lipkin directed her to go to the emergency room immediately, and indeed Marianne had diverticulitis, an inflammation of the intestine for which she needed an operation. "It was interesting how well she handled things when a real emergency struck, and I think the experience gave her confidence. She finally had been successful in recognizing the language of her body, and a doctor whom she had grown to trust had come through for her."

The struggle to overhaul the way medicine is practiced in this country has paved the way for some intense soul-searching that may yet salvage the uniqueness of patients. If all goes according to the most optimistic forecasts, medicine in the twenty-first century will be an equitably financed, cost-effective system providing humane care, universal coverage, and the best of alternative and traditional know-how. Its doctors, compassionate men and women of diverse ethnic origins, half choosing careers in family medicine, internal medicine, and pediatrics, will be as sensitive to the psychological and social needs of patients as they are to the bottom line. The passive patient/authoritarian doctor relationship will become a relic, replaced by a model of mutual participation in which doctor and patient discuss medical choices and share decisions as equal partners.

Serendipitously, medicine's renewed interest in the mind-body phenomenon and the popularity of preventive care and low-tech therapies dovetails nicely with economic reality. It is almost always easier to promote health than to treat sickness. In recent years, medical insurance companies have begun to reimburse subscribers who participate in treatment programs that employ only a combination of diet, meditation, exercise, and support groups to reverse heart disease. Insurers have also shown a greater willingness to cover alternative therapies and preventive measures like wellness examinations, which investigate not just how you feel physically but how you are doing in all aspects of your life.

Whether they are called biopsychosocial, mind-body, holistic, alternative, or behavioral, these approaches are good news for medical consumers, especially those of us who somatize stress. As a matter of fact, the present may be the best time in the history of medicine to be a hypochondriac. Medical students of the next generation are, for the most part, socially conscious, altruistic, and unafraid of dramatic reform. And they are setting an example for their uncertain mentors, who more and more are coming to realize that by treating only biological disease, medicine has given patients short shrift. Many of these older physicians are taking somatizing patients more seriously, recognizing that their suffering is every bit as real as that of patients with chronic diseases, and they are reaching out to help them.

Gerald Weissmann, a professor of medicine at New York University Medical Center and head of its Department of Rheumatology, is among these doctors. Although he is vocally skeptical of any government plan for national health or managed care, Dr. Weissmann can't help but applaud what he sees as a return of medicine to "a more pastoral vision" in which doctor and patient together seek to understand the experience of illness—the severity of pain, the degree of anxiety, and the impact of an illness on family life.

This is a vision in which sick people can afford the best weaponry medicine has to offer together with counseling and support to help them cope with their illnesses, and healthy people in emotional turmoil are protected from invasive procedures. In this system, rather than have their complaints dismissed or taken at face value, hypochondriacs and somatizers would get the chance to address and resolve the issues symptoms may mask. For, as Dr. Weissmann says, "The symptom is never invented by the patient, it is a mark of a deeper hurt." These patients really suffer from their illnesses—in body or mind or both—and "they deserve not only the attention of doctors, but their compassion."

Working with Your Doctor

The family doctor you choose will be not only your primary physician but your medical navigator, guiding you to appropriate care. Especially if you are prone to health worries, establishing a long-term, dependable relationship of trust and confidence is crucial. Here are some suggestions on how to make that relationship work.

CHOOSE THE RIGHT DOCTOR

The key is to invest the time to find the right match from the start. Unfortunately, hypochondriacs tend to wait until they feel ill and frantic to begin their search. The best time to start is *before* a flare-up, when you feel calm and in control.

Do the research. Buy a notebook and start collecting names. Relatives and friends can be a good source for recommendations because they have a sense of whom you might feel comfortable with. Call your local medical society or ask other health professionals in your community for referrals. To check credentials you can consult the *American Medical Directory of Physicians in the United States* and the *Directory of Board Certified Medical Specialists* in your library. If you have doubts about a physician, the state medical licensing board will tell you if he or she has ever been disciplined for unprofessional conduct.

Interview two or three physicians. Telephone their offices and offer to pay for a fifteen-minute interview visit. This is time and money well spent. No matter what you discuss, you'll learn a lot: about the office—its appearance and the courtesy and professionalism of the staff, and about the doctor—whether he makes eye contact, has warmth and humor, listens, and addresses your concerns.

Ask questions. Don't forget that you are the consumer and this is *your* examination. Here are some questions you might want to ask: How often will I need screening exams? How are emergencies handled? What is the telephone call policy of the practice? Are you willing to discuss medical articles I bring in and cite others so I can do my own reading? If you, or another doctor, advise a procedure, are you willing to discuss the pros and cons and suggest alternatives? Do you object to a friend or family member's being present during my appointment?

Assess the style that best suits you. Whether you choose a doctor who is male or female, young or old, gregarious or reserved, it is well to keep in mind that it is more important for a doctor to be trustworthy, compassionate, or just plain decent than to have a sparkling personality. It may take some time to find Dr. Right, but once you define the relationship you want, you are in a better position to create it.

Doctor-patient relationships tend to fall into the following three types, although the ideal relationship has the flexibility to change from one type to another according to circumstances and emotional requirements.

Active-passive. This is the old-fashioned, authoritarian provider-patient model. The physician tends to be paternalistic and the patient acts like a well-behaved child, accepting a diagnosis without question and "following doctor's orders." Hypochondriacs, who perceive themselves as weak and helpless, tend to fall into this type of relationship, although it may not be best. Patients who relinquish responsibility for medical choices are more apt to distrust treatment decisions down the line than those who take a more active role in their care.

Collegial. In this type of relationship doctor and patient are pals, perhaps calling each other by their first names, sharing confidences, even socializing. Though such closeness can be reassuring, ideally it is best if there is a certain distance between them. For the good of both, a patient should not be able to reach his physician on a whim or for a quick telephone fix.

Mutual participation. This is a contractual relationship between two equals. You and your doctor function as a team with each of you having specific duties to perform to accomplish your mutual goal: to promote growth and development and keep you as healthy physically, emotionally, and mentally as possible. In this type of relationship, patients are entitled to know as much about their condition as they're intellectually and emotionally capable of absorbing; they should also expect to collaborate in decisions and participate in treatment and care.

WHAT TO EXPECT OF A DOCTOR

A kind "bedside" manner. Hypochondriacal patients need a sensitive, patient, and competent doctor undaunted by uncertainty, ambiguity, and fear. Your doctor should help you understand your illness and symptoms, perceive your needs, express empathy, care as much about your health concerns as your health. He should never embarrass you, confuse you, or make you feel foolish.

A complete medical history. The majority of diagnoses are made on the basis of history, the symptoms and story of the illness as the patient describes them. During the initial interview, which should last forty-five minutes to an hour, the doctor should not only be listening to you describe your symptoms, family history, and what you think and feel about your condition, but observing, looking for visual clues and facial expressions. A doctor who does not give you her full attention, seems distracted or pressed for time, is probably not giving you the best care.

A thorough, gentle physical. The physical examination is not merely a tool to detect disease but a method of establishing a therapeutic alliance. The doctor should examine various body parts — head, face, neck, chest, stomach, perhaps genitals and rectum. You are entitled to privacy; the exam should be behind closed doors and your body, except for the area being examined, covered. You also have a right to know what the doctor is doing and why every step of the way. If you're anxious, ask the doctor to go slowly and explain the purpose behind the pushing and prodding.

WHAT DOCTORS EXPECT FROM YOU

It is not always easy to talk to a doctor. You may feel frightened or confused, or simply unwell and not be inclined to do any work yourself. But it is part of your responsibility to help your physician learn everything she can about your condition.

Tell the doctor how you feel. Tell the whole story: what your symptoms are, what you think they are, medications you're taking, diagnoses you've received, and doctors you've seen. Tell the doctor everything you know about your family health background and your own. Discuss any lifestyle risks or unusual situations that worry you.

Marty, an anxious health worrier, has a policy for any new

physician he sees. He says up front, "I need to take a few minutes to describe myself. I'm a person who tends to mistrust and doubt what physicians tell me. If we decide to work together, I need you to address not only my symptoms, but the anxiety I have about them."

Be prepared. Make a list of your questions and concerns. Talk about the most troubling issues first. Studies have shown that a patient's most serious complaint tends to be his third. Never spring a new ailment on a physician at the end of a session.

Be specific about ailments. Try to be as descriptive as you can about your symptoms and pain—the onset, intensity, and duration. One of the biggest challenges doctors face is getting clear, precise information. They speak of patient exaggeration, denial, and forgetfulness. By reporting symptoms inaccurately and editing complaints, patients complicate the difficult task of making a correct diagnosis.

One doctor gave the example of asking a patient whether her exhaustion was more pronounced during exercise or at rest, to which the patient responded, "I exercise very sensibly and always have." Although the doctor rephrased the question several times, he never got a clear answer. "Her agenda might be to show me that she's not crazy or that she is not causing her fatigue or that she's a good girl," the doctor says. "But my goal of getting the necessary information to make a diagnosis is thwarted."

Don't overload. Any diagnostician worth his degree wants to get to the bottom of a patient's complaint—identify it, understand it, and treat it. But patients can so overwhelm them with data that the doctors do not have time to process the information. A doctor must attend to each complaint individually, even though he may eventually conclude that the complaints are symptomatic of the same illness. Some patients, once they have a doctor's attention, bombard him with every discomfort they are suffering at once.

Have reasonable expectations. Don't expect symptoms or worry to disappear immediately. Rather than anticipating a complete cure, think about symptom reduction, having increased feelings of control over symptoms, or becoming a little more active.

Follow recommendations. Listen to the doctor's responses and assessment of your health status without feeling defensive or guilty. Be sure you understand his advice. If you are still confused or worried, say so.

By the time Dara consulted a dermatologist about her three-year-old, she was a nervous wreck. Her son had been born with several large café au lait spots, which her pediatrician had said were nothing. But one summer she noticed more and more raised marks on his back and began to read medical texts. "I got it into my head that this was an indication of elephant man's disease. I even called the association for its literature," Dara says. The specialist examined the boy and told her that while the condition had a clinical name, it was absolutely benign. "Are you certain this isn't elephant man's disease?" she asked, to which the doctor responded that it wasn't even something she should consider. Not convinced, Dara ventured, "What if it was your child? Would you be concerned?" With a gentle hand pat and a reassuring smile, he answered, "No, Dara. If it were my son, I wouldn't give it another thought" — and she could tell he meant it.

Don't *always* expect a doctor to say what you want to hear. But if the doctor *never* says anything you want to hear and you find yourself uncomfortable with her — move on. But remember: doctor-shopping inevitably leads to poor medical care. Switch early but not often.

CHAPTER TEN

....

The Steps to Successful Treatment

It is part of the cure to wish to be cured.

— Seneca

NO ONE CAN DECIDE for you whether to seek treatment for hypochondria. Not your spouse, not your mother, not your physician. Unless a person is considered a threat to others or deemed dangerous to himself, treatment is a personal decision. Treatment in this case refers to professional help from a mental health practitioner. This is help for which you pay both psychically and financially and to which you must be willing to commit for an indefinite period of time.

For many, recognition of hypochondria may be enough. Knowing that there are others out there who feel as you do and that you are *not* crazy or sick can be of positive value. Hypochondria may exist in the Psychiatric Association's *Diagnostic and Statistical Manual,* but it is also a problem of everyday life, one so common, in fact, that calling it a psychiatric disorder at all may do sufferers injustice. After all, the dividing line between a mental disorder and a mild neurosis is frequently hazy. The decision to seek assistance may depend on your perception of your distress, the degree of intensity, persistence, and duration of the problem and how disruptive it is to your life. If this book has delivered its message, you know that most of us, to varying degrees, have or will experience doubts and fears about health and inexplicable pains that preoccupy us, more than we'd like, at some point in our lives.

That said, perhaps you can take a fresh look at your own tendency toward this age-old affliction borne by so many. Those with only occasional bouts of hypochondria may be able to "talk themselves off the ledge," as one sufferer puts it, by reasoning with themselves, sharing their angst with a friend, maybe even joking—yes, joking—about the problem. Humor is something that I have purposely avoided in this book because of the derogatory way in which writers of comedy have generally treated hypochondriacs. But poking gentle fun at oneself is an effective way of coping. Laughing at one's tendency to brood and obsess over what is uncontrollable and made worse by worry can help keep things in perspective.

Still, there are several reasons for choosing to seek treatment. Having struggled with health fears and symptoms for a long time, you may have reached a point at which the struggle seems endless. Family members and friends may be complaining that they are sick of hearing you talk about illness and tired of reassuring you. Your doctors may have advised you to seek help because "stress" seems to be contributing to the severity of your physical symptoms. Or you may have picked up this book, found much in it that resonates for you, and noted on the self-assessment questionnaire, the Illness Attitude Scale in the Appendix, that you have some prominent hypochondriacal features. If so, what should you do next?

Effective treatment begins with an empathic person who understands and validates your physical and emotional distress. You may want to talk over the problem with a spouse, friend, parent, or member of the clergy. The problem may be worked through with your physician or another trustworthy health professional whom you trust, whether a general practitioner, nurse practitioner, or homeopathic healer. Support groups are another possibility, but beware of self-help networks that concentrate primarily on legitimating a questionable ailment without focusing on coping techniques. Many have found relief and comfort through chronic pain programs and support groups in which sufferers learn to control pain and reinterpret symptoms through cognitive and behavioral methods.

Phobia self-help groups can be helpful for the anxiety-prone who wish to break destructive behavioral and thought patterns, and specialized clinics treating hypochondria are beginning to be available. For example, White Plains Hospital Center in New York offers a health anxiety program as part of its phobia clinic, and Brigham and Women's Hospital in Boston has cognitive education groups to help patients who have difficulty coping with symptoms and illness. Help for hypochondriacs is also available through support groups that exist for overlapping psychiatric disorders like depression, panic disorder, or obsessive-compulsive disorder, in which sufferers often struggle with germ and disease phobias.

You may also want to seek therapy, at the very least to obtain a diagnosis. What kind of treatment works best? Should you take medication? Try a cognitive behavioral approach? Go back to uncover pain in your childhood or look toward someone for support and just to talk things through?

Since the 1960s, there has been a proliferation of therapies — psychodynamic techniques, behavior modification, cognitive approaches, family and group dynamics — a smorgasbord of schools and orientations — and a parallel deluge of new psychiatric medications touted for a host of mental problems. The array of alternatives can be confusing. Just as there is no one cause of hypochondria, so there is no one "right" treatment for hypochondria, or most psychiatric disorders, though particular approaches may be more appropriate for some individuals than for others. For example, the patient who presents aches and pains dramatically and uses illness to "manage" relationships probably doesn't benefit from the same course of treatment as the obsessional "closet" hypochondriac who fears developing a specific disease or is fixated on a part of his body. Other factors to take into account when considering therapy include motivation, finances, time constraints, and readiness to change. No matter what the approach, people who are ambivalent about therapy usually don't do as well as those who are clear about their choice of treatment.

So how should a person who wants help with hypochondria proceed? The first step should be at least one consultation with a psychiatrist. Unlike other mental health clinicians, psychiatrists have been trained in medicine. They have completed four years of medical school and three years of psychiatric training. They have practiced at least one year of general medicine in a hospital, taking care of patients with strokes, brain tumors, heart attacks, gastrointestinal bleeding. They have learned to identify the cause of unusual, mysterious illnesses. Just like other medical doctors, they are trained to be investigators of disease. If they suspect a hidden physical cause for a patient's symptoms, they know which of a vast array of tests might be appropriate. If the diagnosis is hypochondria, the two of you can assess the extent of the problem and come up with a treatment plan that best suits your needs, which may mean medication, a behavioral therapy program, a referral to a psychologist or social worker, or a combination of approaches.

The psychiatrist you choose need not specialize in hypochondria or somatic behavior. You can obtain a psychiatric referral through many sources — your family doctor, relatives and friends, a local hospital, or by contacting the American Psychiatric Association in Washington, D.C. Or you can telephone a leading figure in the field whose name you have come across in your reading and ask for a referral in your geographic area.

During the initial consult with the psychiatrist, you must be honest about what is troubling you. The doctor needs to know the extent of your discomfort, response to any previous type of treatment, why you choose to engage in therapy, and what your goals and expectations are. She may administer a questionnaire similar to the Illness Attitude Survey. Any information you can supply helps the psychiatrist to clarify the problem and gain insight into your symptoms and whether any physical conditions are involved.

Among the issues a psychiatrist might wish to address are the following:

1. Is the patient excessively worried about dying or contracting a serious illness, or does he believe he has one now? In other words, is it hypochondria, and if so, how does it play itself out?

2. If the patient is hypochondriacal, how long has the condition been going on? Hypochondria that lasts less than six months, called transient hypochondria, probably represents stress or unaddressed issues in one's life rather than deep-seated emotional problems or chronic obsessional worry. If a new patient complains of extreme health concern for a year or two but has no history of hypochondria prior to that period, the psychiatrist may probe more immediate areas of that patient's history. People are often unaware of events or situations that might trigger their illness fears. A fifty-year-old married man became obsessed with fears of AIDS and death, an obsession that began following a one-night stand and persisted for two years despite repeated negative HIV tests. Psychotherapy targeted at unresolved guilt and marital issues lessened his excessive fears and brought about other positive changes in his life.

3. Has the patient had a thorough medical workup to exclude hard-to-diagnose medical conditions that might cause the symptoms? The psychiatrist must be satisfied that all the necessary tests have been conducted and that all reasonable physical possibilities for the persistent symptoms and fear have been excluded. After reviewing the patient's medical history, the psychiatrist may contact the patient's personal physician or order laboratory tests to rule out a serious medical illness. If the patient has a medical illness, the psychiatrist, in consultation with the patient's personal physician, has to assess whether the patient's fears and symptoms are excessive or appropriate.

4. Are there concurrent psychiatric disorders? If one is present, treatment of that disorder might very well lead to a cure for the hypochondria. Does the patient have elements of panic disorder, obsessive-compulsive disorder, or major depression? Effective treatments for each of these problems are described in this chapter.

5. Are there cultural reasons why a patient might be more likely to express emotional conflict as bodily preoccupation? For many immigrants, attempts and expectations to assimilate are a common source of emotional anguish, which is experienced differently by varying cultures. Latin Americans, for example, express emotions largely through physical maladies and complaints, while feelings of guilt and depressed mood are more common among Americans of northern European background. Another important question is whether there is a history of childhood trauma or severe emotional neglect that might predispose someone to express feelings through the body rather than through words. In these situations, psychotherapy may be particularly helpful.

6. What is the symbolic meaning of the illness fear? The particular content of any fear is usually shaped by experience and strengthened by unconscious forces. For example, a thirty-year-old woman became terrified of developing breast cancer shortly after her boyfriend cheated on her. Her fear, which at times became paralyzing in intensity, was connected with a conscious awareness that she felt she was dying and an unconscious fear that a killer was destroying her feminine self. The feelings of inadequacy and invasion reminded her of her critical father, who berated her during her emerging adolescence and often teased her about her developing breasts. Her father became emotionally distant as she became sexually mature. As the unconscious determinants of the breast cancer fear became conscious during the course of a psychodynamic therapy, the intensity and frequency of the fear diminished as well.

7. Is there a family history of psychiatric disorders, such as depression, panic attacks, hypochondria, obsessive-compulsive disorder, psychosis? Family history might suggest that a certain hypochondriacal problem is genetically linked to states of anxiety or depression. Families can also "infect" their members with attitudes and behavior. A psychiatrist's job is to separate the influences of body and mind, which interact with each other to create one's vulnerability to hypochondria.

Treatment of Hypochondria with Accompanying Psychiatric Disorders

If the psychiatric assessment determines that there are signs of an underlying psychiatric condition which might respond readily to medication or a specific psychotherapy, treatment of that disorder might result in a dramatic decrease in hypochondria. Typical treatments for such concurrent disorders follow.

MAJOR DEPRESSION

Depression, the most treatable of all psychiatric disorders, in many cases resolves itself within a six-month period. However, studies show that combined psychotherapy and medicine helps lift depression sooner and makes its recurrence less likely or frequent. The primary effect of the dozen or so most commonly used antidepressants is to restore the proper balance of neurotransmitters in the brain, which promote a feeling of well-being, to natural levels. These include the tricyclics, imipramine (Tofranil), desipramine (Norpramin), and nortriptyline (Pamelor), and the newer selective serotonin reuptake inhibitors (SSRIs), fluoxetine (Prozac), Sertraline (Zoloft), paroxetine (Paxil), and fluvoxamine (Luvox). Many people who take tricyclics experience unpleasant side effects, such as dry mouth and constipation and perhaps sleepiness and weight gain, and the drugs are not generally recommended for people with a history of urinary retention or conduction problems with the heart. SSRIs are less likely to affect the heart than the tricyclics and are better tolerated in general, though some who use them experience nausea or headaches at the beginning of treatment and later a decrease in sexual desire or function. As with most antidepressants, patients have to stay on the medication for six to eight weeks before the full effect is achieved. Other effective medications for depression include venlafaxine (Effexor), bupropion (Wellbutrin), nefazodone (Serzone) and monoamine oxidase inhibitors (MAOIs) like phenelzine (Nardil); the MAOIs are not widely prescribed because users run the risk of developing high blood pressure from the drugs' interaction with certain food and drugs. You and your doctor may have to experiment before finding what works for you.

Studies indicate that when depression and hypochondria coexist, pharmacologic treatment of the depression often results in resolution of the hypochondria. Psychotherapies, particularly interpersonal therapy (which explores past and ongoing relationships linked to the depression) as well as cognitive behavioral treatments (in which specific behavioral changes are sought), are also helpful in the treatment of less severe depressions. In many cases, psychotherapy and medication are combined.

Finally, for severe and unresponsive depressive illness, electroconvulsive therapy is an alternative. The treatment, which has changed dramatically since the 1950s, when it went out of favor, is making a comeback. It is now considered generally safe, rapid and extremely effective: studies show that it relieves depression 75 to 85 percent of the time.

PANIC DISORDER

Two main categories of medicines have been successful in treating panic disorder: tricyclic antidepressants such as imipramine (Tofranil), and benzodiazepines such as alprazolam (Xanax) or clonazepam (Klonopin). The benzodiazepines, prescribed for approximately 15 percent of the U.S. population, are advantageous in that they work quickly to curtail anxiety and panic attacks. The problem is that they can cause dependence and must be taken two or three times a day. If one abruptly stops taking a benzodiazepine, severe withdrawal symptoms can occur, including nausea, tremors, sleep problems, agitation, and increased anxiety. Imipramine is not associated with withdrawal symptoms and requires only one dose a day. In the treatment of panic disorder, the initial dosage of imipramine starts very low (10 milligrams) and is gradually increased to approximately 125 to 150 milligrams daily. While benzodiazepines work within hours to days of starting treatment, imipramine's effects might not be noticed for a month or more. Studies indicate that cognitive behavior therapy, either alone or combined with medication, is also effective for breaking the imprisoning cycle of panic. When panic disorder is treated, associated hypochondria may resolve completely.

OBSESSIVE-COMPULSIVE DISORDER (OCD)

Since the mid-1980s, rapid progress has been made in the pharmacologic treatment of OCD. The serotonin reuptake inhibitors—fluoxetine (Prozac), fluvoxamine (Luvox), and clomipramine (Anafranil)—can help 60 to 70 percent of patients decrease the frequency and intensity of obsessions as well as the related need to perform endless rituals. Successful treatment requires attaining the proper dosage and a therapeutic trial of at least twelve weeks. Behavior therapy, when conducted by a therapist with expertise in treating OCD patients, is also very effective for patients who can tolerate rigorous exposure to feared situations as well as the demand of not engaging in the compulsive responses.

TREATMENT OF HYPOCHONDRIA WITHOUT ACCOMPANYING PSYCHIATRIC DISORDERS

As recently as a decade ago, patients with so-called primary or pure hypochondria were considered difficult to treat, if not hopeless. They did not respond well to either medication therapy or psychotherapy. Doctors were left with the advice "Give the patient kindly support, schedule monthly follow-up visits, and try to avoid ordering unnecessary diagnostic tests."

Contrary to the belief of many family medicine doctors, internists, psychologists, and psychiatrists, effective treatments do exist for patients whose hypochondria is not accompanied by other psychiatric disorders and is not consequent to a recent loss or stressful event. New medications and innovative approaches to curbing health anxiety are helping many of these sufferers find relief.

Three main methods of treatment—psychodynamic, cognitive-behavioral, and psychopharmacological—have been used to combat hypochondria. Despite the dogmatic stance of some therapists, the best treatment in many cases is one that interweaves strategies and techniques from a variety of approaches. For instance, once medication has helped diminish hypochondria, a patient may be encouraged to risk a more intensive psychodynamic exploration of her illness fears. Choosing a systems approach within a family setting doesn't preclude one from using behavioral techniques to cope with hypochondriacal fears. And so forth. The goal is pragmatic—whatever works best.

Nevertheless, as you search for a therapist, be aware that each has a theoretical and technical bias to some degree. The goal of all therapies, of course, is to reduce symptoms, gain control over fears, and replace them with new, more effective, and satisfying ways of coping. But the therapist's orientation, whether eclectic or absolute, guides thinking and practice, influences the kind of information he or she seeks, and dictates how the therapist will work with you to bring about desired change.

What type of therapy? What follows are descriptions of the most common approaches to hypochondria. Each treatment strategy is accompanied by an illustrative case of a patient who believes the particular process helped him or her overcome health preoccupation and illness fears. Still, it is well to bear in mind that each person is uniquely complex and that therapy is far from an exact science. A treatment that works for one person may not work for another, even one with a similar background and symptoms.

PSYCHODYNAMIC THERAPY: THE TALKING CURE

This approach is best suited to a person who wants to make fundamental character changes, in effect, to transform himself. Most psychodynamic therapies take the view that hypochondria results from deep-seated, childhood-rooted psychic injury— early trauma, negative parenting experiences, and the like. These problems adversely affect self-esteem, impede functioning, and prevent a person from pursuing desirable goals like independence, happiness, a loving relationship, or a satisfying career.

At the heart of psychodynamic therapy is the therapeutic relationship, which relies specifically on verbal and nonverbal communication between client and therapist. Over time, the therapist works with the patient to disconfirm maladaptive beliefs.

Perhaps the most famous and ambitious form of psychodynamic therapy, classical psychoanalysis as it was practiced a century ago, is no longer popular. Nevertheless, its principles and methodology live on, a legacy to American psychiatry and psychology. The psychoanalytic technique, developed by Sigmund Freud in late nineteenth-century Vienna, seeks to uncover repressed material so that it can be integrated into the conscious structure of personality. The method consists primarily of exploration of transference—the patient's reactions to the therapist as they are colored by important relationships from the patient's past—and resistance—the patient's unconscious defenses against progress toward health. The route to emotional health is through the examined life: change is thought to arise as unconscious conflicts are made conscious and faced. In the therapy's purest form, patients typically meet with the analyst four to five times a week for four years or longer.

The effectiveness of psychoanalysis is difficult to measure. While anecdotal reports suggest that hypochondria may resolve with psychoanalysis, there has been no systematic study of the success rate of this technique.

More widely accepted than psychoanalysis, psychodynamic therapy relies on many of the same principles, also seeks to uncover unconscious conflicts, but because sessions are less frequent the process is less intense. In the treatment of hypochondria, psychotherapy may focus on unraveling the symbolic significance of health preoccupations and gaining insight into unexpressed conflicts. Support and education in the context of the therapeutic setting may also help diminish worries and loosen controls. Many practitioners believe that change can be achieved by meeting with a patient one to three times weekly for two to five years. Typically in psychodynamic therapy, the therapist takes a more active and verbal role than in psychoanalysis, and the dialogue is more directly focused on current issues in the patient's life.

How effective is psychodynamic therapy? What little research has been conducted is contradictory, ambiguous, and subject to debate. Critics of this approach claim that whatever success it achieves merely reflects the placebo effect—the positive results produced by the patients' expectation that they will improve—not the treatment itself (see Chapter 9). Nevertheless, data from meta-analytic studies—those which combine research findings from many smaller studies into one large one—indicate that many patients in psychotherapy make appreciable gains. One meta-analysis of data from more than two thousand cases found that approximately half improved by the eighth psychotherapy session and three-quarters were substantially better at six months. Nevertheless, not everyone who goes into therapy is helped, or helped as much as others. In fact, 10 percent in therapy get worse instead of better.

Research on the effectiveness of psychoanalytic psychotherapy in the treatment of hypochondria is scanty, and in the few studies conducted in the 1960s, only a small percentage of hypochondriacal patients in analytically oriented therapy improved. But some experts believe the potential for success of hypochondriacal patients in psychotherapy has been underestimated. Clinicians, they say, have formed opinions about the poor prognosis from chronic, unrepresentative patients, and traditional methods are different from newer strategies that combine insight with identifying stresses that precede symptoms and penetrate internalized representations and feelings which triggered illness fears.

What seems probable is that some patients with hypochondria benefit from psychoanalytic work, and many do not. While other areas of life, such as self-esteem and overall well-being, may improve with psychodynamic therapy, hypochondriacal concerns may remain. But where the hypochondria appears to be linked to a recent trauma or loss, psychodynamic therapy can be very helpful.

Greg: High Cholesterol and Damaged Goods

Greg developed hypochondria when he was forty-one, about the same time he received a doctor's report of a slightly elevated cholesterol level. The news was loaded with psychic dynamite. Greg's beloved grandfather, who suffered a heart attack at forty-three, had been a cardiac cripple until his death from a second attack at sixty-four. For Greg, a professor at a major university and married father of three, the report set off months of stomach pains and intense worry that at any moment he would keel over from cardiac arrest.

Pain and fear continued despite a stress test, an MRI (magnetic resonance imaging), a barium enema, and a sonogram, all of which revealed little. "Get on with your life," said his internist, cardiologist, and gastroenterologist. Given his family history, Greg knew his fears were not completely irrational, but he also recognized the signs of depression and negative thought patterns from having once been in therapy. His wife was losing patience. Things had become so bad, Greg recalls, "I was taking my blood pressure at the office and paying my doctor bills from cash." He realized it was time to resume therapy.

At a friend's recommendation, he consulted an analytically trained psychologist and immediately felt a rapport. The therapist was a man in his sixties who displayed equanimity and poise. Greg thought him trustworthy, genuine, and nonjudgmental and admired the therapist's optimism and humor about life. He was given a choice between lying on a couch and sitting up; he chose the couch to help him free-associate. What did he want from the therapist? Not medical reassurance; it had never worked. Greg wanted to probe deeply but not with the intensity of analysis, which he couldn't afford financially or in terms of time. He wanted to understand why the laboratory report had wreaked such havoc in his life. Clearly, the doctor's message had great symbolic meaning. In therapy, Greg talked about his identification with his grandfather, one of the few people in his life who had given him unconditional love, and the fear that he might suffer a similar fate.

It became evident that although the threat of heart disease had some reality, Greg experienced his physical problem as one of character. "Until the report, I'd been able to keep my cholesterol in check with diet and exercise. Now my health was out of my control. I shared with the therapist my sense of degradation, humiliation, and feelings of worthlessness. The high cholesterol wasn't just a physical finding; it meant I, as a person, was defective." Within six months of therapy, his gut pains essentially vanished and the amount of time given to worry about a heart attack decreased by 75 percent.

The therapy involved treading over some painful ground that Greg thought he had worked through fifteen years previously when, out of graduate school and unemployed, he suffered a depression that led him into analysis. Three times a week for two years, he explored the many confusing, charged issues from the past. His was a typically dysfunctional family: remote father, overbearing mother, a younger brother who suffered panic attacks. Before entering therapy, Greg had moved from the Midwest of his youth to the Northeast, where he found himself alone, an inhibited, underdeveloped twenty-five-year-old who had difficulty establishing his sexuality and disengaging from his family. The issues Greg had discussed with his former therapist involved autonomy, separation, and sexuality, but not hypochondria. This time around it became clear that both his grandfather and mother had suffered from the illness, but it was his mother who had projected hypochondria on Greg. For the first time he realized how extraordinarily sensitive she had been to the nuances of his body. "The message my mother gave me was that I was weak and fragile, not like other kids."

For example, when Greg was five, his mother became convinced that he urinated too frequently. She dragged him to doctors, talked about "the problem" incessantly on the phone. Probably to placate her, the physicians performed a cystoscopy, in which a probe is inserted through the penis to examine the bladder. "The doctor said, 'Pull down your pants.' Mom was holding my hand. 'It won't hurt,' she told me. Two days later it felt as if I was peeing razor blades." No abnormality except for posterior urethra valves, a benign condition in some children.

With the guidance and wisdom of his therapist, Greg has been able to separate a less than perfect lab test from the person he is and to disentangle his health from self-esteem. "I actually feel something that previously I knew only intellectually: it's juvenile to believe you are invulnerable, invincible, or immortal. We all go downhill. But if you allow this reality to paralyze you rather than make you appreciate what you have, you might as well be dead."

Therapy has also helped to improve Greg's marriage. Greg's wife has little tolerance for whining. "Illness is pooh-poohed in her family. The belief is that one should suffer in silence and die with dignity. In the best of all possible worlds, I'd like her to be more supportive, but I've learned to accept the way things are. My wife treats my medical problems and symptoms with benign indifference. She supports the therapy, but not the hypochondria."

Once in a while, when he least expects it, fear bubbles up, and Greg thinks about medication. He has read about the miracle drugs. He has seen friends transformed by them. But to him, pharmacology smacks of "smoke and mirrors." "I guess I'm a Calvinistic sort of fellow who believes one ought not to take shortcuts and get too much happiness out of life." But there's more. "I feel a great deal of pride in being able to do this through my own blood, sweat, and tears. It can be painful, but the process of making connections is also rich, even fun. Where else but in therapy could one talk about sexual fantasies, inhibitions, anger, disappointments, one's mother, the bizarre but normal feelings all of us have, that would be offensive to anyone else?"

A BIOLOGICAL APPROACH

Neuropsychiatry: it's new, effective, exciting, and controversial. Since the introduction of Prozac, the first of the selective serotonin reuptake blockers (SSRIs), we have found ourselves in the midst of a revolution—and a lot of hype. Even without fully understanding how these "brain drugs" function to regulate the level of serotonin with a minimum of side effects, doctors have found the SSRIs to be effective in ameliorating symptoms of more problems than their developers ever expected. The Food and Drug Administration currently approves these drugs for depression and obsessive-compulsive disorder (OCD), but dramatic evidence suggests that they are also useful in treating eating disorders, alcoholism, panic disorder, anxiety, premenstrual syndrome, body dysmorphic disorder, and hypochondria, as well as such milder psychic problems as low self-esteem, sensitivity to rejection, and inhibition.

Since Prozac came onto the market in 1988, millions of Americans have tried the tiny green and white capsules. The drug has enjoyed the fastest acceptance of any psychotherapeutic medicine ever. To date, Prozac has been taken by more than 10 million people, is the nation's best-selling drug after the ulcer medication Zantac, and has spawned a family of sister medications—Zoloft, Paxil, Luvox—whose sales are steadily increasing each year.

Nevertheless, there has been a backlash. The potential for overprescription, along with a philosophic abhorrence among some for the way these "feel good" pills have produced a legal drug culture, has led to a nationwide debate over the medications. First came the accusations that Prozac caused some patients to attempt suicide or commit violent acts. The scientific case, never more than flimsy, was later discounted—the main source of the uproar turned out to be the Church of Scientology. Then psychiatrist Peter Kramer wrote *Listening to Prozac*, with its dramatic accounts of the drug's ability to make certain people "better than well."

Kramer introduced the concept of "cosmetic pharmacology," a vision of existence in which "normal" people must use drugs to keep up. The media had a heyday with these stories: a farming town in Washington gained notoriety as the "Prozac capital" after a psychologist dubbed the Pied Piper of Prozac, in conjunction with a local doctor, put most of his seven hundred patients on the drug; pet owners confessed to feeding the medication to their ill-tempered dogs and cats; and any number of professionals were found to be taking Prozac to give them a business "edge." Seeking damage control, Prozac's creator, Eli Lilly, launched an advertising campaign to deplore the media's role in exaggerating Prozac's power and for trivializing the serious nature of depression, for which the drug was specifically promoted. The campaign failed to stem the tide of negative reporting: that a study found the SSRIs no more effective in treating depression than an older generation of antidepressants; that 40 percent of those on the drug experienced negative sexual side effects; that preliminary research from Canada found Prozac hastened tumor growth in mice.

For any potential SSRI candidate, the physical issues surrounding Prozac are certainly worrisome. But the moral ones, like whether the drugs should be taken for minor symptoms or given to pets, are not really important for someone paralyzed by illness fears. These new medications are among the first to show real promise for treating hypochondria.

The effort to treat hypochondria biochemically began with Dr. Brian Fallon's Heightened Illness Concern study at Columbia University, the first clinical trial for hypochondriacs who did not suffer from major depression. Seventy percent of the patients who took daily doses of Prozac showed improvement after twelve weeks, with some completely free of their hypochondriacal worries. Although a few patients benefited from the lower dosages of 20 to 40 milligrams effective for depression, most required the higher dosages of 60 to 80 milligrams typically prescribed for OCD. In 1993, the National Institute of Mental Health awarded Dr. Fallon a half-million-dollar grant to conduct a five-year study on the impact of fluoxetine on hypochondria and whether patients relapse after medication is withdrawn. It is the first federally funded effort involving treatment for hypochondria.

Elsewhere in the United States, Dr. Robert Wesner and Dr. Russell Noyes, Jr., have found the antidepressant imipramine helpful for patients with illness phobia, a subtype of hypochondria. Patients with illness phobia are leery of getting a disease, but they have good insight into the irrational nature of their fears. Whether imipramine is also helpful for the group of hypochondriacs who are more strongly convinced of their illnesses is open to question. Imipramine also appears to benefit patients with undiagnosable pain syndromes. A study of patients who had chronic chest pain despite structurally normal hearts and normal coronary angiograms found that those who took imipramine experienced chest pain half as often as they did before treatment.

Janet: A Prescription for Lead Fears

Janet can pinpoint the exact moment in childhood when the fear set in. She was eight or nine, watching *My Three Sons*, when a television spot advertising a kidney disease foundation appeared. "I was horrified by the photographs of sick little children," says Janet, a petite twenty-nine-year-old mother of a four-year-old. That night Janet remembers crawling into bed with her mother, asking if her kidneys would get sick. After that, disease fears arose constantly. One week it was a brain tumor, the next leukemia. Thoughts of death preoccupied and frightened her. By fifth grade she added to her disease fears worries about what would happen to her after death. "Is there heaven? Reincarnation? Would I go to hell?"

Although her parents tried to convince her that she wasn't sick and that everything would be fine, she could tell they were concerned. Her mother had always been, and to this day is, a worrier. Not about illness, but other kinds of catastrophes. Janet recalls that during the Persian Gulf War her mother worried constantly that the war would go on and on and that her son, as well as her two sons-in-law, would be drafted, shipped overseas, and killed.

When she was eleven, Janet enrolled in ballet classes. She quickly fell in love with dance — the music, the movement, the serious discipline — and she had talent. She didn't mind devoting herself to hours of rigorous practice each day. Her world then was filled with rehearsals, recitals, and ballerina costumes. There wasn't much worry about illness and death. High school was about the happiest time she can remember, but it was also the beginning of an insidious eating disorder. For days in a row she would eat nothing but salad with vinegar, then pig out and be filled with self-hate.

The problem got worse whenever she went away from home, and toward her senior year the fears again began popping up. She vividly recalls a week in Los Angeles when she spent the entire time worrying about dying in an earthquake. After high school, Janet received an offer to join a midwestern ballet company. She took the job and moved to her first big city and apartment. She didn't socialize much; life was work and dieting. Her eating disorder got worse. "I always felt I was fat, that my stomach looked big, or I was ugly. I had a terrible self-image," Janet recalls.

After two years with the company, Janet found herself without energy, crying all the time, and finally sought help. She consulted a social worker with whom she talked about her weight fixation and how dancing had gone sour. "We didn't dig into my childhood, but the therapy helped me make a decision to quit dance for a while." She had an Achilles tendon injury and informed the company that she was in too much pain to perform.

Janet left the Midwest for New York City and stayed with a high school friend. There she became a waitress and met Tim, a musician. She and Tim were married in a civil ceremony and had a small reception at Janet's home. This was the beginning of a happier period. When Janet wasn't waiting tables, she found work choreographing for a neighborhood dance studio. But when she became pregnant, everything changed. "I didn't feel that with all my troubles I should bring a child into the world," Janet says. "But Tim wanted this child, and I couldn't show him my doubts."

The couple moved into a new apartment when Janet was in her fourth month, and the bad thoughts returned. They began innocently enough, with a remark to Tim about paint chips falling off the ceiling and the suggestion that they do something about it before the baby came. She had read about lead poisoning and it frightened her. Soon Janet became hyperaware of the peeling paint. She saw it everywhere: on doorjambs, window casings, flaking from walls. A lead inspector who took samples told her that the problem was minimal and could easily be fixed; but by then Janet was going full tilt, reading voraciously about levels of micrograms, about how lead exposure could stunt a child's growth and lead to brain problems. To protect her fetus, she took to wearing rubber gloves and a mask. Never an obsessive cleaner, she washed the floors every day. Finally, believing she was going crazy, she left the apartment to stay with her sister in Pennsylvania. Her family and husband thought she was overreacting, but not everyone did.

"I didn't know if I was being rational or irrational because many people fanned my fears—the media, a few friends who were antilead fanatics, even my gynecologist thought lead was something to be concerned about." There were other fears, too: of being a terrible wife, of being an incompetent mother. "I became extremely depressed. At one point, I remember thinking that if I had a gun I would shoot myself."

After six weeks in Pennsylvania, she returned to New York with her parents. She was in her final trimester and a little calmer. The family worked together to make the apartment acceptable. They papered over the walls and ceilings. Rather than strip wood, they replaced it to lessen the likelihood of ingesting lead-contaminated dust. In 1991, a beautiful daughter, Chloe, was born; Tim and Janet were overjoyed, and the baby motivated her to take better care of herself.

Her gynecologist had given her a referral to a psychiatrist, whom she went to see. He diagnosed her problem as disease phobia with OCD-related tendencies. Drug therapy was out of the question because she wanted to nurse Chloe. She decided to try cognitive behavior therapy. It was helpful. "I was a good student," Janet says. "I kept a diary of my thoughts and emotions. The combination of a good therapist, knowledge I had something other people had, and therapeutic exercises kept me stable."

But when Chloe was nine months old, Janet had a setback, which started at a dinner party. A male guest who was chewing a pretzel took it out of his mouth to give Chloe a piece. Before Janet could retrieve it, Chloe had eaten it. The incident wouldn't leave her mind. "I kept thinking: Oh my God, the man has AIDS. He had a cut on his mouth, and now Chloe has AIDS." She talked about it with Tim, who tried to be understanding. He even got some background on the man, who appeared to be in perfect health. But AIDS had become an obsession. Not so much the fear she'd get it, but that Chloe or Tim would. Janet forced Tim to switch from a barber who used old-fashioned razors she didn't think he sterilized. "I began to think I was nuts, that I'd never be able to take care of my child. I told my husband he should leave me, take Chloe, and remarry."

Around this time she became friendly with another mother in the park, a woman who had been diagnosed with OCD a few months previously. She had had intermittent trouble since she was a teenager, but in the past few years she had developed an obsession about animals. She would awake in the middle of the night and worry about how animals were being abused. She had terrible fantasies, going from country to country, continent to continent. She couldn't stop them. After starting Prozac, she experienced enormous relief.

That was when Janet decided to get back to therapy. She had become sloppy about her emotional health. She returned to her psychiatrist and told him she wanted to try Prozac. At first, it didn't work. The doctor kept increasing the dose—20 milligrams, 40, then 60. By six weeks, the effect kicked in, and when it did it was amazing. "For the first time ever, a worry would pop into my mind and if I wanted it to go away, I'd just banish it, whoosh. Like that. Tim and I started getting along better. I have always been high-strung and excitable; if we had an argument, I'd become hysterical. Now if we argue, it's not such a big deal. It's just a disagreement. I don't stew about it."

The lead fear is gone, too. In the old days, if workmen were sanding a building, she would go around an entire block to avoid the site. "Now I walk on by and think nothing of it except how far I have come." She is thinking of buying and redecorating the apartment she had hated because of the lead paint. "The best thing is I'm back to ballet after ten years. I say now what my psychiatrist tells me a lot of people say: if only Prozac had been around ten years earlier. But I mean it, I probably would never have quit dancing."

Janet's one remaining fear is that someday she may wake up to find that Prozac no longer works. "I know that if it suddenly came out that by taking Prozac you risk dying ten years sooner, I would still stay on it. I'm happy, and I have *never* been just plain happy."

COGNITIVE AND BEHAVIOR THERAPY

This approach is based on two different but compatible traditions, and whether applied individually or together, cognitive and behavior therapy have gained many converts. Both therapies, sharing an emphasis on fixing symptoms in the here and now, are used to treat a wide variety of medical and psychiatric conditions. Behavior therapy, introduced in the 1960s, addresses actions one can take to overcome fears and accomplish one's goals. Cognitive therapy, which followed shortly, focuses on changing the way one thinks about problems; by transforming maladaptive thoughts and feelings, it seeks to change behavior as well.

These therapies are especially attractive to those who wish to avoid medications, to target specific problems and goals, and to engage in relatively brief treatment — improvement can often be seen in six to twelve sessions. The approach also fits nicely with the concept of managed care, which favors more economical and efficient mental health treatments.

From a behavioral perspective, hypochondria is learned through a series of positive and negative reinforcements, rewards and punishments that occur through life. Positive reinforcement might come from increased attention from doctors or loved ones. Negative reinforcement occurs with the loss of care or affection when someone feels happy or strong.

Some hypochondriacs suffer from fearful avoidance of, for instance, hospitals, visiting sick people, or having a physical exam. Unconfronted fear intensifies; each avoidance confirms the danger of the situation. With such patients, the principles of exposure and response prevention, which are the bulwark of behavior therapy, must be applied. A patient might be asked to visit a cancer ward, work with AIDS patients, read articles about breast cancer, or visit a doctor. By allowing oneself to be flooded with fear and discomfort and refusing to give in to rituals or routines — self-examination, long-lasting discussions about fears with friends and relatives — one learns through experience that exposure, while temporarily increasing fear, can eventually result in its conquest.

The cognitive hypothesis of hypochondria is that bodily signs and symptoms are perceived as more dangerous and a particular illness more probable than they really are. At the same time, hypochondriacs believe they are helpless to prevent the illness and affect its course. Cognitive therapy focuses on the hypochondriac's automatic dysfunctional thoughts and misinterpretations of physical sensations. For example, a patient who knows that one sign of a brain tumor is headaches may begin to have catastrophic thoughts whenever a headache occurs — "If I have a headache, then that means it's a brain tumor." There are no in-betweens. Intrusive thoughts of possible negative consequences of not taking action are also common — "If I do not get this test the stomach pains (assumed to be caused by cancer) will metastasize and become inoperable."

Cognitive behavior therapy works by teaching hypochondriacs a new way of thinking about and responding to symptoms. It encourages patients to curtail the emotional storm of fear by being more rational, for example, arguing back to oneself that headaches might also be a sign of eye strain or of stress. It also teaches about the role of attention — the more one attends to a symptom, the worse it gets.

Dr. Paul Salkovskis and his colleagues at Oxford University have had a 90 percent success rate in curing or diminishing panic attacks with cognitive behavior techniques, which they are finding effective for hypochondria as well. The theory is that both panic and hypochondria sufferers interpret bodily sensations as catastrophic, but panic patients believe that a heart attack or impending doom is happening or is about to happen, whereas hypochondriacs presume that the symptoms indicate a more insidious course. In panic attacks, mounting anxiety produces shortness of breath, chest pain, and sweating, which further intensify terror. Similarly, hypochondriacs selectively attend to and process information. Once health anxiety has developed, health worry leads to a bias toward observations that are consistent with illness beliefs. There may be heightened perception of normal bodily changes, for example, a bloated stomach after eating, previously unnoticed bodily features, physical manipulation of sore areas, or selective attention to illness-related information. This keeps anxiety focused on fears about health and increases the scope of catastrophic misinterpretations.

Research is beginning to reveal that while both cognitive and behavioral methodology can lead to a reduction in hypochondriacal complaints, behavioral techniques may be more effective. In a study comparing the two treatments, behavior therapy sessions of exposure and response prevention appeared to account for improvement more often than the cognitive sessions. In addition, the sequence of behavior therapy followed by cognitive therapy tended to be more successful than vice versa.

Stephen C. Josephson, a psychologist affiliated with Cornell University Medical College's Department of Psychiatry who specializes in behavioral treatment, believes that it is the treatment of choice for problems like OCD, body dysmorphic disorder, and hypochondria.

Dr. Josephson believes that with hypochondria, the therapist must help the patient break two patterns: fear, the hypochondriac's panicky overreaction to internal sensations and health information, and the compulsion to relieve health anxiety with repeated self-inspection, compulsive doctor-shopping, and so on. "The challenge lies not only in providing a rationale for treatment—the reason for keeping people in contact with the source of their distress—but in establishing a rapport with the patients so that you can increase the likelihood that they will stick to the course, which in itself may seem anxiety provoking," he says.

In Dr. Josephson's estimate, about 75 percent of patients who have been given this treatment show lasting significant improvement—a decrease in severity and frequency of symptoms, and anxiety that doesn't last as long as it used to. How does he evaluate successful treatment? "When someone cuts back on obsessing about freckles from five hours to one, when a person afraid to move his limbs begins to exercise, or when you get someone to stop spending valuable time and energy worrying about his health."

According to Dr. Josephson, this is what you can expect should you decide to pursue behavioral treatment for hypochondria:

1. The therapist will review your medical status with your physician and help you to evaluate the extent of your fears, compulsions, and avoidance behaviors.

2. You will be taught strategies for evaluating whether you are sick, learning to discriminate between health fears and real health problems.

3. Your therapist, with your physician's approval, will ask you not to contact medical professionals for the purpose of reassurance, examination, testing, or surgery for ninety days, with obvious exceptions.

4. You will be asked to keep a journal in which to record situations when health fears arise and explore thoughts that you avoid or make you anxious.

5. You may be taught anxiety-reducing skills such as breathing techniques or relaxation exercises, as well as cognitive coping strategies—what to think about when health anxiety hits and how to control it.

6. With the help of the therapist, you will gradually be encouraged to do some of the things you have been avoiding. The emphasis will be on building successes so that you will start seeing your body as strong and less fragile.

7. Some patients may be taught specialized techniques to stop compulsive health behaviors, such as playing back audiotapes of their worries, a powerful way of reducing anxiety—"It gets real boring after a while," Dr. Josephson says. Exposure and response prevention is often carried out gradually through a series of assignments. For example, instead of taking your temperature you might begin to feel your forehead.

8. Patients who may require additional pharmacotherapy to get started will be asked to consult with a psychiatrist or psychopharmacologist.

Anne: A Leap of Faith

For as long as Anne can remember, her body was a burden. Chubby and unpopular as a young girl, teased by other children, she made a pact with God at age twelve: she would not become a woman. Whittling her stout frame from 130 to 90 pounds, she prided herself on her youthful Peter Pen look. When her breasts began developing, she found them disgusting, like "cow udders."

Early adolescence was an internal battle against torturous fantasies she couldn't control. She imagined a young girl who couldn't make her nose stop growing, a person with feces coming out of her mouth. She made all kinds of bargains with herself to make these horrifying visions stop. They made her feel weak and guilty, filling her with self-loathing, but she could not suppress them.

Anne's parents knew she was troubled and tried to help, but they had their own problems. Her father was a workaholic attorney who, though accomplished in his field, had never felt successful. Her mother tended to be self-effacing, unhappy in the role of a 1950s housewife, taking her three daughters, when they were small, to a psychiatrist to make sure she was bringing them up properly. Anne, quiet and well-behaved, managed to fool everyone. The psychiatrist told her parents that her problems were "normal childhood troubles."

Anne made it through a small private high school and decided to go to college in the West. During her freshman year, she found herself confused and frightened. The previous year she had started to menstruate, which disgusted her, and she continued to despise her breasts. She didn't have many friends and purposely chose men to whom she couldn't get close. One night Anne took LSD and had a very bad acid trip. "It was one of the most idiotic things I've ever done. I had this horrible, existential vision that the suffering would never end, that even after I died I would be condemned to eternal misery."

After this episode, she sought help at the college counseling office. A counselor said she was depressed and wanted her to consult a psychiatrist for medication. She refused. "To me, having to take a drug every day was like being an alcoholic." A little while later her back problems began. She had been walking across campus in the cold, carrying a heavy suitcase, when she heard something snap. The next morning she could hardly sit up. Anne dragged herself to an emergency room and was told she had just pulled some muscles, to rest for a few weeks and she'd be better. But the condition did not improve, and back pain would follow her off and on for the next fifteen years. "I remember feeling that I had been given a death sentence. It was as if the doctor had said something completely different from what he had, like 'You have a slipped disk, you will never go back to your activities, you will lose your ability to walk.' "

For months Anne was disabled with pain and terrible cramps in her lower spine. "I focused on them every second. My life revolved around my pain." An aunt and uncle from California came to get her. Ostensibly, she was going to their apartment to recuperate, but what she was really doing was quitting school. During her stay with them, she saw specialists at Stanford, rheumatologists, orthopedists, chiropractors. She underwent CAT scans, MRIs, bone scans, physical therapy. She told her story again and again. "I was lifting, it was cold . . ." The mainstream doctors said it was strained muscles, pulled ligaments, a disk rubbing against a nerve, nothing serious. She also saw holistic and homeopathic healers, a hypnotist, massage therapist, reflexologist. "People preyed on me," she says. "One of these so-called experts told me he intuited breast cancer down the line. It scared me out of my mind."

Anne moved back East and into her parents' apartment. The entire decade of her twenties is a blur of low-paying jobs, night classes, long periods of agony and depression, lying on a mattress on her bedroom floor, getting up only to go to the bathroom. The back pain was constant. She developed a pain in her bladder and several times rushed to a hospital emergency room to be catheterized. She underwent several procedures for these problems, but nothing serious was ever found. Her parents made sure she saw a psychologist, who treated her for depression.

Then her father told her a family secret. Her grandmother,

whom she had never met, had committed suicide. She killed herself because of a mental disorder. She couldn't stop counting her dishes or the dresses in her closet. Anne was certain she was destined to the same fate. Her psychologist, in whom she confided about not wanting to be a woman, about her fears of being fat, about becoming blind, getting AIDS or a terrible disease, about suffering unhappiness forever and ending up like her grandmother, sent her to a psychiatrist for antidepressants. Some worked better than others, but nothing made her well. She functioned at a minimal level and certainly not as an adult.

At twenty-nine, she met a man at a party. She liked him but couldn't enjoy his company for fear he would leave. Finally, she tried to scare him off, acting crazy, being sick. Three months went by and he didn't go away. She was just beginning to see the possibility of happiness when her back went out again. At the recommendation of her psychiatrist, she sought the help of a behavioral therapist. He accepted the reality of her back pain but told her that what she needed was a change in medication and behavior therapy.

Anne began a trial of Anafranil, which helped reduce her health obsessions but made her sleepy. She honestly believes it was behavior therapy that finally did the trick. "What I learned is a new way of coping, something that will always be with me and has become me." She worked intensively for two years in therapy, then off and on for another three. She had a good feeling about the behavioral approach from the beginning and adored her psychologist. Other professionals had been cautious about her back, nervous to take a stand, on the fence about medication, exercise, operations. But this guy made it clear: reassurance is a killer. If I give it to you, it's just like an addictive drug. You'll keep coming back for more. He made her do crazy things. First, he forbade her to see a doctor or talk to anyone for reassurance. Another "homework" assignment was to bang her back against the wall. "I would stand there and suffer the most intense anxiety and not be allowed to go through my routines. I had these complicated rituals, difficult to describe, a whole sequence of thoughts and feelings all revolving around guilt, self-loathing, and terror. The thought process went something like: my pain is a punishment, it hurts because something's wrong with me; I will ruin my body because I won't be able to exercise; I'll get fat and my boyfriend won't be attracted to me."

It's hard for Anne to pinpoint why the therapy worked. "You have to do every little thing the therapist tells you to. You have to be willing to expose yourself to fears that are so powerful, you think they might destroy you. The whole thing is one giant leap of faith. On faith, I began to trust my therapist and believe him. I did the terrifying things he told me to. And when you see small improvements, you realize it really does work. You begin to believe you are healthy. You realize that you can tolerate your feelings. You somehow believed that all the things you did before would help or redeem you, that you'd alleviate guilt and stop something from happening to you. Then you begin to discover another way and don't believe in your own system anymore. You see it as something like poison."

Today Anne is married—to that same boyfriend—and has been off all medication for three years. She has her college degree and a profession in the social services. "I'm very grateful to my husband for sticking through it. We're looking forward to having children. I believe I'm really going to be a good mother. I won't pass these things down to my children because I have learned to control my anxieties. They come back, but I have the power to chase them away."

Epilogue

NOT SO LONG AGO, I had a dream, a true hypochondriac's nightmare. I am in a hospital room following brain surgery. A doctor grimly approaches my bedside, leans down, and whispers into my ear. "Sorry. We weren't able to get it all." In the next frame, my head bandaged, I am frantically informing friends, acquaintances, anyone who will listen, that it is over for me. "It's not fair, I haven't lived enough," I whimper. "There hasn't been enough happiness." I need them to soothe me, care for me, make me well. But the crowd is powerless. They stand mute, pitying me, yet wishing I would go away.

Waking with a shudder, I instantly recognize that raw confluence of emotions — terror, rage, isolation, despair, and self-absorption — which seemed both foreign and familiar. The strange thing about the dream is that at the time of its conception, I hadn't experienced such feelings in nearly two years. I made note of the dream in my journal, but did not realize its significance until later. Not only had the dream carried me back to the hypochondriacal torment that had inspired me to write this book and reconnect me viscerally to my fellow sufferers, it revealed something else: that while the dark terror of hypochondria no longer held a grip on the major fabric of my life, its fiendish spirit was not far away. It abided within the shadowy territory of the unconscious, shielded from daily existence perhaps by the safety net of a pill, the absence of immediate trauma, an absorbing work project, or maybe, I wanted to believe, a more solid barrier of maturity and personal growth.

The reexperience of an old psychic wound has a strange power. For as with physical pain, like cutting your finger with a knife, once the healing sets in, it becomes nearly impossible to duplicate the sensory experience. And that compressed, vivid missive, perhaps a gift from the unconscious, confirmed for me this: I will never go back.

Because once you discover it is within your power to chase away fears, put a halt to fixations, let go of worry, the void gradually fills with something else: an ability to focus, become more productive, enjoy relationships. Dare I call this happiness? When you finally get that glimpse of a better way, it becomes addictive. So you'll bring to bear whatever strengths you possess to beat back the old, whether that means fiddling with neurotransmitters, peering into family dynamics, improving your connection with loved ones, learning to trust your doctor, or opening up to others like yourself.

One thing I am sure of is that people who are so sensitive to the reality of human frailty and the inevitability of death that they sabotage the only life they possess can never be happy. Paralyzed and incapable of giving or taking pleasure, they are unable to grasp that life can be lived another way.

It's like when I find myself driving, grouchily listening to a noxious heavy metal tune on the radio or one of my children's saccharine-sweet story tapes, and I think, God this is awful. Suddenly it dawns on me that I have the power to push the stop button or change the station. But sometimes people get so caught up in what is going on that they lose the ability to hear a better kind of music.

I believe that when hypochondriacs recognize what their mindset is doing to them and their loved ones and that it is possible to change, they will do something about it.

The concept of embarking on a journey from trauma and self-destruction to recovery in this age of self-improvement has become almost trite, a point hammered home by Wendy Kaminer in *I'm Dysfunctional, You're Dysfunctional*. Kaminer rails at twelve-step support groups, quick-fix techniques, and television talk shows in which dysfunctional people reveal their innermost secrets. What she really worries about is the trivialization of suffering: the idea that you're either in recovery or denial, that we must all be kind and good to ourselves, discover our inner child, and take charge of our lives. She decries the notion that a codependent relationship could possibly be akin to the agony of surviving the Holocaust.

The cheapening of psychic pain is a valid concern that has troubled me from the outset of this undertaking. I didn't want to produce what Kaminer calls a "how to be happy" book comprised of "slogans, sound bites, and recipes for success." "This isn't a self-help book," I kept telling people, almost apologetically. I didn't think I had the answers, yet I knew that what I had learned from my own experience and that of others could be prescriptive in its own way, without step-by-step solutions. After three years of studying and contemplating hypochondria in its various guises, I have become something of an expert on it. Still, I have trouble pinning the malady down: each time I put my finger on some tangible, universal truth, it slips away from me. The modern, psychiatric definition of hypochondria as a mental disorder comes in handy because it conveniently simplifies the issues, but the problem is greater than the sum of its DSM criteria.

For as perverse and destructive as hypochondria can be, it is more than a disturbance of the mind-body relationship; it is also a natural response to the human condition. Its very ordinariness accounts for that smile of recognition people give at its mention, why its clinical picture over two millennia has remained so constant. If you are a sensitive, intelligent, and thinking person, you have to be at least a tad hypochondriacal merely by being alive. Otherwise, you are oblivious, in denial, an automaton.

Sometimes, even to the most resilient of us, life must seem a preposterous and cruel joke. To come into a world filled with so much magnificence and beauty, to nurture relationships, build careers, all for what? I've always been a little envious of the pious with their certainty of belief in a Supreme Being and a life hereafter, those who believe that suffering, illness included, represents a special pact with God and a call to a deeper and purer realization of that relationship. Religion provides liberation from the temporal world, a submission to something outside of self. We all need to escape from our existential concerns; the healthiest accomplish this through love, faith, and work; others take flight into cults, alcoholism, binge eating, and sickness. Hypochondria may be the most authentic realization of our fears: we stare directly into the abyss, facing life's uncertainty and perils, but without a shield of self-defense.

When I first recognized this fragility in myself, I thought I was the unusual one, feeling my vulnerability so acutely, fixating on what I fixated on, suffering the way I suffered. I thought I might even know why. When I was seventeen, I was involved in a fatal car accident. I was a new driver behind the wheel of my parents' Chevy, my friend Toby beside me in the passenger seat. We were on our way to the ski slopes. Then I missed a curve on a winding mountain road obscured by a snowbank and in a flash had a fiery collision with a tractor-trailer. Fate let Toby die while I survived with barely an injury.

The accident was the worst thing that ever happened to me. Even twenty-four years later it is difficult for me to say that without guilt and without hearing a condemning voice over my shoulder: "Bad for you, huh? But so much worse for her."

The sense of culpability in the accident's aftermath which filled me with shame, despair, and self-hate was so intense that it endures to this day. Directly afterward, I was numb, and then for many years punitive: I wouldn't allow myself to feel healthy, happy, and strong. I carried the guilt in my body, exorcising it during my early twenties in the rebuking self-starvation of anorexia, and later in a constant certainty of being struck down by illness or death. I couldn't connect the symptoms on any emotional level with the earlier event, but years afterward in psychotherapy, my therapist drew the links and tried to make me see. I worked diligently at insight and even achieved the connection intellectually, but knowledge wasn't powerful enough to allow me to let go of the punitory system I had created, or of the hypochondriacal fears.

Then two things happened: a drug changed some essential biological substrate within me, and in writing this book I met other people who had suffered and are suffering in a way I completely understood. These were not necessarily people who had survived an accident, but nonetheless they had lived their own version of survivor syndrome that had caused them to be emotionally frail, unable to withstand the irony of our peculiar existence. There had been an alcoholic father, a depressed mother, physical or emotional abuse, some trauma, or a series of smaller blows, which had burst upon already weakened ground. I was not the only one who experienced the phenomenon of getting symptoms when things were going well, who couldn't juggle too many stressful events, who didn't let joy in too easily.

Meeting these people made me realize that we humans are boundlessly complex, and that my "accident equals hypochondria" insight was only one clue to an ever more intricate puzzle. No one walks away from trauma unscathed, but not everyone who is traumatized starves herself or develops hypochondria. Why I became more afraid of living and of dying than others will forever remain an enigma. I can point to the car accident. I can point to my father's tendency to brood and be hard on himself, which I have internalized. I can point to a very early preoccupation with my body, not liking my nose, my wispy curls, my bushy eyebrows, which I perceived as too dark. I can also point to a certain naive recklessness I have displayed in my life; a tendency to flirt with disaster—hitchhiking alone through Europe and Central America, putting trust in unworthy relationships, experimenting with more drugs than I should have—a side of myself for which hypochondria may have provided a balance. Other events have had their impact: a distant cousin, beautiful, sweet, and courageous, dies of lymphoma at twenty-five; a childhood classmate gets married and is dead of a brain tumor within a year; my great uncle Charlie, who shortly after his acceptance to medical school diagnoses his own leukemia and dies before his graduation.

You can't help but be touched and terrified by such events. If they can happen to others, why not to you or me? The well-defended can tuck this question away with "hope for the best" that it will not happen to them or their loved ones. The hypochondriac tries to but can't. Morbid preoccupations surface in a habit of checking your neck for swollen lymph nodes, in a tendency to seek too many biopsies and see too many doctors, in an inability to forget your mortality for too long.

If you're lucky, as I was, you finally wake up, not just intellectually but deep in your soul, to a simple paradox: if you are going to live out the rest of your life preparing for the day the tumor arrives, when you get the report of that terrible blood test, when you collapse in crushing pain, what's the point? Why would anyone want to live to 120 as a hypochondriac?

You will realize that the day will ultimately come, that vigilance won't stave it off, and that the best control we have over early illness disasters is minimal: stay away from cigarettes, drink in moderation, exercise, eat nutritiously, wear a seat belt, have checkups every so often.

The possibility always exists that it could happen in the way it did for Uncle Charlie. Or for Jackie O. or Audrey Hepburn, who presumably took good care of themselves but to whom death came suddenly and too early. But for a greater number of us, chances are that when the bad report comes, it will not be a death sentence but something we'll live and cope with for a long time. Because as our life spans lengthen, the risk of chronic illness is higher than it has ever been. One third of the population lives with constant ailments: cancer, heart disease, diabetes, arthritis. And while some fall apart under the stress of a long-term ailment, that's the moment others wake up. Sometimes it takes a heart attack or another life-threatening illness to make roses smell.

As I come to the close of my odyssey, I hope I have succeeded in accomplishing what I set out to do: erase a stigma, debunk some myths, lend some illumination to a puzzling, perpetually elusive malady. If reading this book helps people feel more kindly toward themselves or toward someone they know or bolsters a relationship between doctor and patient, then I will feel that the effort has been worthwhile.

If we continue to stay hypochondriacally miserable, in the end we will doubtless have won the ability to proclaim what people have joked belongs on a hypochondriac's tombstone: "I told you I was sick." But it will be neither funny nor satisfying, for when serious illness strikes a hypochondriac, it has to be more tragic than for the person who has loved, enjoyed, and lived a full life. It is nearly impossible for the hypochondriac to go gently into that good night because, like the person of my nightmare, he has never been happy.

As for that person, we continue to have some things in common: I still detest blood tests, obituaries both intrigue and unnerve me, and my doctor-shopping habit has tilted a bit toward avoidance, but I'm working on it. I can't remember the last time I dwelled on lupus, but I worry sometimes about cancer, and once in a great while, I admit, I reach for my neck, looking for a swollen lymph node . . . but it's different now. Rather than being accompanied by those old desperate emotions, I have a more transient feeling of hey, just checking.

At first I thought that allowing a little more joie de vivre into my life would make me *more* afraid to be struck down, but it seems to work in the opposite way. If I did get that bad news now, it would be utterly terrifying and tremendously sad, but not quite as frightening or tragic as it would have been four years ago when I was hypochondria's prisoner. Because using your energy in less destructive, more gratifying ways puts a whole lot more life under your belt; you become an older, more satisfied person. On a few occasions I have driven by the hospital where I spent that pivotal night and stared up at the place and wondered: Was there *really* a time when I thought that life could possibly be better inside, cooped up, away from my family, than out?

For most of you the road to overcoming hypochondria will not be paved with epiphanies or critical events; rather, it will evolve with a series of small steps, sometimes unnoticeable. The real mark of success may come when you least expect it, like being ready to kiss a child good night or chatting with a friend on the porch and suddenly realizing: I haven't thought about it for a while. Or sharing a bottle of wine with your spouse at the waterfront restaurant where you became engaged more than a decade ago and you wishing you could live forever, not because you're afraid but because you're so happy.

Such moments may be fleeting, but the contentment they bring can be permanent and worth striving for. Because when the time comes to say goodbye, you want to do it serenely, not kicking and screaming, "I haven't lived!"

Sure, I'd love to make it to ninety. Who wouldn't? But I have come to realize that quality is, indeed, a more worthwhile pursuit than quantity. And whether I have ten more years or fifty, the texture of my life is one of the few variables over which I have some control.

When my number is up, I don't want to be hooked up to oxygen machines and breathing tubes in a cold, sterile hospital but surrounded by loved ones at home. I hope not to feel sorry for myself or want others to pity me, but to sense how blessed my life has been, how much I've come through, how many people I've cared for and have cared about me. And when I'm gone, I want my children to say "Boy, she loved life." That's the way I hope they remember me. Their mom the hypochondriac.

Maplewood, New Jersey
October 1995

....

A Self-Diagnostic Test for Hypochondria

HOW CAN YOU TELL whether you worry about illness too much? Let's say that you have an illness like diabetes or asthma—Who can decide how much worry is too much? Even if you don't have an illness, isn't a certain amount of careful health awareness desirable? For example, if a healthy woman in her forties switches from examining her breasts monthly to every two weeks, is she being overanxious or merely sensible?

To deal with such questions, consider taking one of the tests psychiatrists employ to identify at-risk populations in their studies. The Illness Attitude Scale (IAS) was developed in the 1980s by Dr. Robert Kellner, a professor of psychiatry at the University of New Mexico School of Medicine and a leader in hypochondria research. A well-standardized and reliable scale, the IAS has been found useful in examining health attitudes and behavior and in discovering whether concerns about illness fall in the range of normal apprehension or pathological vigilance.

The following fifteen questions represent a modified version of the Illness Attitude Scale. In answer to each one, describe how you generally feel, not only how you have felt recently. If you have a serious illness that a physician has diagnosed, de-

A Word of Caution about Psychological Testing

Before you begin, you should know that the Illness Attitude Scale is only one among dozens of measures used to identify hypochondria and other somatizing-type behaviors. There are also hundreds of instruments that gauge obsessiveness, depression, panic disorder—virtually every form of behavior that deviates from the so-called norm. Just as nonpsychiatrists have such routine screening procedures as blood tests and urinalysis, psychiatrists and psychologists have their tools of the trade to determine the right therapy for a patient.

Some say that the effort to study human behavior scientifically has led to overreliance on psychological testing to the point that clinicians may forget that the person being tested and the assessments based on paper-and-pen self-reporting aren't dependable. Mental health researchers appear to be aware of such criticisms, commonly apologizing in journal articles for scale weaknesses and investigative pitfalls such as faulty recall, limited sample, interviewers' bias, and the like. Still, while flawed, diagnostic testing, like the classification of mental illnesses, is a recognized means for assessing and tracking mental and emotional problems in the community and devising treatment strategies.

The greatest obstacle in probing for hypochondria is the possibility of skewed results attributable to the presence of undetected physical illness. Of course, as we are aware, hypochondriacs can suffer from genuine diseases. Nevertheless, when a medical condition is undiagnosed, the frustration of not knowing can lead to all sorts of distortions. Therefore, your score on this questionnaire will be more reliable if, after appropriate examination, you've been given a clean bill of health, and any medical condition you may have is under control.

scribe how you felt *before* you became ill. When you complete the questionnaire, you can compare your results with those of three other groups of people who have taken it.

Questionnaire: Are You at Risk for Hypochondria?

Read each question, but don't think too long about your answer. Score each answer as follows:

> No = 0
> Rarely = 1
> Sometimes = 2
> Often = 3
> Most of the time = 4

1. Do you worry about your health? _____
2. Do you worry that you may get a serious illness in the future? _____
3. Does the thought of a serious illness scare you? _____

Total for questions 1–3 _____

4. When you have a pain, do you worry that it may be caused by serious illness? _____
5. If a pain lasts a week or more, do you see a physician? _____
6. If a pain lasts a week or more, do you think you have a serious disease? _____

Total for questions 4–6 _____

7. Do you believe you have a physical disease that doctors have not diagnosed correctly? _____
8. When your doctor tells you that you do not have a physical disease, do you refuse to believe her? _____
9. Shortly after your doctor reports on the results of your examination, do you begin to believe that you may have contracted a new illness? _____

Total for questions 7–9 _____

10. Are you uncomfortable about news of death—obituary notices, funerals? _____
11. Does the thought of death scare you? _____
12. Are you afraid that you may soon die? _____

Total for questions 10–12 _____

13. When you read or hear about an illness, do you develop symptoms similar to those of the illness? _____
14. When you feel a strange sensation in your body, do you find it difficult to think about anything else? _____
15. When you feel a strange sensation in your body, do you worry about it? _____

Total for questions 13–15 _____

Scoring Your Illness Attitude Scale

Enter your total score for each category of hypochondria in the score sheet below.

SCORE SHEET	
Category of Hypochondria	**Your Score**
Questions 1–3: Worry about Illness	
Questions 4–6: Concern about Pain	
Questions 7–9: Hypochondriacal Beliefs	
Questions 10–12: Fear of Death	
Questions 13–15: Bodily Preoccupation	

Now compare your score in each category with those of patients from the three other populations: a group that fits the diagnostic criteria for hypochondria; a group of patients who visit a family practitioner; and a random group of employees. The first figure in each category is an average score, and the figures in parentheses show the ranges of the scores.

HOW DO YOU COMPARE?						
Category of Hypochondria	**Hypochondria**		**Family Practice**		**Employees**	
	Avg	(Range)	Avg	(Range)	Avg	(Range)
Worry about Illness	9	(6–12)	4	(1–7)	2	(0–4)
Concern about Pain	10	(8–12)	5	(2–8)	3	(1–5)
Hypochondriacal Beliefs	8	(5–11)	2	(0–4)	1	(0–3)
Fear of Death	8	(4–12)	1	(0–3)	1	(0–3)
Bodily Preoccupation	8	(5–11)	4	(2–6)	2	(0–4)

If you find that many of your scores fall within the typical range for hypochondriacs, you suffer from hypochondria. If you score within the typical range in only one or two categories, you probably do not have a severe case of hypochondria.

NOTES

Prologue

page

1 It is easy: William Styron, *Darkness Visible: A Memoir of Madness* (New York: Vintage, 1990), 44.

10 *The Merck Manual:* 16th ed. (Rahway, N.J.: Merck, Sharp, and Dohme Research Labs, 1992), 1591.

Chapter 1: A Much Maligned Malady

14 I have always felt: F. E. Kenyon, "Hypochondriasis: A Survey of Some Historical, Clinical, and Social Aspects," *British Journal of Medical Psychology* 38 (1965): 120.

15 Meet Fred: David Blum, "Listening to Advil," *New York Magazine* 26 (November 1, 1993): 20.

17 standard medical text: Arthur J. Barsky, "Overview: Hypochondriasis, Bodily Complaints, and Somatic Styles," *American Journal of Psychiatry* 140 (March 1983): 273.

18 "Hypochondria carries": Arthur Barsky, personal interview, October 19, 1993.

19 One British researcher: Kenyon, "Hypochondriasis," 125.

19 "Perhaps no other": Donald R. Lipsitt, "Psychodynamic Considerations of Hypochondriasis," *Psychotherapy and Psychosomatics* 23 (1974): 132–141.

page

20 *Morbus hypochondriacus:* Robert Kellner, *Somatization and Hypochondriasis* (New York: Praeger, 1986), 1.

20 English malady: Kenyon, "Hypochondriasis," 118.

21 symptoms as so "ambiguous": Robert Burton, *The Anatomy of Melancholy*, ed. Holbrook Jackson (London and Toronto: J. M. Dent, 1977), 410–411.

21 Elizabethan attitude toward: Robert Meister, *Hypochondria: Toward a Better Understanding* (New York: Taplinger, 1980), 95–98.

21 "greatest medical treatise": *The Anatomy of Melancholy*, xi.

21 "sharp belchings": Ibid., 411–412.

22 "some sudden commotion": Ibid., 380–381.

22 "If one wheel": Ibid., 171.

22 watched public hangings: Kristin McMurran in an interview with Susan Baur, *People*, August 29, 1988, 81.

22 physical disabilities seem: John Wain, *Samuel Johnson: A Biography* (New York: Viking, 1974), 253–254. See also Judith L. Rapoport, *The Boy Who Couldn't Stop Washing: The Experience and Treatment of Obsessive-Compulsive Disorder* (New York: Dutton, 1987), 3–5.

23 controversial theories of evolution: McMurran, interview with Baur, 81–82.

23 "He was always": Linda H. Davis, "The Man on the Swing," *New Yorker* 69 (December 27, 1993–January 3, 1994): 90–104.

24 How did hypochondriacal complaints: Susan Baur, *Hypochondria: Woeful Imaginings* (Berkeley: University of California Press, 1988), 28–29.

25 doctors resorted to savage: Edward Shorter, *From Paralysis to Fatigue: A History of Psychosomatic Illness in the Modern Era* (New York: Free Press, 1992), 83.

25 "Any woman whose": David B. Morris, *The Culture of Pain* (Berkeley: University of California Press, 1991), 109.

25 Then, in 1895: James Strachey, *The Standard Edition of the Complete Psychological Works of Sigmund Freud*, vol. 2, "Studies on Hysteria," edited by Josef Breuer and Sigmund Freud (London: Hogarth Press, 1957, 1st ed., 1991, revised).

26 Fits and paralysis: Shorter, *From Paralysis to Fatigue*, 267.

page

26 "Toward the end": Baur, *Hypochondria*, 28.

26 once psychoanalysis came: Shorter, *From Paralysis to Fatigue*, 193.

27 "Consultation with a psychiatrist": Ibid., 261.

27 "a fateful chapter": Ibid., 244.

27 "fashionable" diseases: Ibid., 305.

28 "an extremely difficult": Arthur Kleinman, *The Illness Narratives: Suffering, Healing and the Human Condition* (New York: Basic Books, 1988), 40.

28 "A single-minded quest": Ibid., 42.

28 new generation of drugs: Jeffrey M. Jonas and Ron Shaumburg, *Everything You Need to Know about Prozac* (New York: Bantam, 1991), 32.

29 "Only a very small proportion": *The Merck Manual*, 16th ed. (Rahway, N.J.: Merck, Sharp, and Dohme Research Labs, 1992), 1591.

30 "These were the patients": Nicholas Cummings, personal interview, April 25, 1994.

30 "in the United States": *Mind–Body Medicine: How to Use Your Mind for Better Health*, edited by Daniel Goleman and Joel Gurin (Yonkers, N.Y.: Consumer Reports Books, 1993), 224.

31 Of one thousand patients: Kurt Kroenke et al., "The Prevalence of Symptoms in Medical Outpatients and the Adequacy of Therapy," *Archives of Internal Medicine* 150 (1990): 1685–1689.

31 two Montreal clinics: Laurence J. Kirmayer, "Three Forms of Somatization in Primary Care," *Journal of Nervous and Mental Disease* 179 (November 1991): 647–655.

31 consult physicians four times: Epidemiological studies sponsored by the National Institute of Mental Health indicate that patients diagnosed with somatization disorder typically make six outpatient visits in a six-month period; the average American patient sees his or her doctor three times a year. See "National Ambulatory Care Survey," National Center for Health Statistics, 1990, and G. Richard Smith, "Somatization Disorder in the Medical Setting," a U.S. Department of Health and Human Services publication, 1990, 23.

3 1 medical bills: Daniel Goleman, "Patients Refusing to Be Well," *New York Times*, August 21, 1991, C-10.

3 1 about $20 billion: T. Michael Kashner, personal interview, May 8, 1994. Kashner, an economist in the Department of Psychiatry at Southwestern Medical Center in Dallas and a career scientist in Health Services Research and Development with the Dallas Veterans Administration Medical Center, believes this estimate is conservative. The $20 billion figure is not the total cost of health care that somatizers use; it represents only the amount of money that could be saved if minimal attention were given to the problem of persons who consistently present complaints to doctors for which no medical cause can be determined. See Kashner et al., "The Impact of a Psychiatric Consultation Letter on the Expenditures and Outcomes of Care of Patients with Somatization Disorder," *Medical Care* 30 (September 1992): 811–820. See also Kashner et al., "Enhancing the Health of Somatization Disorder Patients," *Psychosomatics* 36 (October 1995): 462–470.

3 2 Viennese analyst: Shorter, *From Paralysis to Fatigue*, 259–260.

3 3 Textbook Cases: American Psychiatric Association, *Diagnostic and Statistical Manual of Mental Disorders*, 4th ed. (DSM-IV)(Washington, D.C.: APA, 1994), 445–468.

Chapter 2: The Many Faces of Somatization

3 5 To some, ill health: W. H. Auden, "The Art of Healing," in *Epistle to a Godson and Other Poems* (New York: Random House, 1969), 8.

3 6 study of Briquet's: The modern concept of somatization disorder is a direct descendant of the Washington University–Renard Hospital studies on Briquet's syndrome, named for the French doctor Pierre Briquet, who first described its symptoms. The group's "family studies" on hysteria during the 1960s and 1970s led researchers to conclude that conversion symptoms, e.g., unexplained blindness, and Briquet's, a polysymptomatic condition occurring early in life and mainly in women, were

separate diagnostic entities. Today this distinction is widely accepted. See Samuel B. Guze, "The Diagnosis of Hysteria: What Are We Trying to Do?" *American Journal of Psychiatry* 124 (October 1967): 491–498, and Guze et al., "Sex, Age, and the Diagnosis of Hysteria (Briquet's Syndrome)," *American Journal of Psychiatry* 129 (December 1972): 745–748.

36 "There is obviously": Ian Pilowsky, "Abnormal Illness Behaviour," *British Journal of Medical Psychology* 42 (1969): 347–349.

36 third edition of: American Psychiatric Association, *Diagnostic and Statistical Manual of Mental Disorders*, 3d ed. (DSM-III) (Washington D.C.: APA, 1980).

40 During the 1960s: I. Pilowsky, "Dimensions of Hypochondriasis," *British Journal of Psychiatry* 113 (1967): 89–93.

40–51 The patients speak: Abir, Julie, and Peter, and the names of all the sufferers I interviewed, are pseudonyms. I changed occupations and, with the exception of gender, other identifying characteristics.

51 "beauty hypochondria": Katherine A. Phillips, "Body Dysmorphic Disorder: The Distress of Imagined Ugliness," *American Journal of Psychiatry* 148 (September 1991): 1138–1149.

51 precise gender ratio: Katharine A. Phillips, "An Ugly Secret: Body Dysmorphic Disorder," *Medical and Health Annual* (Chicago: Encyclopaedia Britannica, 1993), 364.

53 Somatization disorder is relatively rare: DSM-IV, 447.

53 Across the nation: *Psychiatric Disorders in America*, edited by Lee N. Robins and Darrel A. Regier (New York: Free Press, 1991), 228.

55 "That's something the chronic pain": Robert Dworkin, personal interview, November 3, 1993.

Chapter 3: Digging Beneath Symptoms

60 The sorrow that: Joyce McDougall, *Theaters of the Body* (New York: Norton, 1989), 139.

page

61 "The great secret": Lewis Thomas, *The Lives of a Cell: Notes of a Biology Watcher* (New York: Viking, 1974), 85.

61 "A large portion": Charles V. Ford, personal interview, May 13, 1994.

62 a herniated disc: John E. Sarno, *Healing Back Pain: The Mind–Body Connection* (New York: Warner, 1991), 103.

62 A study conducted: Julia E. Connelly et al., "Healthy Patients Who Perceive Poor Health and Their Use of Primary Care Services," *Journal of General Internal Medicine* 6 January/February 1991): 47–51.

63 "Unlike the hypochondriac": Suzy Szasz, *Living with It: Why You Don't Have to Be Healthy to Be Happy* (Buffalo and New York: Prometheus, 1991), 7, 10.

64 "It's all right": Anatole Broyard, *Intoxicated by My Illness* (New York: Fawcett Columbine, 1992), 23.

64 "There is, let us confess it": Virginia Woolf, "On Being Ill," in *Collected Essays*, vol. 4 (New York: Harcourt, Brace and World, 1925), 196, 199.

64 The Romantic poets: Susan Sontag, *Illness as Metaphor* (New York: Farrar, Straus and Giroux, 1977), 33–34.

65 called a common task: Stephen A. Green, *Feel Good Again* (Yonkers, N.Y.: Consumer Reports Books, 1990), 105.

65 "disease plus meaning": Larry Dossey, *Meaning and Medicine* (New York: Bantam, 1991), 18.

65 "the lived experience": Arthur Kleinman, *The Illness Narratives: Suffering, Healing, and the Human Condition* (New York: Basic Books, 1988), 3–4.

67 Angela Farnum: Steve Salerno, "High Price of Managed Care," *Wall Street Journal*, January 18, 1994, A-16.

67 Rhode Island laboratory: "19,000 Cancer Tests Rechecked after Misreading," *New York Times*, September 27, 1993, A-12.

68 One physician told Hanner: Linda Hanner, *When You're Sick and Don't Know Why* (Minneapolis: DCI Publishing, 1991), 143.

69 one of every two adults: Daniel Goleman, "1 in 2 Experiences a Mental Disorder," *New York Times*, January 14, 1994, A-20. This University of Michigan study found major depression to

page

be the most common disorder, with 10 percent of Americans experiencing the problem in a given year. The second most common disorder was alcohol dependence. Original study in *Archives of General Psychiatry*, January 1994.

70 "Regardless of whether": Charles Ford, personal interview, April 13, 1994.

70 research conducted at McGill University: Nancy Wartik, "Hypochondria: Real Treatments for a Real Disorder," *American Health*, May 1994, 70.

71 study of forty-two hypochondriacal patients: Brian A. Fallon et al., "Hypochondriasis," in *Obsessive-Compulsive-Related Disorders*, ed. Eric Hollander (Washington, D.C.: American Psychiatric Press, 1993), 79.

71 during the course of any given year: Statistics on depression, panic disorder, and OCD taken from July 1993 "Update," a fact sheet prepared by National Institute of Mental Health's Office of Scientific Information.

72 Nearly 50 percent: Robert Fisch, "Masked Depression: Its Interrelations with Somatization, Hypochondriasis, and Conversion," *International Journal of Psychiatry in Medicine* 17 (1987): 367–379.

72 A Viennese psychiatrist: Edward Shorter, *From the Mind into the Body: The Cultural Origins of Psychosomatic Symptoms* (New York: Free Press, 1994), 130.

73 "numbness, an enervation": William Styron, *Darkness Visible: A Memoir of Madness* (New York: Vintage, 1990), 43–44, 50.

73 Patients who experience: Nancy Wartik, "Taking Depression to Heart," *American Health*, January/February 1994, 30.

74 researchers at Columbia University: Robert H. Dworkin, et al., "A High-Risk Method for Studying Psychosocial Antecedents of Chronic Pain," *Journal of Abnormal Psychology* 101 (1992): 200–205.

74 John: A Case: Mack Lipkin, Jr., personal interview, September 15, 1993.

76 Consider a 1994: American Psychiatric Association, Annual Meeting, Philadelphia, May 21–26, 1994.

page

76 Are Your Symptoms Related: *The Diagnostic and Statistical Manual* divides anxiety into thirteen categories. They include generalized anxiety disorder, when a person worries about everything much of the time; acute stress disorder, which follows a major stress or life crisis, for example, a heart attack or an impending divorce; simple phobia, a fear of places or situations from which escape might be difficult or in which help might not be available in the event of sudden symptoms; the two anxiety syndromes, in addition to panic disorder, that have the strong connection to somatization and hypochondria, are post traumatic stress disorder (PTSD) and obsessive-compulsive disorder.

77 Each year 100,000 people: According to a fact sheet, "Key Facts about Mental Illness," published by the National Institute of Mental Health, unnecessary angiograms performed because of panic symptoms waste more than $32 million annually.

77 Patients with cardiophobia: Georg H. Eifert, "Cardiophobia: A Paradigmatic Behavioural Mode of Heart-Focused Anxiety and Non-anginal Chest Pain," *Behaviour Research Therapy* 30 (1992): 329–345.

78 Generally, people have seen: In a study of seventy-one patients with panic disorder, each averaged 7.5 test procedures, most commonly EEG, ECG, and upper GI series. "Panic Disorder: "The Great Masquerader," *Internal Medicine News*, November 15–30, 1990, 20.

80 "These people aren't crazy": Eric Hollander, personal interview, April 21, 1994.

83 "When an event": Debra Neumann, personal interview, January 27, 1995.

84 "in symbols, body problems": A. G. Britton, "The Terrible Truth," *Self*, October 1992, 188–202.

Chapter 4: Are Hypochondriacs Born or Made? The Nature–Nurture Debate

page

86 How shall a man: R. W. Emerson, *Conduct of Life* (New York: Hurst, 1959), 9.

87 taint of "black blood": Kay Redfield Jamison, *Touched with Fire* (New York: Free Press, 1993), 196–201.

88 has been "remedicalized": Alfie Kohn, "Back to Nurture," *American Health*, April 1993, 29–31.

89 "To be able to do so": William Styron, *Darkness Visible: A Memoir of Madness* (New York: Vintage, 1990), 38.

90 irresistible as a classic: Peter D. Kramer, *Listening to Prozac* (New York: Viking, 1993), 73.

90 "It is not within the scope": Donald R. Lipsitt, "Psychodynamic Considerations of Hypochondriasis," *Psychotherapy and Psychosomatics* 23 (1974): 132.

91 George A. Ladee: Susan Baur, *Hypochondria: Woeful Imaginings* (Berkeley: University of California Press, 1988), 73–74.

91 "substitutes illness": Ibid., 5.

91 "an overwhelming sense": Donald R. Lipsitt, personal interview, October 18, 1993.

92 "capable of safeguarding": Baur, *Hypochondria*, 74.

93 "Pity me that": Edna St. Vincent Millay, "Pity Me Not," *A Treasury of Great Poems*, ed. Louis Untermeyer (New York: Simon and Schuster, 1942), 1167.

94 heterosexual students with: David Brody et al., "AIDS Concerns among Low-risk Heterosexuals: The Other Side of the Epidemic," *Medical Care* 30 (March 1992): 276–281.

95 In *Worried Sick*: Arthur J. Barsky, *Worried Sick: Our Troubled Quest for Wellness* (Boston: Little, Brown, 1988), 23–36.

97 Serotonin, especially plentiful: Jeffrey M. Jonas and Ron Schaumburg, *Everything You Need to Know about Prozac* (New York: Bantam, 1991) 36–39.

99 evaluated nineteen anorectic patients: *Obsessive-Compulsive-Related Disorders*, ed. Eric Hollander (Washington, D.C.: American Psychiatric Press, 1993), 55.

99 "an internal alarm": Eric Hollander, personal interview, April 21, 1994.

page

100 Research supports the idea: An oft-cited study on brain response to OCD treatment was conducted by Lewis Baxter and colleagues at the University of California at Los Angeles. See Baxter et al., "Caudate Glucose Metabolic Rate Changes with Both Drug and Behavior Therapy for Obsessive-Compulsive Disorder," *Archives of General Psychiatry* 49 (September 1992): 681–689.

101 to study twins and adopted children: Philip Elmer-Dewitt, "The Genetic Revolution," *Time*, January 17, 1994, 46–53.

101 The exceptions are schizophrenia: Aubrey Milunsky, *Heredity and Your Family's Health* (Baltimore: Johns Hopkins University Press, 1992), 382–391, and personal interview, January 10, 1993.

102 One study of twenty-four pairs: Robert Kellner, *Somatization and Hypochondriasis* (New York: Praeger, 1986), 63–65.

103 "The truth is": Keith Russell Ablow, "The Overselling of Biological Psychiatry," *Washington Post Health*, August 4, 1992, 9.

103 The view that all is genetic: Martin Seligman, *What You Can Change and What You Can't: The Complete Guide to Successful Self-improvement* (New York: Knopf, 1993), 4.

104 "Quite often, a hypochondriac": Laurence Kirmayer, personal interview, April 14, 1994.

105 "The patient, call her Susie": Eric Hollander, personal interview, April 21, 1994.

106 Ironically, biological theories: David Stipp, "Brain Flicks: Doctors Film an Obsession," *Wall Street Journal*, December 2, 1992, B-1, B-7.

106 Freud himself was never: Judith L. Rapoport, *The Boy Who Couldn't Stop Washing: Experience and Treatment of Obsessive-Compulsive Disorder* (New York: Dutton, 1989), 100.

106 "In view of the intimate": Harold H. Bloomfield and Peter McWilliams, in *How to Heal Depression* (Los Angeles: Prelude, 1994), 83.

107 "Symptoms have a social": Edward Shorter, *From the Mind into the Body: The Cultural Origins of Psychosomatic Symptoms* (New York: Free Press, 1994), ix.

page

107 "don't account for": Ibid., 202.

107 Talk to cultural anthropologists: Baur, *Hypochondria*, 34–35.

109 "Hysterical pain": David B. Morris, *The Culture of Pain* (Berkeley: University of California Press, 1991), 121.

109 "Live as domestic a life": Ibid., 113.

109 By World War I: Tom Lutz, *American Nervousness, 1903: An Anecdotal History* (Ithaca: Cornell University Press, 1991), 19–37.

110 "physicians were far more comfortable": Charles V. Ford, personal interview, April 13, 1994.

110 Cultural explanations of hypochondria: Shorter, *From the Mind into the Body*, 207.

Chapter 5: Healthism: A Symptom of Our Time

111 For each disorder: Marcel Proust, *The Guermantes Way*, trans. C. K. Scott Moncrieff (New York: Modern Library, Random House, 1952), 415.

111 The faces stare: Colleen Drischler, letter to the editor, in *USA Weekend*, January 1–3, 1993, 12.

112 Middle-aged baby boomers: Arthur J. Barsky, "The Paradox of Health," *New England Journal of Medicine* 318 (February 18, 1988): 414–418.

112 "We fear the worst": Norman Cousins, "A Nation of Hypochondriacs," *Time*, June 18, 1990, 88.

113 "My clinical impression": Donna Stewart, "The Changing Faces of Somatization," *Psychosomatics* 31 (Spring 1990): 154–155.

114 "A public in dogged pursuit": Clifton K. Meador, "The Last Well Person," *New England Journal of Medicine* 330 (February 10, 1994): 440–441.

115 Lewis Thomas: *The Lives of a Cell: Notes of a Biology Watcher* (New York: Viking, 1974), 82.

115 Americans spend about $60 billion: Interview with staff members of Towne-Oller & Associates, a subsidiary of Information Services, Chicago. See also N. R. Kleinfield, "The

page

Do-It-Yourself Armamentarium," *New York Times Magazine*, October 3, 1993, 70–78, and Elyse Tanouye, "Home Medical Tests Post Healthy Sales," *Wall Street Journal*, November 12, 1992, B-1, B-11.

117 "To tell us": Lynn Payer, "The Great Sickness Scam," adapted from *Disease Mongers*, *Redbook*, January 1993, 47.

118 In an experiment: Morton Lebow and Elaine Bratic Arkin, "Women's Health and Mass Media: The Reporting Risk," *Women's Health and the Mass Media* 3 (Winter 1993): 185.

119 Yet they're the ones: Gina Kolata, "Mammography Campaigns Draw In the Young and Healthy," *New York Times*, "Week in Review," January 10, 1993, 6. One survey found that a third of women in their thirties were "very worried" about getting breast cancer, in contrast to 16 percent of women in their sixties.

120 "ambiguity of uncertain wellness": Delia Cioffi, "Asymmetry of Doubt in Medical Self-Diagnosis: The Ambiguity of 'Uncertain Wellness,'" *Journal of Personality and Social Psychology* 61 (1991): 969–980.

121 the risk of death: Elisabeth Rosenthal, "Deaths after Surgery Prompt Inquiry at a Queens Hospital," *New York Times*, August 1, 1995, A-1, B-2. In 1994, for example, hospitals in New York State reported seventy-eight deaths that were potentially related to anesthesia.

121 synthetic jaw implants: Bruce Ingersoll and Rose Gutfeld, "Implants in Jaw Joint Fail, Leaving Patients in Pain and Disfigured," *Wall Street Journal*, August 31, 1993, A-1, A-4.

121 Consider tryptophan: Patricia Long, "The Vitamin Wars," *Health*, May/June 1993, 54.

121 Even something as wholesome: Kevin Helliker, "Some Mothers, Trying in Vain to Breast-Feed, Starve Their Infants," *Wall Street Journal*, July 22, 1994, A-1, A-4.

123 Judging the Medical News: This advice is culled from three sources: Gina Kolata, "Amid Inconclusive Health Studies, Some Experts Advise Less Advice," *New York Times*, May 10, 1995, C-12; Marilyn Chase, "How to Put Hyped Study Results under a Microscope," *Wall Street Journal*, January 16,

page

1995, B-1; and "Ten Tips for Judging the Medical News, *Harvard Women's Health Watch*, October 1993, 6.

125 "Beauty's shelf life": Patricia Volk, *New York Times Magazine*, September 4, 1994, 49.

125 Demi Moore: Michelle Stacey, "Women Who Exercise Too Much," *Elle*, August 1994, 184.

126 according to one study: Joni E. Johnston, *Appearance Obsession* (Deerfield Beach, Fla.: Health Communications, 1994), 187.

126 Each year approximately 2.5 million: "1994 National Statistics on Cosmetic Surgery," fact sheet (Chicago: American Academy of Cosmetic Surgery, 1995).

126 "There's a difference between health and healthism": Barbara Ehrenreich, "The Morality of Muscle Tone," reprinted from *Lear's, Utne Reader*, May/June 1992, 65–68.

128 "It's a depressing reality": Kathy LaTour, *The Breast Cancer Companion: From Diagnosis through Treatment to Recovery: Everything You Need to Know for Every Step Along the Way* (New York: Avon, 1993), 258, 307–308.

128 "Grant study": Martin E. P. Seligman, *Learned Optimism* (New York: Pocket Books, 1990) 179–181.

129 two Yale psychologists: Ibid., 169. See also E. J. Langer and J. Rodin, "Effects of Choice and Enhanced Personality Responsibility for the Aged: A Field Experiment in an Institutional Setting," *Journal of Personality and Social Psychology* 34 (1976): 191–199.

129 What is unclear and still unknown: Denise Grady, "Think Right. Stay Well?" *American Health*, November 1992, 50–54.

Chapter 6: It's Never All in Your Head

131 "Words cannot express": Dorothy, who after being diagnosed with chronic fatigue syndrome returns to chastise a doctor who had humiliated her, in a scene from the television situation comedy *Golden Girls*, from Dennis Jackson, "So I

page

Really Have Something Real," *CFIDS Chronicle*, Summer/ Fall 1989, 108–111.

135 "bacterial pneumonia would": Robert Meister, *Hypochondria: Toward a Better Understanding* (New York: Taplinger, 1980), 17.

135 Even the shamans: Kat Duff, *The Alchemy of Illness* (New York: Pantheon, 1993), 52.

136 the medical profession lost: Larry Dossey, *Meaning and Medicine* (New York: Bantam, 1991), 111.

137 the psychosomatic concept has been slow to die: Nearly twenty years ago, the American Psychiatric Association dropped from the *Diagnostic and Statistical Manual* the classification "psychophysiological disorders," which included migraines, ulcers, asthma, among others. The concept was replaced by "psychological factors affecting medical condition," a category that theoretically can be applied to all physical illnesses but is reserved for cases in which psychosocial factors play an overriding role in causing or aggravating a condition. Or when, as the manual stipulates, "there is reasonable evidence to suggest an association between the psychological factors and the development or exacerbation of, or delayed recovery from, the medical condition." American Psychiatric Association, *Diagnostic and Statistical Manual of Mental Disorders*, 4th ed. (DSM-IV) (Washington, D.C.: APA, 1994), 675–677.

138 "the frustration of dependent": Franz Alexander et al., *Psychosomatic Specificity*, vol. 1 (Chicago: University of Chicago Press, 1968), 16–17.

138 "constant pressure and an unwillingness": Jean Rosenbaum, *The Mind Factor: How Your Emotions Affect Your Health* (Englewood Cliffs, N.J.: Prentice-Hall, 1973), 100.

139 About 30 percent of thirty-year-olds: "Debugging the System," *Harvard Health Letter* 19 (June 1994): 5.

139 "I welcome the new finding": John W. Anderson, letter to *The New Yorker*, October 19, 1993, 10, in response to Terrence Mahoney, "Marshall's Hunch," *New Yorker*, September 20, 1993, 64–73.

139 according to a Harvard Medical School survey: D. M.

page

Eisenberg et al., *New England Journal of Medicine*, January 28, 1993.

140 Vicki Perryman: Lucinda Harper, "Mental-Health Law Protects Many People but Vexes Employers," *Wall Street Journal*, July 19, 1994, A-1, A-5. Ms. Perryman, who has since become a speech pathologist in Albuquerque, is suing her former employer for discrimination against people with mental disorders.

142 The latest thinking: Robin Marantz Henig, *A Dancing Matrix: Voyages Along the Viral Frontier* (New York: Knopf, 1993), 120–129.

143 "So much human suffering": Anthony L. Komaroff, "Chronic Fatigue Syndrome: An Alternative View," *Harvard Mental Health Letter* 9 (May 1993): 4–5; see also Katie Baer, "Still Puzzling after All These Years," *Harvard Health Letter* 18 (September 1993): 4.

143 "Should we have to figure out": Peter Manu, personal interview, August 16, 1993.

145 patients must make the mind-brain connection: Duff, *The Alchemy of Illness*, 29–31.

146 "If you experience: Robert M. Sapolsky, *Why Zebras Don't Get Ulcers: A Guide to Stress-related Disease and Coping* (New York: W. H. Freeman, 1994), 13.

146 "We do not all collapse": Ibid., 251.

146 "Stress has a great clinical advantage": Laurence J. Kirmayer, "Mind and Body as Metaphors: Hidden Values in Biomedicine," in *Biomedicine Examined*, edited by M. Lock and D. R. Gordon (Boston: Kluwer Academic Publishers, 1988), 57–93.

147 One in five Americans: Gina Kolata, "Study Says 1 in 5 Americans Suffer from Chronic Pain," *New York Times*, October 21, 1994, A-20.

147 Nearly 12 million: *Mind-Body Medicine: How to Use Your Mind for Better Health*, edited by Daniel Goleman and Joel Gurin (Yonkers, N.Y.: Consumer Reports Books, 1993), 111.

148 pain physiologists Patrick Wall and Ronald Melzack: Ronald

page

Melzack and Patrick D. Wall, *The Challenge of Pain* (New York: Viking, 1989).

150 The prevailing view: Ronald V. Norris, *Premenstrual Syndrome: A Doctor's Proven Program on How to Recognize and Treat PMS* (New York: Berkley, 1984), 3.

151 "is a physical event": Oliver Sacks, *Migraine: Understanding a Common Disorder* (Berkeley: University of California Press, 1985), 8.

152 This doesn't mean: David B. Morris, *The Culture of Pain* (Berkeley: University of California Press, 1991), 76.

153 Dr. Sarno's treatment strategy: John E. Sarno, *Healing Back Pain: The Mind-Body Connection* (New York: Warner, 1991), 77–78.

154 "biochemical hyper-response": Neil Solomon and Marc Lipton, *Sick and Tired of Being Sick and Tired* (New York: Wynwood Press, 1989), 33.

154 "We sometimes label people: Ibid., 78.

Chapter 7: The Susceptibility Factor

156 I believe my consumption: Woody Allen, *Without Feathers* (New York: Random House, 1975), 3.

157 Every year a small percentage: Mack Lipkin, Jr., and Gerri S. Lamb, "The Couvade Syndrome: An Epidemiologic Study," *Annals of Internal Medicine* 96 (April 1982): 509–511. In this controlled study, 60 of 267 expectant fathers (22 percent) sought care for symptoms related to pregnancy that could not otherwise be explained.

157 A typical case: Gary W. Small et al., "Mass Hysteria among Student Performers: Social Relationship as a Symptom Predictor," *American Journal of Psychiatry* 148 (September 1991): 1200–1205.

158 "These people are under": Gary W. Small, personal interview, February 7, 1995.

160 "Women speak and hear": Deborah Tannen, *You Just Don't*

Understand: Women and Men in Conversation (New York: Ballantine, 1990), 42.

161 mapping of brain differences: Gina Kolata, "Man's World, Woman's World? Brain Studies Point to Differences," *New York Times*, February 28, 1995, C-1, C-7.

161 men rely on such visceral: James W. Pennebaker, personal interview, March 19, 1995. See also James W. Pennebaker, *The Psychology of Physical Symptoms* (New York: Springer-Verlag, 1982), 4–9.

162 Men also tend to make passive patients: Sherrie H. Kaplan, personal interview, April 10, 1995. Kaplan, a social psychologist, and her husband, Sheldon Greenfield, an internist, developed an "assertiveness coaching session" for patients waiting to see their physicians. Trained aides reviewed the patients' medical charts with them in the waiting room, offering advice and encouragement on becoming active medical consumers. Four months later, coached patients had missed less work, reported fewer symptoms, and rated their overall health as significantly better than those who had simply "followed doctors' orders."

163 female victimization the hidden factor: Douglas Drossman, "Psychosocial Factors in Chronic Functional Abdominal Pain," in *Basic and Clinical Aspects of Chronic Abdominal Pain*, edited by E. A. Mayer and H. E. Raybould (New York: Elsevier Science Publishing, 1993), 271–280. See also Drossman et al., "Sexual and Physical Abuse in Women with Functional or Organic Gastrointestinal Disorders," *Annals of Internal Medicine* 113 (December 1990): 828–833. When the women with irritable bowel and other nonstructural GI disorders were compared with a group of patients with organic diagnoses, such as Crohn's disease or peptic ulcer, they reported significantly greater frequency of abuse, both sexual and physical — 53 versus 37 percent and 13 versus 2 percent, respectively — than the women with medical illnesses.

163 A study at two Boston hospitals: "Doctors Rarely Ask Patients about Abuse," *Washington Post Health*, July 21, 1992. the American Medical Association: Cynthia Costello and

page

Anne J. Stone, eds., *The American Woman 1994–95*: Where
We Stand (New York: Norton, 1994), 60–61, 122.

164 demanding, bitchy, and noncompliant: Leslie Laurence and
Beth Weinhouse, *Outrageous Practices: The Alarming Truth
about How Medicine Mistreats Women* (New York: Fawcett
Columbine, 1994), 338.

164 Studying gender differences: Jacqueline M. Golding et al.,
"Does Somatization Disorder Occur in Men?" *Archives of
General Psychiatry* 48 (March 1991): 231–235.

165 "she has a body": John M. Smith, *Women and Doctors: A
Physician's Explosive Account of Women's Medical Treatment, and Mistreatment, in America Today and What You
Can Do about It* (New York: Atlantic Monthly Press, 1992),
27–28.

165 A growing awareness: Ibid., 14–15. In 1990, the AMA's
Council of Ethical and Judicial Affairs adopted a report,
based on a review of forty-eight studies in journals from 1970
to 1990, that documented disparities in a number of areas.
Among the findings: women are 25 to 30 percent less likely
than men to receive kidney transplants; doctors test men
twice as often as women for lung cancer; and angiograms are
ordered for men at a disproportionately higher rate.

166 Physicians continue to see: Robin Marantz Henig, "Are
Women's Hearts Different?" *New York Times Magazine*, October 3, 1993, 60.

166 When Rigdon, a surgical nurse: Ibid., 58–60.

168 "Saying 'I'm sick' ": Sylvia Pollack, personal interview,
March 10, 1995.

168 ongoing study of Volvo employees: "We're Not Like Men,"
Harvard Women's Health Watch, October 1994, 6.

169 "flooders" —a term employed: Richard Restak, *The Brain
Has a Mind of Its Own: Insights from a Practicing Neurologist* (New York: Harmony, 1991), 121–122.

170 *ataques de nervios:* Interestingly, the highest rates of somatization in males can be found among Hispanics, particularly in
Puerto Rico, one of the few cultures in which men's unexplained medical complaints are on a par with women's.

page

Puerto Rican men, whose complaints are nearly ten times those of the U.S. population, also have high rates of hidden depression, panic disorder, and overall disability. See Javier I. Escobar, "Somatic Symptom Index: A New and Abridged Somatization Construct," *Journal of Nervous and Mental Disease* 177 (1989): 140–146. See also Escobar, "Transcultural Aspects of Dissociative and Somatoform Disorders," *Psychiatric Clinics of North America* 18 (September 1995): 555–569.

170 regions of New Guinea: Arthur Kleinman, *The Illness Narratives: Suffering, Healing, and the Human Condition* (New York: Basic Books, 1988), 14.

170 "The British patient": Lynn Payer, *Medicine and Culture: Varieties of Treatment in the United States, England, West Germany, and France* (New York: Henry Holt, 1988), 103.

171 The Navajos of the American West: Andrew Weil, *Health and Healing: Understanding Conventional and Alternative Medicine* (Boston: Houghton Mifflin, 1983), 43.

171 eastern Africa, for instance: Laurence J. Kirmayer, "Somatization and Psychologization: Understanding Cultural Idioms of Distress," prepared for *Clinical Methods in Transcultural Psychiatry*, ed. S. Okpaku, forthcoming from American Psychiatric Press, 12.

171 *Koro*, or *suk-yeong*, a frightening: Robert E. Bartholomew, "The Social Psychology of 'Epidemic' Koro," *International Journal of Social Psychiatry* 40 (1994): 46–60.

172 spirits or ghosts: Raymond Prince, "Koro and the Fox Spirit of Hainan Island," in *The Vulnerable Male*, ed. Laurence Kirmayer, *Transcultural Psychiatric Research Review* (Montreal: McGill–Queens University Press, 1992), vol. xxix, 2, 128–129.

172 Cultural Diversity in Medicine: Monique P. Yazigi, "Curing Sick Stereotypes," *New York Times*, "Education Life," April 10, 1994, 7. Forty-three percent of noncitizens lack health care coverage compared with 16 percent of the overall population. See also *New York Times*, January 25, 1995, A-13.

173 neurasthenia, the once-popular syndrome: Kleinman, *The*

page

Illness Narratives, 108–110. Mental illness is so stigmatized in Chinese culture that having a psychiatric diagnosis makes it difficult to marry off children and maintain status in the community. Similarly, psychiatrists in China are accorded very low social status because of their role in treating mentally ill patients.

174 Anthropologists interviewed patients: Craig Kaplan et al., "Somatization in Primary Care: Patients with Unexplained and Vexing Medical Complaints," *Journal of General Internal Medicine* 3 (March/April 1988): 183.

174 a smattering of studies: Italians and Greeks also tend to experience problems in physical terms, at least in comparison with white Anglo-Saxon Protestants or Irish Catholics. For a review of ethnic studies, see Robert Kellner, *Somatization and Hypochondriasis* (New York: Praeger, 1986), 75–82.

175 Jews are prone to hypochondria: Edward Shorter, *From the Mind into the Body: The Cultural Origins of Psychosomatic Symptoms* (New York: Free Press, 1994), 92–117. This section, "The Psychosomatic Symptoms of Jews," is devoted entirely to this one issue.

177 "world's greatest entertainer": Michael Freeland, *Jolson* (New York: Stein and Day, 1972), 142, 94.

177 Jerzy Kosinski, the tortured intellectual: David Owen, "Betting on Broadway," *New Yorker*, June 13, 1994, 70.

178 Mark Zborowski, a staff anthropologist: Morris, *The Culture of Pain*, 52–56.

178 early Jewish Scripture: Ibid., 34, 54.

179 In Western Europe, medicine: Shorter, *From the Mind into the Body*, 115. Perhaps in response to the fact that prestigious professorships were off-limits to Jews, as were positions in finance, engineering, and law, the number of Jewish physicians in Berlin climbed from 5 percent at the turn of the century to 50 percent in 1933.

179 "high involvement speakers": Tannen, *You Just Don't Understand*, 206–207.

181 "The public's impression": Paul T. Costa, Jr., personal interview, February 16, 1995.

page

181   the teenage diaries: Martin E. P. Seligman, *Learned Optimism*
      (New York: Knopf, 1990), 178–179.
182   "Ruminators who are pessimists": Ibid., 82.
183   The Baltimore Longitudinal Study: Paul T. Costa, Jr., and
      Robert R. McCrae, "Hypochondriasis, Neuroticism, and
      Aging," *American Psychologist* 40 (January 1985): 19–28.
      See also Arthur J. Barsky et al., "The Relation between Hypo-
      chondriasis and Age," *American Journal of Psychiatry* 148
      (July 1991): 923–928.
183   Henny Youngman factor: Stephen Crystal, personal inter-
      view, April 17, 1995.

Chapter 8. Family Ties — In Sickness and in Health

185   "The reason so many": Salvador Minuchin, *Family Healing:
      Tales of Hope and Renewal from Family Therapy* (New York:
      Touchstone, Simon and Schuster, 1993), 43.
187   Infants also vary: Jerome Kagan, personal interview, Octo-
      ber 2, 1995. See also Jerome Kagan, *Galen's Prophecy* (New
      York: Basic Books, 1994).
189   pediatric office visits are unnecessary: Robert S. Mendelsohn,
      How to Raise a Healthy Child . . . In Spite of Your Doctor
      (Chicago: Contemporary Books, 1984), 7.
189   between 2 and 10 percent: Daniel Goleman, "Childhood De-
      pression May Herald Adult Ills," *New York Times*, Janu-
      ary 11, 1994, C-1, C-10.
190   By ninth grade: Mina K. Dulcan and Charles W. Popper,
      Concise Guide to Child and Adolescent Psychiatry (Washing-
      ton D.C.: American Psychiatric Press, 1991), 115.
190   Half of all adult: Judith L. Rapoport, *The Boy Who Couldn't
      Stop Washing: Experience and Treatment of Obsessive-
      Compulsive Disorder* (New York: Dutton, 1987), 7.
190   "they cannot be soothed away": Norma Doft, *When Your
      Child Needs Help: A Parent's Guide to Therapy for Children*
      (New York: Harmony, 1992), 33.
191   Researchers say that youngsters: Michael Vasey et al., "Worry

page

in Childhood: A Developmental Perspective," *Cognitive Therapy and Research* 18 (1994), 529–549.

191 A realistic concept of death: Dulcan and Popper, *Concise Guide to Child and Adolescent Psychiatry*, 167.

192 In her essay: Perri Klass, *A Not Entirely Benign Procedure: Four Years as a Medical Student* (New York: Plume, 1987), 125–126.

193 "Ask Mom and Dad": David Sherry, personal interview, May 15, 1995.

194 A 1991 survey: Herbert A. Schreier and Judith A. Libow, *Hurting for Love: Münchausen by Proxy Syndrome* (New York: Guilford Press, 1993), 62–63.

195 "exquisite sense of what is going on": Berney Goodman, "The Body's Mind," *Thinking Allowed*, PBS Television Series (Berkeley: Thinking Allowed Productions, 1994).

196 "The overanxious parent": Schreier and Libow, *Hurting for Love*, 14.

197 "family scapegoat, whipping boy": Augustus V. Napier with Carl A. Whitaker, *The Family Crucible* (New York: Harper and Row, 1978), 54.

199 Dramatic improvements or remissions: Salvador Minuchin et al., "A Conceptual Model of Psychosomatic Illness in Children," *Archives of General Psychiatry* 32 (August 1975): 1031–1038.

199 four transactional characteristics: Ibid., 1033–1034.

200 Other research has found: Richard Livingston, "Children of People with Somatization Disorder," *Journal of the American Academy of Child and Adolescent Psychiatry* 32 (May 1993): 536–544, and Livingston, Amy Witt, and G. Richard Smith, "Families That Somatize," *Journal of Developmental and Behavioral Pediatrics* 16 (February 1995), 42–46.

200 In a three-year study: David Sherry et al., "Psychosomatic Musculoskeletal Pain in Childhood," *Pediatrics* 88 (December 1991): 1093–1099.

202 William Whitehead, a psychologist: William Whitehead et al., "Modeling and Reinforcement of the Sick Role during Childhood Predicts Adult Illness Behavior," *Psychosomatic Medicine* 56 (1994): 541–550.

page

203 The French novelist: Berney Goodman, *When the Body Speaks Its Mind* (New York: Putnam, 1994), 33.

207 "Pregnancy's most powerful weapon": Susan Baur, *Hypochondria: Woeful Imaginings* (Berkeley: University of California Press, 1988), 83.

211 The Humpty-Dumpty syndrome: Charles V. Ford, *The Somatizing Disorders: Illness as a Way of Life* (New York: Elsevier Biomedical, 1983), 192–193.

216 the most successful marriages: Jane E. Brody, "Illness as a Marriage Threat," *New York Times*, June 8, 1994, C-11.

Chapter 9: Between Doctor and Patient

223 To write prescriptions: Franz Kafka, "A Country Doctor," in *Franz Kafka: The Complete Stories* (New York: Schocken Books, 1946), 223.

224 "You could often tell"; Mack Lipkin, Jr., personal interview, September 15, 1993.

225 Whether or not the doctor: Eric J. Cassell, *The Nature of Suffering: And the Goals of Medicine* (New York: Oxford University Press, 1991), 68.

226 "By far, the most frequently used": Michael Balint, *The Doctor, His Patient, and the Illness* (New York: International Universities Press, 1957, rev. ed., 1972), 1.

226 The placebo response: Daniel Goleman, "Placebo Effect Is Shown to Be Twice as Powerful as Expected," *New York Times*, August 17, 1993, C-3. Even a worthless treatment can work much of the time, provided both doctor and patient believe in it. In an uncontrolled 1993 study, investigators followed nearly seven thousand patients who received experimental therapies for asthma, ulcers, and herpes; all these treatments, initially hailed as promising, later proved useless. More than two thirds of the patients improved, 40 percent with "excellent" results and 30 percent with "good" ones, double the benefits reported in previous studies.

226 Because placebo responses originate: Andrew Weil, *Health and Healing* (Boston: Houghton Mifflin, 1988), 207, 218.

page

227 "They may hope for miracles: Jay Katz, *The Silent World of Doctor and Patient* (New York: Free Press, 1984), 192.

227 "Medicine, after all": Ibid.

227 "the promise of nonabandonment": Ibid., 194.

228 "No guidance whatever": Balint, *The Doctor, His Patient, and the Illness*, 1. During the 1960s, Balint and his wife, Enid, began offering seminars, known as Balint groups, in which physicians and mental health experts met weekly to explore attitudes and responses to patients. The popularity of the groups — the first effort to merge primary care and psychiatry systematically — spread through Western Europe, and in recent years they have gained a following in the United States, particularly among family practitioners. A national organization, the American Balint Society, headquartered in Santa Rosa, California, supports the development of Balint research and training nationwide.

229 Think tanks began churning out: The prestigious Rand Corporation announced that at least one third of what goes on in medicine provides little or no benefit to patients. See Robert H. Brook, "Quality of Care: Do We Care?" *Annals of Internal Medicine* 115 (September 15, 1991): 486–490.

230 In a well-known study: Daniel Goleman, "All Too Often, the Doctor Isn't Listening, Studies Show," *New York Times*, November 13, 1991, C-1, C-15.
Patients get the chance: In publications for the American Academy on Physician and Patient, a professional society dedicated to research, education, and professional standards in doctor-patient communication.
the typical general practitioner: *Mind-Body Medicine: How to Use Your Mind for Better Health*, edited by Daniel Goleman and Joel Gurin (New York: Basic Books, 1988), 432.

231 "It won't work": Edward E. Rosenbaum, *A Taste of My Own Medicine: When the Doctor Is the Patient* (New York: Random House, 1988), 69, 72.

234 "all too unquestionably": Katz, *The Silent World of Doctor and Patient*, 200.

234 One half of those who consult: Kurt Kroenke, personal interview, September 21, 1993.

page

235 "whom most physicians dread": James E. Groves, "Taking Care of the Hateful Patient," *New England Journal of Medicine* 298 (April 1978): 883–887.

235 In a 1993 study: S. R. Hahn et al., "Psychopathology and the Difficult Patient in Primary Care: Recognition, Prevalence, and Impairment," research paper presented at Seventh Annual NIMH International Research Conference on Mental Health Problems in the General Health Care Sector, September 20–22, 1993.

235 "in an intense way": Donald R. Lipsitt, personal interview, October 19, 1993.

236 "The hypochondriac's doubt": Arthur Kleinman, *The Illness Narratives: Suffering, Healing, and the Human Condition* (New York: Basic Books, 1988), 197.

236 make them prey for hypochondriacs: Edwin Cassem, "When Symptoms Seem Groundless," *Emergency Medicine*, June 15, 1992, 191–199.

236 inhibit personal gratification: Charles V. Ford, *The Somatizing Disorders: Illness as a Way of Life* (New York: Elsevier Biomedical, 1983), 210, 223–225.

237 The system abets: Terry Mizrahi, *Getting Rid of Patients: Contradictions in the Socialization of Physicians* (New Brunswick, N.J.: Rutgers University Press, 1986), 36, 68–76.

238 "rare diseases are somehow": Perri Klass, *A Not Entirely Benign Procedure: Four Years as a Medical Student* (New York: Plume, 1987), 70.

241 While many may pine: Robin Toner, "The Family Doctor Is Rarely In," *New York Times*, "Week in Review," February 6, 1994, 1.

242 "Suddenly I began to wonder": Gilda Radner, *It's Always Something* (New York: Simon and Schuster, 1989), 67.

244 when doctors are trained: Debra L. Roter et al., "Improving Physicians' Interviewing Skills and Reducing Patients' Emotional Distress: A Randomized Clinical Trial," *Archives of Internal Medicine* 155 (September 25, 1995): 1877–1884.

244 Kurt Kroenke: personal interview, September 21, 1993.

245 consultation letters to physicians: G. Richard Smith et al., "Patients with Multiple Unexplained Symptoms," *Archives of*

page

Internal Medicine 146 (January 1986): 69–72. Why did the patients' functioning improve? One theory is that somatizing patients had received such invasive testing before the letter that they had had to reduce activities to recuperate. But Smith, the psychiatrist who led the study, believes it is more probable that "the well-intended but fruitless diagnostic procedures" increased the patients' perception that they were sick. For further analysis of data, see T. Michael Kashner et al., "An Analysis of Panel Data," *Medical Care*, September 1992, 811–820, and Kashner et al., "Enhancing the Health of Somatization Disorder Patients," *Psychosomatics* 36 (October 1995), 462–470.

246 "We try to impart": Joseph Connelly, personal interview, February 15, 1994.

247 "When a doctor feels": Robert Feinstein, personal interview, February 15, 1994.

249 he is vocally skeptical: See Gerald Weissmann, *The Doctor Dilemma* (Knoxville, Tenn.: Whittle Direct Books: Grand Rounds Press, 1992).

249 "The symptom is never invented": Gerald Weissmann, "The Flight into Sickness," *New Republic*, April 6, 1992, 41.

250 Working with Your Doctor: Sources consulted: Paul J. Donoghue and Mary E. Siegel, *Sick and Tired of Feeling Sick and Tired* (New York: Norton, 1992); Donald M. Vickery and James F. Fries, *Take Care of Yourself: The Complete Guide to Medical Self-Care* (Reading, Mass.: Addison-Wesley, 1993); and Peter H. Berczeller, *Doctors and Patients: What We Feel about You* (New York: Macmillan, 1994).

250 you can consult: American Medical Association, *Directory of Physicians in the United States*, 34th ed., 4 vols. (Chicago: Division of Survey and Data Resources, AMA, 1994), and *The Official Directory of Board Certified Medical Specialists*, 4 vols. (New Providence, N.J.: Marquis Who's Who, 1995).

Chapter 10. The Steps to Successful Treatment

page

266 One meta-analysis of data: Frederic I. Kass, John M. Oldham, and Herbert Pardes, *Columbia University College of Physicians and Surgeons: Complete Home Guide to Mental Health* (New York: Henry Holt, 1992), 83.

267 In fact, 10 percent in therapy: Jack Engler and Daniel Goleman, *The Consumer's Guide to Psychotherapy* (New York: Fireside, Simon and Schuster, 1992), 30.

271 "better than well": Peter D. Kramer, *Listening to Prozac: A Psychiatrist Explores Antidepressant Drugs and the Remaking of the Self* (New York: Viking, 1993), x.

272 Prozac hastened tumor growth: Lorne Brandes et al., "Stimulation of Malignant Tumor Growth by Antidepressant Drugs at Clinically Relevant Doses," *Cancer Research* 52 (July 1, 1992): 3796–3800. Investigators found that rodents which received doses of amitriptyline (Elavil) and fluoxetine (Prozac) equivalent to those for humans experienced an increase in the rate of growth of breast cancers and increases in the weight of other tumors. Presently there is no evidence of any carcinogenic effect of antidepressants on humans. Additional research is in progress.

272 first federally funded: Results from Dr. Fallon's pilot study were reported in the *Journal of Clinical Psychopharmacology*, December 1993. In this NIMH-sponsored study, patients begin a twelve-week trial on either fluoxetine or a placebo in conjunction with supportive weekly therapy; those who respond to the treatment continue with the same prescription in a twelve-week, double-blind maintenance phase, their progress assessed by an independent psychiatrist. Participants — men and women eighteen to seventy-five who believe they worry too much about sickness — are recruited through newspaper ads, television, medical bulletins, and referrals from physicians. Those who score above a certain threshold for hypochondria on structured interviews and agree to take part in the study receive free treatment at one of three sites: the Anxiety Disorders Clinic of the New York State Psychiatric Institute; within the family medicine practice at St.

Josephs Medical Center, Stamford, Connecticut; and at the Freedom from Fear Clinic, Staten Island, New York. Dr. Fallon's aim is to enroll 124 participants, half of whom have hypochondria without other complicating psychiatric conditions and half of whom suffer from hypochondria in conjunction with a range of underlying conditions.

272 Elsewhere in the United States: R. Wesner and R. Noyes, "Imipramine: An Effective Treatment for Illness Phobia," *Journal of Affective Disorders*, 1991, 43–48.
chronic chest pain: Richard O. Cannon III et al., "Imipramine in Patients with Chest Pain Despite Normal Coronary Angiograms," *New England Journal of Medicine*, May 19, 1994, 1411–1417.

279 90 percent success rate: Hilary M. C. Warwick and Paul M. Salkovskis, "Hypochondriasis," *Behavior Research Therapy* 28 (1990): 105–117. See also Hilary M. C. Warwick and Isaac Marks, "Behavioural Treatment of Illness Phobia and Hypochondriasis," *British Journal of Psychiatry* 152 (1988): 239–241, and Richard Stern and Margaret Fernandez, "Group Cognitive and Behavioural Treatment of Hypochondriasis," *British Medical Journal* 303 (November 16, 1991): 1229–1232.

279 account for improvement: Sako Visser and Theo K. Bouman, "Cognitive-Behavioural Approaches in Treatment of Hypochondriasis," *Behaviour Research Therapy* 30 (May 1992): 301.

280 "The challenge lies": Stephen Josephson, personal interview, February 11, 1994.

280 this is what you can expect: See Stephen C. Josephson and Eric A. Hollander, *OCD Newsletter* 4 (1990): 5–8.

Epilogue

288 "how to be happy" book: Wendy Kaminer, *I'm Dysfunctional, You're Dysfunctional: The Recovery Movement and other Self-help Fashions* (Reading, Mass.: Addison-Wesley, 1992), 5, 8.

ACKNOWLEDGMENTS

THOSE WHO KNOW ME have heard me describe this book as "blessed," not in any divine sense but in the number of talented and wonderful people who helped to shepherd the project from conception to the final stages of production. Without them, *Phantom Illness* simply would not have been.

The book was merely an unsent proposal for a magazine article languishing in a desk drawer in 1992, when Max Gartenberg, a dear friend who happened to be a literary agent, paid our family a visit. Max had been suggesting for some time that I expand my journalistic horizons beyond newspapers and magazines and embark on a book project. That day I showed him the hypochondria proposal. Max was interested; his wife, Pat Gartenberg, a former head of the English department at Rutgers University, found the topic fascinating. Discussions ensued. Perhaps we should leave out the word *hypochondria*, because of the associated stigma. Would hypochondriacs, who may not see themselves as such, buy the book? Did I need to team up with a medical expert?

The collaboration issue was resolved with a phone call to Brian Fallon, a psychiatrist I knew who was conducting cutting-edge research on hypochondria. It took a few meetings to determine the scope of the book, but early on it was clear we were on our way to what proved to be a rewarding collaboration. I can't thank Brian enough for his unflagging support of the project, for his careful reading of the manuscript, and for the trust in me he displayed, bringing me together with many of the patients I interviewed.

Brian joins me in thanking Max Gartenberg for his invaluable assistance in shaping the book proposal and getting it into the right people's hands. I am especially indebted to Max for his deft line editing of the manuscript, a courtesy that went beyond the call of any agent.

I owe a huge debt of gratitude to Betsy Lerner, my first editor at Houghton Mifflin, who acquired the book. Betsy, whose vision for the work dovetailed with mine, gave me great support during the early stages of research. But just as I began writing in January 1994, Betsy left for Doubleday, and responsibility for my manuscript fell to her colleague Gail Winston. Betsy did all she could to allay my anxiety. "In some ways," she told me, "Gail will be a better editor for you." (Gail's background is in editing psychology and medical books, while Betsy is known for her interest in women's issues, psychology, and anything quirky that falls between the cracks.)

From the moment I met Gail I knew all was okay. She seemed to have so much enthusiasm for the project that I completely forgot she had inherited it. ("Orphaned" manuscripts, as authors well know, can be ripe for disaster.) Gail was warm, encouraging, and unfailingly generous with her knowledge and time. She provided latitude and a firm hand in just the right proportions and was always there to point me in the right direction when I got into a quagmire. I can still envision her incisive comments in the margins: "I'm not convinced. Do we have to say this twice? This doesn't work." Nine out of ten times I even listened.

There are so many others whose contributions were invaluable. Lynne Smilow, at whose kitchen table I would invariably end up once a month in tears, saying "I can't do it," provided coffee and chat, after which I'd come away convinced that just maybe I could. My loyal friend Beth Halliday's intelligent criticism was tempered by encouragement and cheer. My parents charted the ups and downs of my progress from Florida and Massachusetts, and lent the wisdom accumulated during years spent in publishing. Also deserving mention are Tina Pohlman, Gail's intelligent, helpful assistant; Gerry Morse, for her adroit copy editing of the final manuscript; Becky Saikia-Wilson, for her calm handling of production crises; Richard Lavenstein, who saved the day with his suggestion of the title *Phantom Illness*; Rabbi John Schecter; Nick Nichols, M.D.; Estelle Abrams; my caring babysitters, Jennifer, Molly, and Sherry; Aunt Mary Anne, who graciously housed our children whenever necessary; and my ever-supportive parents-in-law.

No less important are the physicians, mental health professionals, and assorted experts whom I interviewed; the research librarians who assisted me; and the well-stocked libraries in Maplewood, South Orange, Millburn, Newark, and Seton Hall University, which provided solace and sheltered me in heat waves and in cold. Special thanks to Robert Meister, Susan Baur, and Edward Shorter, the writer-historians who cut a swath through the hypochondria research jungle before me and made my job that much easier.

Most of all, I want to thank the individuals who entrusted their stories and struggles to me. I will be forever indebted to them for their generosity and candor. Without them, *Phantom Illness* would be without its heart.

My deepest gratitude I save for my family. I thank my husband, David, for his encouragement, patience, and the pride and delight he took in this project each step of the way. I am also grateful to him for agreeing *not* to read the manuscript until its completion. David, who makes his living as a writer too, has journalistic standards he knows I have found intimidating at times.

Last, I thank my children for enduring three years of life with "Mommy's book," sometimes without Mommy for chunks of time. Just how much of a fixture the book became in our lives — the project has been in existence more than half of five-year-old Michael's life — came home to me one night at bedtime hour. Danielle, our eight-year-old, was getting ready for a reading session with her father. I heard her call out, "Daddy, Daddy, I know what I want to read! Let's read *Phantom Illness!*" Of course, she meant the children's book *Phantom Tollbooth* — and we all had a good laugh.

Thank you, Danielle, Michael, and David, for your love — and for providing that extra incentive to stay well in both heart and mind. I cherish you all.

INDEX

Abir, anecdotal account of
  hypochondria by, 40–43
Ablow, Keith Russell, 102–3
Abnormal illness behavior, 65–66
  somatizing and, 66–67
Abuse
  guidelines for physicians, 164
  sexual, 84
Acid-blocking drugs, 138
Acronyms, medical, 114
Adolescents, 191
  depression and, 190
Adopted children, studies of,
  100–101
Advertising. *See* Media
Age, 108
Aging, 180–84
  successful, 129
AIDS, fear of, 58, 93–94, 158,
  209
Alarm, sense of, 94–95
Alchemy of Illness, The (Duff),
  144–45
Alcohol abuse. *See* Substance abuse
Alexander, Franz, 137–38
Alexithymia, 72
Allen, Woody, 91, 156, 175
"All in the head" reasoning, fallacy
  of, 131–55

Alprazolam (Xanax), 262
Alternative medicine, 68, 139–40,
  241
American Academy of Cosmetic
  Surgery, 126–27
American Academy on Physician
  and Patient, 224
American Chronic Pain Outreach
  Association, 149–50
American Medical Association
  (AMA)
  abuse guidelines for physicians,
    164
  alternative medicine and,
    139–40
  on hypochondriacs, 30
  task force on false memory, 84
*American Medical Directory of
  Physicians in the United
  States,* 250
American Nervousness, 1903
  (Lutz), 109
American Psychiatric Association,
  36, 258
  hypochondriasis recognized by, 8
Amplification, 94
  factors in, 95–97
  pain and, 151
Anafranil, 82–83, 100, 263, 283

Anatomy of Melancholy, The (Burton), 21
Anderson, John W., 139
Anecdotal reports, 39–59
on behavior therapy, 280–84
on biological approach, 272–76
on body dysmorphic disorder, 51–54
on conversion disorder, 56–59
on eating disorders, 273
on marriage, 217–20
on pain disorder, 54–56
on psychodynamic therapy, 267–70
on Prozac, 276
on somatization disorder, 53–54
Anger, 90–91
of physicians, 235
Anglo-Saxons, hypochondria and, 108
Anna O., Freud's studies of, 26
Anorexia nervosa, 99, 159, 191
Antacids, 138
Antibiotics
overtreatment and, 120
ulcers and, 138–39
Antidepressants, 82, 261. *See also* Depression; Drugs; Imipramine; Medications; SSRIs; Zoloft
Anti-Semitism
Jewish behavior and, 180
Jewish hypochondria and, 175–76
Anxiety, 70, 91, 93
hypochondria and, 70–71
panic disorder and, 262
predisposition to, 156
Prozac and, 11
skills for reducing, 280
symptoms and, 76–79
Appearance, importance of, 122, 125–26

"Art of Healing, The" (Auden), 35
Ataques de nervios, 170
Attention, as amplification factor, 95–96. *See also* Child development; Childhood
Attitudes
toward health, 62–63
study of, 62
Auden, W. H., 35
Authoritarian families, 200

Baby boomers: health, hypochondria, and, 112–15
Back pain, 153
Balint, Michael, 226, 228–29, 244, 247
Baltimore Longitudinal Study of Aging, 183
Barsky, Arthur, 7, 18, 61, 71, 80, 94
amplification factors and, 95–97
Baur, Susan, 24, 26, 91, 107, 207–8
BDD. *See* Body dysmorphic disorder
Beauty, value of, 125
Beck, Aaron, 93
Bedside manner, 252
Behavior(s). *See also* Behavior therapy; Obsessive-compulsive disorder; Stress
abnormal illness, 66
biological substrate and, 105–6
cognitive-behavioral view of, 93–100
culture and, 106–10
drugs and, 28–29
heredity and, 100–6
obsessive, 79–80
during pregnancy, 208
psychodynamic view of, 89–93
Behavioral approach, 249
Behavioral sciences, nature-nurture debate and, 102–3

Behavior therapy
anecdotal account of, 280–84
cognitive therapy and, 276–84
effectiveness of, 278–80
perspective of, 277–78
Beliefs
as amplification factor, 96–97
health and, 62–63
Benzodiazepines, 262
Biochemistry, PS2 syndrome and, 154
Biological approach, 97–100
anecdotal information about, 272–76
to treatment, 270–76
Biological determinism, 103
Biological markers, for depression, 72
Biological theories, of hypochondria, 88
Biomedicine, 97
Biopsychiatry, 28–29, 102–3
Biopsychosocial approach, 243, 248–49
Biotechnology, promise of, 240
Birth, as trigger, 83–84
Blum, David, 15–16
Body. See also Mind-body connection(s)
obsession with, 122, 125–27
standards of, 122–26
Body dysmorphic disorder (BDD), 33, 35, 51–54
anecdotal report on, 52–53
imagined ugliness and, 52–53
Body language, unconscious and, 136
Boswell, James, 22
Bowen, Murray, 197
Brain. See also Neurological disorders
biological view and, 97–100
circuitry of, 100
depressive disorders and, 72
gatekeeper in, 106

gender and mapping of, 161
hypochondria and, 88
mapping techniques, 100
"Brain fag," 171
Breast Cancer Companion, The (LaTour), 127–28
Breast implants, 121
Breuer, Josef, 26
Brigham and Women's Hospital (Boston), 94
cognitive education groups at, 257
Brighter Side of Human Nature, The (Kohn), 88
Briquet's syndrome, 36
Britton, A. G., 84–85
Broyard, Anatole, 63–64
Bulimia, 191
Bupropion (Wellbutrin), 261
Burton, Robert, 21–22
Business, medicine as, 243

Cancer
fear of, 6, 23, 48, 175, 231
pain treatment for, 148
support groups and, 128
type C personality theory, 127
Cardiophobia, 77, 78–79
Cardiovascular disease. See Cardiophobia; Heart disease
Cartesian dualism, body and, 24
Cartesian split, 155
Castration anxiety, 171–72
Centers for Disease Control and Prevention (CDC), 141
CFS. See Chronic fatigue syndrome
Change, possibility of, 286
Chemical treatments, 97. See also Treatment
Cheyne, George, 21
Chicago Institute for Psychoanalysis, 137
Child abuse, Münchausen by proxy as, 193–94
Child development, 187–93

Childhood
  depression in, 189–90
  parental response to illness and,
    65
China, medicine in, 173–74
Chronic fatigue syndrome (CFS),
    87, 140–45
  treatment of, 144
Chronic illness
  in children, 190
  psychiatric disorders and, 74
Chronic pain, 55, 148
Church of Scientology, 271
Cioffi, Delia, 120
Class, as cultural factor, 92
Classical conversion, 27–28
Classifications, in DSM, 36–39
Clinical depression. *See* Depression
Clomipramine (Anafranil), 263
Clonazepam (Klonopin), 262
Cognitive-behavioral view, 93–100
Cognitive restructuring, 150
Cognitive therapy
  and behavioral treatments, 262,
    276–84
  effectiveness of, 279
  perspective of, 277–79
Columbia University
  Heightened Illness Concern
    study at, 41, 271
  research on psychiatric disorders
    and chronic illness, 74
Common sense, 121–22, 203
Communication
  gender and, 160
  in marriage, 211
Compassion, of doctors, 230, 237
Compulsive behaviors, 99–100.
    See also Obsessive-compulsive
    disorder
  predisposition to, 156
Concentration camp survivors,
    176
Conduct of Life (Emerson), 86
Conflict, 91

symptoms as expression of, 27–28
Conflict resolution, in families, 200
Connelly, Joseph, 246
Conquest Over Pain's Stranglehold
    (COPS), 149
Consultation, with psychiatrist,
    258–60
Consumers, patients as, 229–34
Context, of pain, 179
Control, feeling of, 129
Controversies, over somatoform
    disorders, 36–38
Conversion disorder, 33–34, 56–59
  anecdotal report on, 57–58
Cortisol, 72
Cosmetic pharmacology, 271
Cosmetic surgery, 126
Costa, Paul T., Jr., 181
Counseling. *See* Therapy
"Country Doctor, A" (Kafka), 223
Cousins, Norman, 112–13
Couvade syndrome, 157
Craziness, sickness and, 63–64. *See
    also* Mental illness
Creative people, as hypochon-
    driacs, 22–23
Credentials, medical, 250
Critical illness, experience of,
    63–64
Criticism, of medical profession,
    230–31
Cross-cultural studies. *See also*
    Culture
  of illness behavior, 178
  pain responses and, 171
Crystal, Stephen, 183–84
Cues, parental, 104–5
Cultural anthropologists, 107
Cultural Diversity in Medicine
    (course), 172–73
Culture, 92, 106–10. *See also*
    Greeks; Hindu cultures;
    Italians; Jews; Latin Ameri-
    cans; Navajos
  differences among, 172–73

emotional conflict, bodily preoccupation, and, 260
emotions, sickness, and, 170–74
and pain, 178–79
women vs. men and, 168–69
Culture of Pain, The (Morris), 25,
109, 178
Cummings, Nicholas, 30
Cure, doctors and, 226, 227–28

Darkness Visible (Styron), 1, 73
Darwin, Charles, 23
Davis, Linda H., 23
Death
concept of, 191
depression and, 73–74
fear of, 289–91
Death rates, 116
Deformed body. See Body dysmorphic disorder
Dependency: pregnancy, hypochondria, and, 208
Depression, 70, 71. See also Antidepressants; Drugs; Manic
depression; Medications
in adolescence, 190
biological markers for, 72
brain chemistry and, 72
case study in, 74–75
CFS and, 144
in childhood, 189–90
chronic illness and, 73–74
culture and, 260
death and, 73–74
electroconvulsive therapy and,
262
genetic factors in, 101
hypochondria and, 7, 70–71
masked, 72
pain and, 55
people suffering from, 75
Prozac and, 270–72
of Styron, 73
symptoms of, 71–74
treatability of, 75–76

treatment of, 261–62
Depressive disorder. See Depression
Descartes, René, 24
Desipramine (Norpramin), 261
Deviation, intolerance of, 122, 125
Dhat, 172
Diagnosis
fashionable, 110
misdiagnosis and, 67–68
stress, chronic pain, and, 152–53
therapy and, 239–40
Diagnostic and Statistical Manual
of Mental Disorders. See DSM
Diagnostic studies. See Medical tests
Dietary supplements, 121
Directory of Board Certified Med-
ical Specialists, 250
Disease(s). See also Classifications;
DSM
classical view of, 19–20
fashionable, 27
in Greek medicine, 20
illness compared with, 65
somatoform vs. factitious, 39
Disease conviction, 43–47
Disease labels, 114
Disease mongering. See Health;
Media
Disease Mongers (Payer), 117
Disease phobia, 47–51
Disfigurement. See Body dysmor-
phic disorder
Disorders
psychiatric, 261–63
psychosomatic, 19, 26–27,
134–37
Disposition, health and, 129–30
Doctor, His Patient, and the Ill-
ness, The (Balint), 226, 228
Doctor, The (film), 231
Doctor-patient relationship
choosing a doctor, 250–51
expectations in, 252–54
Radner, Gilda, and, 242
training in, 244

Doctors
  attitudes of, 224, 249
  characteristics of, 236–37
  choosing, 250–51
  compassion and, 237
  consulting, 124
  as drugs, 228
  gender and treatment by, 164–
    69
  guidelines on abuse for, 164
  image of, 227
  interviewing, 250
  loss of faith in, 229–34
  perception of patients, 234–40
  placebo response and, 226–27
  psychiatric training and, 243–49
  role of, 223–54
  women patients and, 163–64
Doft, Norma, 190
Domestic violence, 163
Dossey, Larry, 65, 136
Drischler, Colleen, 111–12
Drossman, Douglas, 163
Drug abuse. See Substance abuse
Drugs. See also Medications;
    Pharmacologic treatment
  acid-blocking, 138
  for depression, 29, 261–62
  doctor as, 228
  "feel good," 271
  overtreatment and, 120–21
  pain-relieving, 149
  serotonin reuptake inhibitors
    (SSRIs), 261
  tricyclics, 261
  Zantac, 206
DSM (Diagnostic and Statistical
    Manual of Mental Disorders),
    36, 38, 173
  panic disorder and, 78
DSM-IV, 37, 38
Duff, Kat, 144–45
Dworkin, Robert, 55
Dysfunction, somatic illness and,
    70

Dysfunctional behavior, family
    and, 196–201
Dysmorphophobia, 51

Eating disorder
  anecdotal information about, 273
  anorexia nervosa as, 99
  bulimia as, 191
Economics, treatment and, 248
Effexor, 261
Ehrenreich, Barbara, 126–27
Elderly. See Aging
Electroconvulsive therapy, 262
Eli Lilly Company, Prozac and, 271
Emerson, Ralph Waldo, 86
Emotional problems, medical train-
    ing in, 244–49. See also Medi-
    cal training
Emotions
  childhood pain and, 191–92
  hypochondria and, 21–22, 88,
    285–86
  physical symptoms of, 61
England
  hypochondria in, 20–21
  stoicism in, 170
English Malady, The, 21
Enmeshment, in families, 199
"Enough to Make You Sick"
    (Klass), 192
Environment. See also Nature-
    nurture debate
  nature-nurture debate and, 102
  parental cues and, 104–5
Epidemiological research. See also
    Research
  catchment area (ECA) survey,
    183
  on psychological-social vs. med-
    ical illnesses, 30–31
  reports on, 124
Epstein-Barr virus, 141
Escape, hypochondria as, 107–8
Ethnic groups, 107
  emotions, sickness, and, 170–74

hypochondria and, 108
pain responses among, 178
Ethnicity, 92
Examination. *See* Physical examination; Psychiatrists
Exercise, role of, 125
Expectations, 96
    treatment and, 266
Expenditures
    on health care, 31
    medical, 115
Explanatory styles, pessimistic, 182
Explosive urges, 98

Factitious disorders, classification of, 39
Fads
    diagnoses as, 110
    health, 121–22
Fallon, Brian, 7, 8, 41, 80, 246, 271–72
False memory, 84
Family. *See also* Child development; Marriage
    conflict resolution and, 200
    connections in, 196–201
    enmeshment in, 199
    home atmosphere and, 193
    hypochondria and, 185–222
    overprotectiveness in, 199–200
    research project on, 198–99
    rigidity in, 200
Family Healing (Minuchin), 185
Family history, of psychiatric disorders, 260
Family life, 92
Family practice, 246
Family systems approach, 197–201, 264
Family therapy, 197
Family tree. *See* Nature-nurture debate
Farnum, Angela, 67
Fear(s)
    dealing with, 94

stopping, 287
symbolic meaning of, 260
"Feel good" pills, 270
Feeling, divided from thought, 135
Feinstein, Robert, 246–47
Females. *See* Girls; Women
Feminism, hysteria and, 108–9
Ferenczi, Sandor, 14
Fibromyalgia, 54, 159
Fight-or-flight response, 145
Fitness, obsession with, 125
Fluoxetine (Prozac), 7. *See also* Prozac
    study of, 271–72
Fluvoxamine (Luvox), 261, 263
Folk illnesses, 174
Food and Drug Administration, 121
    drugs approved by, 270
Ford, Charles, 61, 70, 109–10, 211, 236
Frailty, gender and, 159–60
France, hypochondria in, 20
Free association, 92–93
Freedom from Fear (clinic), 41, 43
Freeland, Michael, 177
Freud, Sigmund, 14. *See also* Psychoanalysis
    biological theories and, 106
    conversion disorder and, 56
    on hypochondria, 90
    psychoanalytic technique and, 265
    psychoanalytic theory and, 24–25
    relevance to present, 27–28
    Studies in Hysteria, 26
    unconscious and, 136
From Paralysis to Fatigue (Shorter), 27
From the Mind into the Body (Shorter), 107, 175–76

Galen, 20, 25
Gastrointestinal (GI) ailments, emotional aspects of, 163

Gate-control theory, of pain, 148–
    49
Gender, 92. *See also* Men; Women
    brain and, 161
    medical treatment and, 163–64
    susceptibility and, 159–64
Genetic factors. *See also* Heredity;
    Nature-nurture debate
    hypochondria and, 88
    Milunsky and, 101–2
    overriding, 103
Geriatric physicians, 184
Getting Rid of Patients (Mizrahi),
    237
Giamatti, Bartlett, 162
Girls, adolescent, 191. *See also*
    Women
Golden Girls (television program),
    131
GOMERs, 238
Grandmother effect, 129
Grant study, of traits and aging,
    128
Greek medicine, 19–20
Greeks, pain tolerance of, 175
GROP (getting rid of patients)
    mentality, 237–38
Guermantes Way, The (Proust),
    111
Guilt, 130, 288–89
    culture and, 260
    Jews and, 177
Gur, Ruben C., 161
Gynecologists, men vs. women as,
    165

Haley, Jay, 197
Hanner, Linda, 67–68
Happiness, 286
    attitudes toward health and, 63
Harvard Medical School, survey of
    alternative medicine, 139–40,
    241
Headaches, 149–50, 151–52
Healing, doctors and, 226

Health. *See also* Stress
    attitudes toward, 62–63
    classical view of, 19–20
    and hypochondria, 111–15
    medical tests and, 119–20
    pitfalls of pursuing, 117–22
    promoting, 121–22
    reasons for, 129–30
    societal preoccupation with, 18
    unrealistic notion of, 97
Health care
    CFS and, 144
    expenditures on industry, 31
    managed care and, 243
Health fads, 110, 121–22, 125
Healthism, 111–30
Health reform, 240–43
Heart disease, gender and, 165–66.
    See also Cardiophobia
Hebraic debility, 176
Henson, Jim, 162
Heredity
    hypochondria and, 86–110
    overriding, 103
High-involvement speaking, 179–
    80
High utilizers, 240
Hindu cultures, 172
Hippocrates, 19
Hispanic cultures, 170. *See also*
    Latin Americans
Holistic medicine, 248–49
    Weil, Andrew, and, 227
Holistic vision, 139
Hollander, Eric, 80, 105
    on biological view, 98, 99
Holocaust, 176
Hormones, depression and, 72
How to Raise a Healthy Child
    (Mendelsohn), 189
Humor, application of, 256
"Humors," doctrine of, 20
"Humpty-Dumpty syndrome,"
    211–12
Hurting for Love (Schreier), 194–95

Hyp, 20–21, 146
Hypochondria. *See also* Hyp;
    Hypochondriasis
  with accompanying psychiatric
    disorders, 261–63
  without accompanying psych-
    iatric disorders, 263–84
  and aging, 181
  amplification scales and, 94
  anecdotal reports on, 40–51
  behavioral perspective on, 276–
    77
  behavior therapy for, 279–80
  bodily preoccupation in (anec-
    dotal report), 40–43
  causes of, 88–89
  change of social attitudes
    toward, 24–27
  cognitive perspective on, 277–78
  controversy over, 37–38
  culture and, 106–10
  current study of, 28–32
  defined, 6, 8–9
  diagnosing, 17
  disease conviction and (anecdo-
    tal report), 43–47
  disease phobia and, 47–51
  doctor-patient relationship and,
    223–54
  environment and, 104–5
  facts about, 16
  family patterns and, 209
  Freud and, 26, 90
  gender and, 161
  hereditary basis for, 102
  heritable nature of, 87
  historical perspective on, 18–23
  incest and, 84–85
  of Jews, 174–80
  link to obsessive-compulsive dis-
    orders or depression, 7
  as marriage threat, 201, 204–16,
    217–20
  medical expenditures and, 115
  misdiagnosis and, 67–68

nature-nurture debate and, 86–
    110
  negative concept of, 19
  neurology and, 29
  as neurotic disorder, 29. *See also*
    Freud, Sigmund; Psychoan-
    alysis
  obsessive-compulsive disorder
    and, 79–80
  panic sufferers and, 77–79
  as phantom of the mind, 19
  preoccupation with body and,
    126–27
  primary (pure), 70–71, 264
  PS2 and, 154–55
  and psychiatric condition, 70–
    71
  as realization of fears, 289
  self-diagnostic test for, 293–97
  sensationalized medical stories
    and, 119
  in 17th-century England, 20–21
  sick role and, 202–3
  as somatoform disorder, 33
  of Styron, 73
  transitory, 14–15, 259
  as weakness, 92
Hypochondria: Woeful Imaginings
    (Baur), 24, 207–8
"Hypochondriack, The" (Boswell),
    22
Hypochondriacs. *See also* Hypo-
    chondria
  attitudes toward, 15
  characteristics of, 16
  Columbia University study of,
    271–72
  doctor personalities and, 232
  impact on doctors, 235–36
  medical training about, 239
  profile of, 108
  as subject of ridicule, 15–16
Hypochondriasis, 8–9, 33
"Hypochondrium," 19
Hypoglycemia, 110

Hysteria
    feminism and, 108–9
    Freud on, 25, 90
    mass, 157–58
Hysterical neurosis, 56. *See also*
    Conversion disorder

IAS, 256, 293–97
Iatrogenic illness, 224
IBS. *See* Irritable bowel syndrome
Idioms of distress, 172
Illness. *See also* Diagnosis; Dis-
    ease(s); Sick role
    as accidents, 115
    dynamics of, 65, 92
    experience of, 63–64
    family dynamics of, 198
    mass, 158
    power of, 186
    preoccupation with, 15. *See also*
        Hypochondria
    reasons for, 129–30
    as relief for women, 168
    sick role and, 63–67
    social setting and, 196–97
    social transmission of, 157
    symbolic meaning of fear, 260
    victimization and, 163
Illness as a Way of Life (Ford),
    236
Illness as Metaphor (Sontag), 64,
    127
Illness Attitude Scale (IAS), 256,
    293–97
Illness Narratives, The (Kleinman),
    27, 65, 236
Illness phobia, imipramine and,
    272
*I'm Dysfunctional, You're Dys-
    functional* (Kaminer), 287
Imipramine (Tofranil), 29, 261,
    262. *See also* Antidepressants;
    Drugs; Medications
    and panic attacks, 79
    study of, 272

Immune system
    CFS and, 143
    stress and, 146
Incest, hypochondria and, 84–85
Incompetence, medical, 230
India, emotions and sickness in,
    171. *See also* Culture
Industrialization, pressures of, 109
Infants, 187–88. *See also* Child
    development
Infection, ulcers and, 138–39
Institute for Health Care and
    Aging Research (Rutgers), 184
Insufficient milk syndrome, 122
Insurance: hypochondria, PS2,
    and, 155
Interpersonal therapy, 262
Interventional studies, 124
Interviews, in choosing doctors,
    250–51
Intolerant role, in marriage, 213–
    15
Intoxicated by My Illness
    (Broyard), 63–64
Intuition, gender and, 161
IQ: heredity, environment, and, 103
Irish-Catholics, hypochondria and,
    108, 178
Irritable bowel syndrome (IBS),
    132, 151
Italians. *See also* Culture
    hypochondria and, 108
    pain and, 178
    pain tolerance of, 175
It's Always Something (Radner),
    242

Jargon, medical, 238
Jews. *See also* Culture
    hypochondria and, 108, 174–80
    medical care and, 179
    pain and, 178
    women and, 179
Johnson, Samuel, 22
Jolson, Al, 177

Josephson, Stephen C., 279–80
Journalism, medical, 116. *See also*
    Media
Journal of Existential Psychiatry,
    134
*Journal of the American Medical
    Association*, 122

Kafka, Franz, 223
Kagan, Jerome, 187–88
Kaiser-Permanente Health Plan,
    mental health program of, 30
Kaminer, Wendy, 287
Kaplan, Sherrie H., 162
Katz, Jay, 227, 234
Kellner, Robert, 293
Kirmayer, Laurence, 105, 146
Klass, Perri, 192, 238–39
Kleinman, Arthur, 27, 28, 65, 236
Klonopin, 262
Kohn, Alfie, 88
Komaroff, Anthony, 143
Koro (suk-yeong), 171
Kosinski, Jerzy, 177
Kramer, Peter, 15, 271
Kroenke, Kurt, 234, 244–45, 246

Ladee, George A., 91–92
Landesman, Rocco, 177
Latin Americans, emotional ex-
    pression by, 260. *See also* Cul-
    ture; Hispanic cultures
LaTour, Kathy, 127–28
Learned Optimism (Seligman), 182
Learned response, hypochondria
    as, 93
Life expectancy, 116
Lipkin, Mack, Jr., 74–75, 224,
    243–44
Lipsitt, Donald R., 19, 91, 92,
    235–36
Lipton, Marc, 154
"Listening to Advil" (Blum), 15–16
Listening to Prozac (Kramer), 15,
    271

Lives of a Cell, The (Thomas), 60–
    61
*Living with It: Why You Don't
    Have to Be Healthy to Be
    Happy* (Szasz), 63
Look good–feel better philosophy,
    122
Lorenzo's Oil (movie), 101
Loss, hypochondria and, 90
Lupus, 2, 3
Lutz, Tom, 109
Luvox, 29, 261, 263, 270

Magic, medicine and, 227
Magic Mountain story, 64
Male menopause, depression and,
    74–75
Malingerers, 39
Managed care, 243
Manhattan (movie), 91
Manic depression, 87, 101. *See
    also* Depression
Mann, Thomas, 64
Manu, Peter, 143–44
MAOIs. *See* Monoamine oxidase
    inhibitors
Marketing, medical, 117
Marriage. *See also* Family
    anecdotal account of, 217–20
    "Humpty-Dumpty syndrome"
        in, 211–12
    hypochondria and, 201, 204–6,
        217–20
    intolerant role in, 213–15
    patterns of discord in, 211–15
    sympathizer role in, 212–13
Masked depression, chronic illness
    and, 73
Mass hysteria, 157–58
Mass illness, 158
Maudsley, Henry, 60
McGill University, research at, 70–
    71
Meador, Clifton K., 114
Meaning and Medicine (Dossey), 65

Mechanic, David, 65
Media, 92
  benefits of vigilance by, 116–17
  disease of the month syndromes
    and, 113
  health, hypochondria, and, 111–
    12, 115–17
  medical news in, 116, 123–24
  warning reports by, 118–19
Medical care
  comfort and, 186
  high utilizers of, 61
  Jews and, 179
Medical community, influence of,
  92
Medical consumers, specialists and,
  241
Medical genetics, 101–2
Medical history, 252
  psychiatric review of, 259
Medical Information Line, 115
Medical news. See also Media
  judging, 123–24
Medical sociologists
  Mechanic as, 65
  Parsons as, 63
  Pilowsky and, 66
Medical tests, 119–20
Medical training
  cultural diversity and, 172–73
  curriculum of, 239
  impact of, 237–38
  in psychiatry, 243–49
Medications. See also Antidepres-
  sants; Drugs; medications by
  name
  Anafranil, 82–83, 100
  Cortisol, 72
  for depression, 261–62
  imipramine, 29, 79
  for panic disorder, 262
  Prozac, 7, 8, 29, 100
  Zoloft, 82
Medicine. See also Biomedicine;
  Child development; Doctors

Cartesian split and, 155
doctor-patient relationship and,
  225–29
expenditures on, 115
family practice in, 246
gender and treatment in, 164–69
health reform and, 240–43
mind-body dualism in, 134–35
patient expectations of, 233
trust in, by women, 166–67
Medicine and Culture (Payer), 170
Medicine and Meaning (Dossey),
  136
Melancholy, 21, 146
Melzack, Ronald, 148
Memories, recovered, 84
Men. See also Gender; Male menopause
  as patients, 162
  symptoms and, 162
Mendelsohn, Robert S., 189, 203
Menopause. See Male menopause
Men's movement, 169
Menstrual cycle, somatization disorder and, 53
Mental health
  Kaiser-Permanente Health Plan
    program for, 30
  neurobiology and, 97
Mental illness
  causes of hypochondria and,
    88
  genetic theories and, 101
  hypochondriasis as, 8
  somatoform disorders as, 32
Mental origin. See also Psychosomatic disorder
  of disease, 137
  of ulcers, 137–40
Merck Manual, The, 10, 29
Migraine: Understanding a Common Disorder (Sacks), 151
Migraine headaches, 151–52
  pain control and, 149
Millay, Edna St. Vincent, 93

Milunsky, Aubrey, 101–2, 103
Mind: health, disease, and, 21–22
Mind-body connection(s), 129–30,
    155. See also Chronic fatigue
    syndrome (CFS); Somatiza-
    tion; Somatoform disorders
    diagnosis and, 152–53
    pain and, 150. See also Pain
Mind-body dualism, 133–35,
    248–49
Mind Factor, The, 138
Minuchin, Salvador, 185
    family systems movement and,
    197, 198–201
Misdiagnosis, 67–68
Mitchell, S. Weir, 109
Mizrahi, Terry, 237–38
Monoamine oxidase inhibitors
    (MAOIs), 261
Mood, as amplification factor, 96
Mood disorders, 29
Moore, Demi, 125
Morality, and bodily preoccupa-
    tion, 127
"Morality of Muscle Tone, The"
    (Ehrenreich), 127
Morbus hypochondriacus, 20
Morris, David, 25, 109, 178
Morrison, Hyman, 176
Mothers, Münchausen's by proxy
    and, 193–94. See also Family;
    Women
Mount Sinai Medical Center (New
    York), 98
Münchausen's syndrome, 39, 66
    by proxy, 39, 193–96

Nardil, 261
National Institute of Mental Health
    epidemiological catchment area
    (ECA) survey, 183
    hypochrondria study at, 7
    research by, 53
    study of fluoxetine and, 272
National Institute on Aging, 181

National Institutes of Health, 241
    Office of Research on Women's
    Health, 165
Nationality, and illness, 175. See
    also Culture
Nature-nurture debate
    adopted children and, 100–101
    hypochondria and, 86–110
    identical twins studies and, 100–
    101
Navajos: emotions, sickness, and,
    171
NDA (no discernible abnormality),
    30
Nefazodone (Serzone), 261
Negative reinforcement, 277
Nervous breakdown, 86
Neumann, Debra, 83
Neuralgia, depression and, 75
Neurasthenia, 109, 173
Neurobiology, 97
Neurological disorders
    hysteria as, 25
    mood disorders and, 29
Neuropsychiatry, 270–73
Neuroses. See also Somatoform
    disorders
    heritability of, 101
    hysterical, 56
    medical training about, 239
Neuroticism, pessimism and, 182
Neurotransmitters, 29, 88, 97
    pain and, 150–51
New England Journal of Medicine,
    114, 122
New England Medical Center, 162
New Guinea, 170
New York, emotions and sickness
    in, 170–71
New York magazine, article on
    hypochondria, 15–16
NIH. See National Institutes of
    Health
NIMH. See National Institute of
    Mental Health

Nontraditional medicine, 241
Norpramin, 261
Nortriptyline (Pamelor), 261
Not Entirely Benign Procedure, A
(Klass), 238
Noyes, Russell, Jr., 272

Obsessive-compulsive disorder
(OCD), 71, 190
disorders related to, 98–99
case study and, 80–83
hypochondria and, 7, 22, 79–80,
99
treatment of, 263
OCD. *See* Obsessive-compulsive
disorder
Office of Alternative Medicine, of
NIH, 241
Office of Research on Women's
Health, 165
"On Being Ill" (Woolf), 64
Optimism
good health and, 128–29
research in, 181
Osler, William, 21
Overanxious parents, vs. Mün-
chausen parents, 195–96
Overprotectiveness, in families,
199–200
Overtesting, 119–20
Over-the-counter medication,
120–21
Overtreatment, 120–21
Oxford University, cognitive be-
havior techniques at, 278

Pain
anecdotal report on, 55–56
back, 153
childhood and, 187–93
chronic, 148
culture and, 178–79. *See also*
Culture
emotional vs. physical, 188
ethnic group and, 108

gender and, 161
internalization of, 176
statistics on, 147
tolerance for, 147–55
Pain clinics, 149
Pain disorder, 34, 54–55
Pain physiologists, 148
Pain specialists, on somatoform
pain, 55
Pain Treatment Center (Columbia
Presbyterian Medical Center),
55
Paleopathology, 147–48
Pamelor, 261
Panic disorder, 71, 77–78, 93, 190
case study in, 78–79
obsessive-compulsive disorder
and, 82
treatment of, 262
Parents. *See also* Child development; Family
cues of, 104–5
empowering, 198–99
Münchausen by proxy and,
193–96
overanxious, 195–96
response to children's illnesses
and, 65
Paroxetine (Paxil), 261
Parsons, Talcott, on "sick role,"
63, 64–65
Pathology
medical tests and, 120
normal concerns as, 113
Patients. *See also* Doctor-patient relationship
anecdotes from, 39–59. *See also*
Anecdotal reports
doctors and, 223–54
expectations of, 233–34
as medical consumers, 229–34
men as, 162
psychosocial stress and, 61
as victims, 234
view of doctors by, 229–34

"Patients Refusing to Be Well, a Disease of Many Symptoms," 6
Paxil, 29, 261, 270
Payer, Lynn, 117, 170
Pediatricians, 189
Peers, and childhood illness, 190–91
Pennebaker, James W., 95–96, 161
People in Pain (Zborowski), 178
Perception
  health and, 157
  of pain, 148
Perfection, obsession with, 122–27
Perryman, Vicki, 140
Personality
  illness and, 128
  theories of, 89. *See also* Behavior(s)
Pessimistic explanatory style, 182
Phantom pains, 187–93
Pharmacologic treatment. *See also* Drugs; Medications
  of depression, 261–62
  of OCD, 263
  of panic disorder, 262
Pharmacology, cosmetic, 271
Phenelzine (Nardil), 261
Phobias
  in children, 190
  disease, 47–51
Phobia self-help groups, 257
Phobic tendencies, Prozac and, 11
Physical abuse, 162–63
Physical distress, psychosocial stress and, 61
Physical examination, 252
  to eliminate medical conditions, 259
Physical symptom, as expression of unconscious conflict, 27–28
Physical trauma. *See* Trauma
Physicianhood, psychology of, 236–37. *See also* Doctors
Physicochemical properties, of stress, 146–47. *See also* Stress

Physiology
  of mind-body connection, 130
  of pain, 179
Pilowsky, Ian, 36, 40
Placebo response
  doctor-patient relationship and, 226–27
  physician's role in, 227
  psychodynamic therapy and, 266
Plastic surgery, growth of, 126
PMS, 114, 115, 131, 150–51
PNI, 129
Political correctness, 172
Pollack, Sylvia, 168
Poor people, risk for illness of, 107
Popular health movement, 155
Positive reinforcement, 277
Post-traumatic stress disorder (PTSD), symptoms and, 83–85
Predispositions, genetic, 103
Pregnancy, hypochondria and, 207–8
Premenstrual syndrome (PMS), 114, 115, 131, 150–51
Prescription medication, 120–21. *See also* Drugs; Medication
Preventive care, 248. *See also* Health care
Primary Care Outcomes Research Institute, 162
Primary hypochondria, 263
PRIME MD (Primary Care Evaluation of Mental Disorders), 246
Profound sensitivity syndrome (PS2), 154
Protetch, David, 35
Proust, Marcel, 22, 111, 203
Prozac, 7, 8, 29, 100, 261, 263, 270–72. *See also* Antidepressants; Drugs; Medication
  anecdotal information on, 276
  impact of, 10–11

PS2, 154
Psychiatric disorders
    CFS and, 141
    diagnosing, 239–40
    family history of, 260
    and hypochondria, 259, 261–63
    hypochondriasis as, 9
    serotonin and, 98
Psychiatrists
    consulting, 258–60
    questions asked by, 259–64
Psychiatry. *See also* Therapy
    hypochondria studies and, 28–
        29
    multicultural dimension of, 173
Psychic pain, 286–87
Psychoactive medications, 88
Psychoanalysis, 24–25, 89. *See also*
    Freud, Sigmund
    as psychodynamic therapy, 265
    psychosomatic illness and, 26–
        27
Psychodynamic therapy, 264–70
    anecdotal information about,
        267–70
    effectiveness of, 266
Psychodynamic view of behavior,
    89–93
Psychogenic musculoskeletal pain,
    193
Psychological causes, of symptoms,
    30–31
Psychological functioning, "sick
    role" and, 63
Psychological illness
    hypochondria as, 87–88
    as sick role, 64–65
    symptoms and, 68–69
Psychological states, pain and, 55
Psychological testing, caution
    about, 294
Psychology, of physicianhood,
    236–37
Psychoneuroimmunology (PNI),
    129

Psychosocial stress, patients and,
    61
Psychosomatic disorder, 19, 26–
    27, 136
    Alexander and, 138
    family patterns and, 199
    myth of, 134–37
    ulcers as, 137–40
Psychotherapy
    and depression, 261, 262
    intervention and, 247
PTSD, 83–85
Public health problems, CFS as,
    142

Questionnaires
    for hypochondriacal beliefs, 36
    Illness Attitude Scale (IAS) as,
        256, 293–97
    psychiatrist-administered, 258

Radner, Gilda, 119, 242
Reality-checking therapy, 94
Recovery process, 11
    sick role and, 64–65
Reference group phenomenon,
    183–84
Reform, of health system, 240–43
Reinforcement, 277
Relationships. *See also* Marriage
    active-passive, 251
    collegial, 251
    doctor-patient, 223–54
    mutual participation, 251
    reacting to hypochondria in,
        221–22
Religion, medicine and, 227
Repression, gender and, 161
Reproduction, bodily changes,
    gender, and, 161–62
Research. *See also* Cross-cultural
    studies; Epidemiological re-
    search
    Baltimore Longitudinal Study of
        Aging, 183

on behavioral and cognitive methodology effectiveness, 279
on choice of doctor, 250–51
on doctor-patient relationship, 229–30
evaluating, 123–24
Fallon's Heightened Illness Concern study, 41, 271–72
on fluoxetine, 272
Grant study of traits and aging, 128
Illness Attitude Scale (IAS) and, 293–97
neglect of women in, 165
on psychiatric disorders and chronic illness, 74
on psychodynamic therapy, 266
on somatoform disorders, 36
Restak, Richard, 169
Rigdon, Elizabeth, 166
Rigidity, in families, 200
Risk factors
diseasing of, 113–14
for mental and physical illness, 107
Roles
"sick," 63–66
of women, 167–68
Rosenbaum, Edward, 231
Roter, Debra, 244
Rusk Institute of Rehabilitation Medicine, 153

Sacks, Oliver, 151–52
Sadomasochistic tendencies, of Münchausen patients, 195
St. Josephs Medical Center (Stamford, Conn.), 246–47
Salkovskis, Paul, 279
Sapolsky, Robert, 146
Sarno, John E., 62, 153
Satir, Virginia, 197
Schizophrenia, 101
Schreier, Herbert A., 194

Scientology, Church of, 271
Selective serotonin reuptake inhibitors. *See* SSRIs
Self, concept of, 103
Self-acceptance, 11
Self-destructive tendencies, 105
Self-help groups, 256–57
pain relief and, 149
Seligman, Martin, 103, 181
Selye, Hans, 145
Seneca, 255
Sensitivity, to physical sensations, 94
Separation, child-family, 198. *See also* Family
Separation anxiety, 188
Serotonin, 97. *See also* SSRIs
Sertraline (Zoloft), 261
Serzone, 261
Sexism, medical profession and, 164–69
Sexual abuse, 163. *See also* Trauma
recovered memories and, 84
Sexual energy, Freud and, 90
Sexual symptoms, somatization disorders and, 53
SF–36 questionnaire, 245–46
Share the Pain, 149
Sherry, David, 193
Shingles
case study and, 74–75
depression and, 73–74
Shorter, Edward, 27, 107, 110, 175–76
Sick and Tired of Being Sick and Tired (Solomon and Lipton), 154
Sickness. *See* Disease(s); Illness
Sick role
avoiding encouraging, 202–3
of child, 193
and illness behavior, 63–67
legitimacy of, 64–65
Parsons on, 63, 64–65

Silent World of Doctor and Patient, The (Katz), 227
Silicone-gel breast implants, 121
Small, Gary W., 158
Smith, John, 165
Social causes, of symptoms, 30–31
Social psychology, of symptoms, 157–58
Social scientists, culture and, 106–7
Society, health concerns and, 112–15
Sociology. *See also* Medical sociologists
abnormal illness behavior and, 66
hypochondria and, 107
sick role and, 63–66
Solomon, Neil, 154
Somatization, 32. *See also* Anecdotal reports; Somatoform disorders
abnormal illness behavior and, 66–67
Minuchin and, 198
sick role and, 64–65
treatment of, 224–25
Somatization disorder, 53–54
Somatizers, 6
medical training about, 239
real illness and, 247
society and, 113
Somatoform disorders, 32, 33
classification of, 39
disagreements over, 36–38
distinguishing among, 35–36
recognizing, 69–70
Sontag, Susan, 64, 127
Spastic colon, 151
Specialists, 241. *See also* Doctors
Speech, gender and, 160
Spiegel, David, 128
Spiritual impoverishment, 126–27
Spitzer, Robert L., 246
Spock, Benjamin, 116
SSRIs (selective serotonin reuptake blockers), 29, 261, 263, 270

Stekel, Wilhelm, 32
Stern, Henri, 176
Stewart, Donna, 113
Stigma
of hypochondria, 15, 18, 24
of psychiatric problems, 69
Strategies, behavior therapy and, 280
Stress
in authoritarian families, 200
coping with, 145–47
post-traumatic, 83–85
psychosocial, 61
role of, 145–46
shingles and, 74–75
and transient hypochondria, 259
ulcers and, 139
women and, 167–68
Stressors, hypochondria and, 104
Stress-related disorders, 146
Studies in Hysteria (Freud and Breuer), 25–26
Styron, William, 1, 73, 89
Substance abuse, gender and, 162
Suicide
depression and, 73
gender and, 162
Suk-yeong (koro), 171
Support groups, 256–57
Surgery
on hypochondriacs, 224–25
unnecessary, 121
Susceptibility, 156–84
ethnic and cultural considerations in, 170–74
Sympathizer role, in marriage, 213–14
Symptoms. *See also* Pain
anxiety and, 76–79
appraisal of, 65
cognitive-behavioral view of, 93–100
cognitive behavior therapy and, 278–79
dealing with, 94

of depressive disorder, 71–74
emotions and, 61
evaluating, 60–85
as expression of unconscious
conflict, 27–28
Freud and, 90
hypochondria and, 15
post-traumatic stress and, 83–85
and psychodynamic view of personality, 90–91
psychological, 68–69
psychological-social vs. medical
causes of, 31
reality of, 249
recognizing somatoform disorders and, 69–70
responses to, 62–63
sick role of child and, 193
social psychology of, 157–58
undiagnosable, 6
Syndromes
chronic fatigue, 141–42
culture and, 170–71
media and, 113
temperomandibular joint, 54,
132
tension myositis, 153
Syndrome X, 166
Systems perspective. See Family
systems approach
Szasz, Suzy, 62

Tagamet, 138
Talk therapy, 105
psychodynamic therapy and,
264–70
Tannen, Deborah, 160, 179–80
Taste of My Own Medicine, A
(Rosenbaum), 231
Teasdale, Sara, 23
Technology, impact of scientific,
136
Temple University School of Med-
icine, fears of AIDS study at,
94

Temperomandibular joint syndrome, 54, 132
Tennyson, Alfred, Lord, 23, 87
Tension myositis syndrome (TMS),
153–54
Test, for hypochondria, 293–97
Therapeutic alliance, doctor-
patient relationship and, 227
Therapeutic approaches, 89
Therapy, 10, 11. See also Depres-
sion; Family systems approach;
Psychiatric disorders; Psycho-
therapy
alternatives in, 257–58
behavior, 262, 277, 279–80
cognitive, 262, 277–78
for depression, 262
psychodynamic, 264–70
talk, 105
types of, 263–84
Thomas, Lewis, 60–61, 115
Thought, divided from feeling, 135
TMS, 153–54
Tofranil. See Imipramine
Tolstoy, Leo, 23
Toner, Robin, 241
Tourette's syndrome, 98
Transference, 265
Transformations (self-help group),
149
Transitory hypochondria, 14–15,
259
Trauma, 83–85
GI ailments and, 163
Treatment. See also Drugs; Medications; Therapy
with accompanying psychiatric
disorders, 261–63
without accompanying psychiatric disorders, 263–84
biological, 97–98, 270–76
for chronic pain. See Pain
of depression, 75–76
gender and, 163, 164–69
overtreatment and, 120–21

Treatment (*cont.*)
  pharmacological, 261–63
  psychiatric consultation as, 258
  psychodynamic, 264–70
  recognition of need for, 255–56
  steps to, 255–85
  support groups for, 256–57
  of symptoms, 65
Trends, biopsychosocial vs. managed care, 243
Trichotillomania, 98
Tricyclic antidepressants
  for depression, 261
  for panic disorder, 262
Triggers, PTSD and, 83–84
Tryptophan, 121
Twiggy, legacy of, 125
Twin studies
  heredity and, 100–101
  hypochondria and, 102

Ugliness, imagined, 52–53
Ulcers
  blame for, 138
  psychosomatic disorders and, 137–40
Unconscious
  body language and, 136
  and psychodynamic therapy, 265
  symptoms as expression of, 27–28
University of Arkansas for Medical Sciences, gender research at, 164
University of Arkansas Medical School, study at, 245
University of Connecticut School of Medicine, CFS study at, 144
University of Pennsylvania School of Medicine, study of gender and feelings, 161
University of Virginia Medical School, study at, 62

Values, appearance as, 125
"Vapours," 20
Venlafaxine (Effexor), 261
Victimization
  illness and, 128–30
  of women, 162–63
Victims, patients as, 234
Violence, Prozac and, 271
Volk, Patricia, 125
Vulnerability, sense of, 94–95

Wall, Patrick, 148
Washington University (St. Louis), 36
Weakness, hypochondria as, 92
Weil, Andrew, 226–27
Weissman, Gerald, 249
Wellbutrin, 261
Wellness, concern with, 112
Wesner, Robert, 272
Western medicine, 135
Wharton, Edith, 109
What You Can Change and What You Can't (Seligman), 103
When You're Sick and Don't Know Why (Hanner), 67–68
Whitaker, Carl, 197
White, E. B., 23
White Anglo-Saxon Protestants, pain and, 178
White-coat hypertension, 86–87
Whitehead, William, 202
White Plains Hospital Center (New York), health anxiety program at, 257
Winfrey, Oprah, 125
Without Feathers (Allen), 156
Wollstonecraft, Mary, 108–9
Women. *See also* Gender; Girls; Mothers
  bodily changes and, 161–62
  hysteria and, 25
  illness as relief for, 168
  Jewish, 179
  medical bias against, 164–65

pregnancy and, 207–8
roles of, 167–68
somatization disorder in, 53
susceptibility of, 158, 159–64
violence toward, 162–63
Women and Doctors (Smith), 165
Women's health, 164–65
Wonder drugs. *See* Drugs
Woolf, Virginia, 64
Worried Sick (Barsky), 18
   amplification factors and, 95–97

Worry
   Jewish hypochondria and, 176
   stopping, 287

Xanax, 262

Yuppie flu, 141

Zantac, 138, 206, 271
Zborowski, Mark, 178–79
Zoloft, 29, 82, 271, 261, 270